DEDICATION

This book is dedicated to my dear friend Jorge L. Alio from Alicante, Spain.

Contents

ACKNOWLEDGMENTS

When I started writing this book, the pen was mine but the power behind it was His. No acknowledgment is enough to thank Him for everything.

ABOUT THE EDITOR

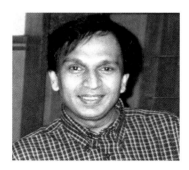

Amar Agarwal, MS, FRCS, FRCOphth is the pioneer of phakonit, which is phako with needle incision technology. This technique became popularized as bimanual phaco, microincision cataract surgery (MICS), or microphaco. He is also the first to remove cataracts through a 0.7-mm tip by the technique called microphakonit. He has also discovered no-anesthesia cataract surgery and FAVIT, a new technique to remove dropped nuclei. The air pump, which was the simple idea of using an aquarium pump to increase the fluid into the eye in bimanual phaco and coaxial phaco, has helped prevent surge. This built the basis of various techniques of forced infusion for small incision cataract surgery. He was also the first to use trypan blue for staining epiretinal membranes and has published the details in his 4-volume textbook of ophthalmology. His latest discovery is a new refractive error called aberropia.

Dr. Agarwal has received many awards for his work in ophthalmology, the most significant being the Barraquer Award and the Kelman Award. He has also written more than 33 books, which have been published in various languages. He also trains doctors from all over the world on phaco, bimanual phaco, LASIK, and retina at his eye center in India.

Contributing Authors

Athiya Agarwal, MD, FRSH, DO
Dr. Agarwal's Group of Eye Hospitals and Eye Research Centre
Chennai, India

Sunita Agarwal, MS, DO
Dr. Agarwal's Group of Eye Hospitals and Eye Research Centre
Chennai, India

Jorge L. Alio, MD, PhD
Instituto Oftalmológico de Alicante
Alicante, Spain
Refractive Surgery and Cornea Department
Miguel Hernández University Medical School
Alicante, Spain

Aritz Bidaguren, MD
Ophthalmology Department
Hospital Donostia
Basque Health Service-Osakidetza
Donostia, San Sebastián, Spain

Ana Blanco, MD
Ophthalmology Department
Hospital Donostia
Basque Health Service-Osakidetza
Donostia, San Sebastián, Spain

Daniel Böhringer, MD
University Eye Hospital Freiburg
Freiburg, Germany

Vatinee Y. Bunya, MD
Cornea Fellow
Cornea Service
Wills Eye Hospital
Philadelphia, Pa

Roy S. Chuck, MD, PhD
Director of Refractive Surgery and Associate Professor, Cornea and External Diseases
Wilmer Eye Institute
Johns Hopkins University
Baltimore, Md

Glenn C. Cockerham, MD
Associate Professor, Ophthalmology
Stanford University
Stanford, Calif

Kimberly P. Cockerham, MD, FACS
Associate Professor
Department of Ophthalmology
University of California
San Francisco, Calif

Kenneth Daniels, OD, FAAO
Adjunct Assistant Clinical Professor
Pennsylvania College of Optometry
CASCLS and Center International Studies
Hopewell-Lambertville Eye Associates
Hopewell, NJ
Affiliated with the Wills-Princeton Laser Eye Group
Series Editor, The Basic Bookshelf for Eyecare Professionals
SLACK Incorporated
Thorofare, NJ

Murat Dogru, MD
Assistant Professor
Department of Ophthalmology
Keio University School of Medicine
Tokyo, Japan

Eric D. Donnenfeld, MD
Founding Partner, Ophthalmic Consultants of Long Island
Rockville Centre, NY
Clinical Associate Professor of Ophthalmology
New York University Medical Center
New York, NY

M. Alaa El Danasoury, FRCS
Chief of Cornea and Refractive Surgery
El Magrabi Eye Hospital
Cairo, Egypt

Akef El-Maghraby, MD, FRCS
Chairman
Magrabi Hospitals and Centers
Jeddah, Saudi Arabia

Ahmad M. Fahmy, OD, FAAO
Minnesota Eye Consultants
Minneapolis, Minn

Ashok Garg, MS, PhD, FRSM, FIAO
Garg Eye Institute & Research Centre
Hisar, Haryana, India

Ane Gibelalde, MD
Ophthalmology Department
Hospital Donostia
Basque Health Service-Osakidetza
Donostia, San Sebastián, Spain

Grant D. Gilliland, MD
Texas Ophthalmic Plastic, Reconstructive, and Orbital Surgery Associates
Dallas, Tex

Oscar Gris, MD
Associate Professor of Ophthalmology
University of Barcelona
Chief of Cornea and Anterior Segment
Hospital Clinic i Provincial of Barcelona
Cornea and External Diseases Unit
Instituto de Microcirugia Ocular
Barcelona, Spain

José Luis Güell, MD
Associate Professor of Ophthalmology
Autonoma University of Barcelona
Director of Cornea and Refractive Surgery Unit
Instituto de Microcirugia Ocular
Barcelona, Spain

Kristin M. Hammersmith, MD
Director, Fellowship Program
Wills Eye Hospital
Instructor, Jefferson Medical College of Thomas Jefferson University
Philadelphia, Pa

David R. Hardten, MD, FACS
Minnesota Eye Consultants
Minneapolis, Minn

Marc J. Hirschbein, MD, FACS
Oculoplastic Service
Krieger Eye Institute
Sinai Hospital of Baltimore
Baltimore, Md

Mahmoud M. Ismail, MD, PhD
Associate Professor
University of Al-Azhar
Chief of Cornea and Refractive Surgery
El Magrabi Eye Hospital
Cairo, Egypt

Soosan Jacob, MS, FRCS, Dip NB
Dr. Agarwal's Group of Eye Hospitals and Eye Research Centre
Chennai, India

W. Barry Lee, MD
Cornea and External Disease Service
Eye Consultants of Atlanta
Atlanta, Ga

Itziar Martínez-Soroa, MD
Ophthalmology Department
Hospital Donostia
Basque Health Service-Osakidetza
Donostia, San Sebastián, Spain

Javier Mendicute, MD, PhD
Chairman Ophthalmology Department
Hospital Donostia
Basque Health Service-Osakidetza
Begitek Clínica Oftalmológica
Donostia, San Sebastián, Spain

M. Emilia Mulet, MD, PhD
Associate Professor
Miguel Hernández University Medical School
Alicante, Spain
Vissum Instituto Oftalmologico de Alicante
Alicante, Spain

Juan Murube, MD
Department of Ophthalmology
University of Alcala
Madrid, Spain

Alexander V. On, MD
Oculoplastic Service
Krieger Eye Institute
Sinai Hospital of Baltimore
Baltimore, Md

Vasudha A. Panday, MD
Cornea Fellow
Wilmer Eye Institute
Johns Hopkins University
Baltimore, Md

Suresh K. Pandey, MD
Director
SuVI Eye Institute & Research Center
Kota, Rajasthan, India
Assistant Clinical Professor
John A. Moran Eye Center
Department of Ophthalmology & Visual Sciences
University of Utah
Salt Lake City, Utah
Visiting Ophthalmologist
Intraocular Implant Unit
Sydney Eye Hospital
University of Sydney
Sydney, Australia

Sanjay V. Patel, MD
Assistant Professor
Department of Ophthalmology
Mayo Clinic College of Medicine
Rochester, Minn

Henry D. Perry, MD
Senior Founding Partner, Ophthalmic Consultants of Long Island
Rockville Centre, NY
Clinical Associate Professor of Ophthalmology
Weill Medical College of Cornell University
New York, NY

Demetrio Pita-Salorio, MD
Professor and Chairman
Department of Ophthalmology
School of Medicine
University of Barcelona
Barcelona, Spain
Deceased, devoted Catholic

Christopher J. Rapuano, MD
Codirector, Cornea Service
Wills Eye Hospital
Professor of Ophthalmology
Jefferson Medical College of Thomas Jefferson University
Philadelphia, Pa

Thomas Reinhard, MD
Professor and Chairman
University Eye Hospital Freiburg
Freiburg, Germany

Johann M. G. Reyes, MD
Cornea Research Fellow
Wilmer Eye Institute
Johns Hopkins University
Baltimore, Md

Ivan R. Schwab, MD
Professor and Director of Cornea and External Disease Service
University of California, Davis
Department of Ophthalmology
Sacramento, Calif

Cristina Simón-Castellví, MD
Simon Eye Clinic
Barcelona, Spain

Guillermo L. Simón-Castellví, MD
Chief Anterior Segment Surgeon
Simon Eye Clinic
Barcelona, Spain
Department of Ophthalmology
School of Medicine
University of Barcelona
Barcelona, Spain

José María Simón-Castellví, MD
Anterior Segment Consultant
Emergency Room
Simon Eye Clinic
Barcelona, Spain

Sarabel Simón-Castellví, MD
Chief Posterior Segment Surgeon
Simon Eye Clinic
Barcelona, Spain

José María Simón-Tor, MD
Chairman
Glaucoma Senior Consultant
Simon Eye Clinic
Barcelona, Spain

Renée Solomon, MD
Fellow, Ophthalmic Consultants of Long Island
Rockville Centre, NY

H. Kaz Soong, MD
Professor
Department of Ophthalmology and Visual Sciences
W. K. Kellogg Eye Center
University of Michigan
Ann Arbor, Mich

Leejee Suh, MD
Resident
Wilmer Eye Institute
Johns Hopkins University
Baltimore, Md

C. Sujatha, DO
Dr. Agarwal's Group of Eye Hospitals and Eye Research Centre
Chennai, India

Rainer Sundmacher, MD, FRCOphth
Professor and Chairman
University Eye Hospital Düsseldorf
Düsseldorf, Germany

Olan Suwan-apichon, MD
Cornea Research Fellow
Wilmer Eye Institute
Johns Hopkins University
Baltimore, Md
Assistant Professor
Khon Kaen University
Khon Kaen, Thailand

Brighu N. Swamy, MBBS (Hons), M Med (Clin Epi)
University of Sydney
Sydney, Australia

Kazuo Tsubota, MD
Professor and Chairman
Department of Ophthalmology
Keio University School of Medicine
Tokyo, Japan

John R. Wittpenn, MD
Partner, Ophthalmic Consultants of Long Island
Rockville Centre, NY
Clinical Associate Professor of Ophthalmology
State University of New York
Stony Brook, NY

Orin Zwick, MD
Oculoplastic Fellow
University of California
San Francisco, Calif

PREFACE

The world is going through a major evolutionary process. We need to presume that this is always for the good of mankind. However, there are some aspects of the environment in which we live that need to be taken in the right perspective. For the last few decades, we have witnessed a major revolution in the way we work, think, and behave. Thus, we live not by the sun's light and warmth, but with artificial lighting and air conditioning. This is coupled with the fact that environmental pollution and global warming are making our living areas far more dry than what they used to be a few decades ago. Notwithstanding the onslaught of computer monitors that have changed the way we behave. Thus, a multifactorial etiology is resulting in our eyes becoming very dry.

We have known that the tears of the eye not only give lubrication, but provide essential nutrition and protection against foreign onslaught. Thus, when the tears start getting deficient the resultant eye is exposed to various onslaughts of aging, allergy, and disease. It has been recorded in one of the first books on ophthalmology that the blink reflex is about 25 per minute. However, with the printing press coming into the picture of human development, this fell to 15 per minute when more and more people started reading and writing, thus keeping their eyes more open. Now with computers, the blinks are down to less than 5 per minute. Classically, the blink reflex works in the same principle as the soap bubble maker children play with, with each blink the tear spreads evenly over the cornea and gives us a better vision. With less blinks, the tear film breaks up very easily and we don't even realize it.

Evolutionary sciences tell us for any one aspect of human evolution, 5000 years are necessary before it can be encoded into the DNA. Yet in the last 100 years, we have grown out of bounds of this time gap. As scientists, we need to wake up to the fact that dry eyes are a spreading reality and we, as eye care practitioners, need to update our patients on a firm footing. Thus, this book hopes to help us do what evolution will do anyway in its own time.

Since this problem has cropped up in a multifactorial manner, quite obviously its management will need to be dealt with also in a multipronged approach. Where some may prefer to be conservative and use medications, other patients may need more intensive therapy of lacrimal plugs, and still others would need surgery. Updating ourselves with the recent trends is what medicine is all about. Stem cell research has opened up a huge new manner of treating our patients. Helping human consciousness to evolve newer trends in the treatment of dry eyes, we will need to know all the methodologies available. This is what this book brings to you. Contributing authors from all over the world have pitched in their knowledge and skill toward a greater camaraderie, all in final pursuit of the removal of human suffering.

I would like to thank John Bond, April Billick, Amy McShane, Jennifer Briggs, Michelle Gatt, and the others at SLACK Incorporated who helped me write this book. I would also like to thank my consultant, Dr. Soosan Jacob, for helping me. At the end, I hope you enjoy this book as much as I did writing it.

Amar Agarwal, MS, FRCS, FRCOphth

Foreword

Tears are an important first line protection for the ocular surface. During infancy, tear quality is at its peak and is associated with very low blink rates. As we add years to our lives, there is an inevitable loss of our tear quantity and quality. With the steady increase in life expectancy, eye diseases caused or exacerbated by tear dysfunction are emerging as some of the most common reasons for patient discomfort and loss of vision. External factors also play a role. Industrial pollutants, indoor air climate control, poor lid hygiene, and prolonged sun exposure wear down baseline tear secretion.

Recent studies point to chronic, low-grade inflammation in the tear gland resulting from popular dietary habits as a common cause of dry eye syndrome. Our experience from treating Sjögren's syndrome patients reminds us of just how destructive this inflammatory mechanism can be to tear production.

We are witnessing an important milestone in eye care. The pathophysiology of tear dysfunction, maybe the most common ocular disease, is finally being unraveled. New methods of avoiding and treating this condition are providing relief to a rapidly growing segment of our patients seeking solutions to their annoying and sometimes sight-threatening disease.

With this text, Dr. Agarwal and his contributing authors have provided well-organized and timely information to guide us to a better understanding of the causes of tear loss and recent breakthroughs in treatment alternatives. Dr. Agarwal, a respected educator and clinician, presents a systemic approach to the assessment of patients with dry eye conditions with special emphasis on the latest treatment options. Discussion of the impact of dry eye syndrome on cataract and refractive patients is of particular importance. As an investigator of a number of multifocal intraocular lenses, I have seen how frequently lack of adequate tear function can affect the quality of vision in this growing population of patients.

Dr. Agarwal has provided ophthalmologists with the right information to better understand and manage patients afflicted by problem dry eye, a condition that continues to affect more people worldwide.

R. Bruce Wallace, III, MD, FACS
Wallace Eye Surgery
Alexandria, La

Section I

Overview

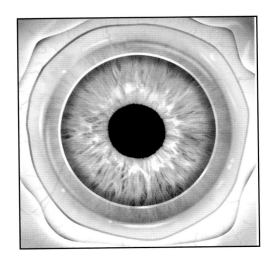

Key Points

1. The chief histological constituents of the ocular surface include the nonkeratinized epithelia and underlying stroma of the entire conjunctiva, the cornea and the corneoscleral limbus, and the tear film.
2. The caruncle is a reddish body (5 mm high by 3 mm wide) that is medial to the plica. It has features of both the conjunctiva and skin. It is lined by conjunctival epithelium and contains cutaneous adnexal structures.
3. It is believed that over a period of time conjunctival epithelium covering the cornea assumes its characteristics by a process referred to as conjunctival transdifferentiation. Stem cells act as a barrier that exerts an inhibitory growth pressure, preventing the migration of conjunctival epithelial cells onto the cornea.
4. The junction of the cornea and sclera is demarcated by a gray, semitransparent area with a dentate border referred to as the limbus. This transitional zone is only 1 mm wide and marks the point of insertion of the conjunctiva.
5. The corneal epithelium has a capacity for rapid regeneration that depends on the self-renewal ability of corneal stem cells. Corneal epithelium consists of corneal stem cells, TAC, postmitotic cells, and terminally differentiated cells. Both stem cells and TAC exhibit an ability to proliferate, whereas postmitotic cells have lost this ability. Stem cells are imbued with the potential for self-renewal and can proliferate extensively. TAC, on the other hand, exhibit a reduced proliferation lifespan compared to stem cells and have lost the ability for self-renewal.

REFERENCES

1. Wolff E. *Anatomy of the Eye and Orbit.* Philadelphia: W.B. Saunders; 1970.
2. Hart WM, ed. *Adler's Physiology of the Eye.* 9th ed. St. Louis, Mo: Mosby Year Book, Inc; 1992.
3. Allansmith MR, Baird RS, Greiner JV. Density of goblet cells in vernal conjunctivitis and contact lens-associated giant papillary conjunctivitis. *Arch Ophthalmol.* 1981;99:884–885.
4. Twining SS, Zhou X, Schulte DP, et al. Effect of vitamin A deficiency on the early response to experimental pseudomonas keratitis. *Invest Ophthalmol Vis Sci.* 1996;37:511–522.
5. Klyce SD, Crosson CE. Transport processes across the rabbit corneal epithelium: a review. *Curr Eye Res.* 1985;4:323–331.
6. Inatomi T, Spurr-Michaud SJ, Tisdale AS, Zhan Q, Feldman ST, Gipson IK. Expression of secretory mucin genes by human conjunctival epithelia. *Invest Ophthalmol Vis Sci.* 1996;37:1.684–1.692.
7. Inatomi T, Spurr-Michaud SJ, Tisdale AS, Gipson IK. Human corneal and conjunctival epithelia express MUC 1 mucin. *Invest Ophthalmol Vis Sci.* 1995;36:1.818–1.827.
8. Price-Schiavi SA, Meller D, Jing X, Carvajal ME, Tseng SCG, Carraway KL. Sialomucin complex at the rat ocular surface: a new model for ocular surface protection. *Biochem J.* 1998;335(Pt 2):457–463.
9. Dilly PN. Contribution of the epithelium to the stability of the tear film. *Trans Ophthalmol Soc UK.* 1985;104:381–389.

10. Watanabe H, Fabricant M, Tisdale AS, Spurr-Michaud SJ, Lindberg K, Gipson IK. Human corneal and conjunctival epithelia produce a mucin-like glycoprotein for the apical surface. *Invest Ophthalmol Vis Sci.* 1995;36:337–344.

11. Pflugfelder SC, Tseng SCG, Yoshino K, Monroy D, Felix C, Reis BL. Correlation of goblet cell density and mucosal epithelial membrane mucin expression with rose bengal staining in patients with ocular irritation. *Ophthalmology.* 1997;104:223–235.

12. Nichols BA, Chiappino ML, Dawson CR. Demonstration of the mucous layer of the tear film by electron microscopy. *Invest Ophthalmol Vis Sci.* 1985;26:464–473.

13. Moll R, Franke WW, Schiller DL, Geiger B, Krepler R. The catalog of human cytokeratins. Patterns of expression in normal epithelia, tumors and cultured cells. *Cell.* 1982;31:11–24.

14. Galvin S, Loomis C, Manabe M, Dhouailly D, Sun TT. The major pathways of keratinocyte differentiation as defined by keratin expression, an overview. *Adv Dermatol.* 1989;4:277–299.

15. Tseng SCG, Hatchell D, Tierney N, Huang AJW, Sun TT. Expression of specific keratin markers by rabbit corneal, conjunctival, and esophageal epithelia during vitamin A deficiency. *J Cell Biol.* 1984;99:2.279–2.286.

16. Schermer A, Galvin S, Sun TT. Differentiation-related expression of a major 64K corneal keratin in vivo and in culture suggests limbal location of corneal epithelial stem cells. *J Cell Biol.* 1986;103:49–62.

17. Pellegrini G, Golisano O, Paterna P, et al. Location and clonal analysis of stem cells and their differentiated progeny in the human ocular surface. *J Cell Biol.* 1999;145:769–782.

18. Schwartz GS, Holland EJ. Iatrogenic limbal stem cell deficiency. *Cornea.* 1998;7:31–37.

2

Lacrimal System: Anatomy and Physiology

*Alexander V. On, MD and
Marc J. Hirschbein, MD, FACS*

INTRODUCTION

Tearing represents a problem that is not only annoying for the patient, but also a diagnostic and therapeutic challenge for the ophthalmologist. Lacrimal problems may be congenital or acquired and may occur at any age. Abnormalities in the flow of tears can adversely affect vision and daily activities or may even result in abscess formation, orbital cellulitis, or sepsis. Knowledge of the anatomy and physiology of the lacrimal system is essential for the accurate diagnosis and treatment of tearing.

ANATOMY

The lacrimal glands are responsible for tear production. The main lacrimal gland is thought to be responsible for reflex tear production. It is located in the lacrimal fossa of the superotemporal orbit and consists of 2 lobes. The orbital and palpebral lobes are separated by the levator aponeurosis. The ducts from the orbital lobe pass through the palpebral lobe and then the ducts from both lobes exit the superior fornix 5 mm above the superior tarsal border. The accessory lacrimal glands of Krauss and Wolfring are believed to be the main contributors to basal tear production. These glands are located in the conjunctiva at the fornices and superior to the upper edge of the superior tarsus, respectively (Figure 2-1).

The lacrimal gland is well vascularized. Its main blood supply is from the lacrimal artery, which is a branch of the ophthalmic artery, or the middle meningeal artery. Venous return is via the superior ophthalmic vein, and lymphatic drainage passes with the conjunctival system to the preauricular nodes.[1]

Figure 2-1. Anatomy of the lids showing various glands. (Reprinted with permission from Agarwal A. *Dr. Agarwal's 4 Volume Textbook of Ophthalmology.* New Dehli, India: Jaypee Brothers Medical Publishers Ltd.)

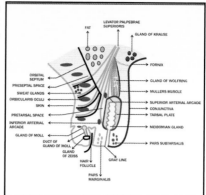

Figure 2-2. Anatomy of the lacrimal apparatus. (Reprinted with permission from Agarwal A. *Handbook of Ophthalmology.* Thorofare, NJ: SLACK Incorporated; 2005.)

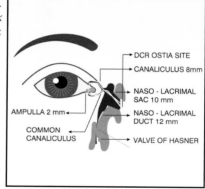

After bathing the ocular surface, tears enter the puncta, which are the beginnings of the lacrimal drainage system (Figure 2-2). The puncta should sit in apposition to the globe, allowing proper collection of tears. The upper punctum is 6 mm and the lower is 6.5 mm from the medial canthus. Each is approximately 0.3 mm in diameter and sits on a papilla, an elevated ridge of tissue. Internally, a ring of connective tissue encircles the lumen of the punctum. This connective tissue ring becomes important during the placement of punctal plugs. It surrounds the narrow portion of a correctly inserted plug, holding the plug in place with the cuff above the opening and flush to the surface. If the plug is properly sized, dilation of the punctum is unnecessary. Dilation will distort the connective tissue ring and can result in placement of the plug too deeply or allow it to slip out before the ring rebounds to its normal shape.

From the puncta, tears pass into the canaliculi. These structures begin with the ampullae, which are 2 mm in length and oriented vertically. An opening is made in the ampullae during punctoplasty to create a larger "drain" for tears to enter. The canaliculi then make a 110-degree turn horizontally for 8 to 10 mm. They measure 0.5 to 1.0 mm internally and are lined by stratified squamous epithelium. The canaliculi join to form a common canaliculus (in 90% of individuals), which runs 3 to 5 mm in length before passing the valve of Rosenmüller.[2]

The common canaliculus then opens into the lacrimal sac. The sac is lined by a multilayered columnar epithelium interspersed with goblet cells.[3] It is external to the periorbita, making it technically outside the orbit.[2] The sac sits within the lacrimal fossa, which is formed by the lacrimal bone and the frontal process of the maxillary bone. The thickness of the lacrimal bone averages 106 μm.[4] Portions of the lacrimal bone and the anterior lacrimal crest of the maxillary bone are removed during dacryocystorhinostomy (DCR) surgery to produce an opening between the lacrimal sac and the nasal cavity. The medial canthal tendon surrounds the lacrimal sac. The fundus of the sac extends 4 mm above the tendon and the body 10 mm below.

The lacrimal sac narrows at its inferior aspect, becoming the nasolacrimal duct. This duct measures 12 mm and runs in an inferolateroposterior direction within the maxillary bone. Blockage of the lacrimal duct results in tearing that requires DCR to bypass the obstruction. The duct exits via the valve of Hasner into the inferior meatus. An imperforate valve of Hasner is most often the cause of congenital nasolacrimal duct obstruction. In most cases, the valve eventually opens, resulting in spontaneous resolution of tearing in 90% of patients at 1 year of age.[2]

Any discussion of lacrimal system anatomy would be incomplete without mentioning the structures surrounding it. Most notably, the anterior cranial fossa is in very close proximity to the lacrimal system. Anatomic studies provide evidence of the cribiform plate being 25.1±2.95 mm from the internal common punctum.[5] Cerebrospinal fluid leak, a known complication of DCR, can result from direct penetration or more often from propagation of cracks created by improper twisting motion during bone removal.[2] The lacrimal fossa sits superiorly to the maxillary sinus and anterolateral to the ethmoid sinus. In 93% of orbits, the ethmoid air cells extend anterior to the lacrimal fossa.[4] The lateral nasal wall is composed of 3 turbinates: the superior, middle, and inferior turbinates. The middle turbinate is medial to the lacrimal sac and duct, and its meatus is where the opening for DCR is made. The nasolacrimal duct exits beneath the inferior turbinate in the inferior meatus as already mentioned. The duct lies medial to the maxillary antrum and can therefore be obstructed by masses located within this sinus.[2]

PHYSIOLOGY OF TEAR PRODUCTION

Recent evidence suggests that the ocular surface, which includes the cornea, conjunctiva, and the lacrimal and meibomian glands, exists as an integrated functional[6] unit (see Figure 13–6 and 13–8).[7] The majority of tear production from both the main and accessory lacrimal glands is reflexive. The afferent signal is carried along the ophthalmic branch of the trigeminal nerve (V1) to the pons. Within the pons, these nerve signals are integrated with emotional inputs from the cortex and other inputs from other central nervous system (CNS) centers. The efferent signal consists of parasympathetic fibers running with the facial nerve (CN VII) and from the paraspinal sympathetic chain. The parasympathetic fibers synapse in the sphenopalatine ganglion where postsynaptic fibers continue to the main and accessory lacrimal glands via the retro orbital nerve plexus. Sympathetic fibers synapse in the superior cervical ganglion and travel with the internal carotid artery to the lacrimal glands. Both systems are believed to elicit tear secretion. Stimulation of the ocular surface or nasal mucosa activates the reflex loop, resulting in the delivery of tears and proteins to the ocular surface.[6]

PHYSIOLOGY OF THE LACRIMAL PUMP

Tear production occurs at approximately 0.8 to 1.2 μL/min, resulting in about 1.5 cc/day.[2] Evaporation eliminates 10% of the produced tears in the young and up to 20% in adults. The lacrimal drainage system clears the rest of the tears.[8] The model of the lacrimal pump introduced by Jones in 1961 was the accepted model for many years. His theory was based upon static anatomical observations and suggested that capillary action, negative intrasac pressure gradients, and lateral to medial closing of the eyelids all combined to allow clearing of tears.[9] However, physiologic studies performed later suggested a better explanation of the tear pump.

The pump suggested by Rosengren-Doane involves a complex cycle involving positive and negative pressures with the orbicularis muscle acting as the motive force. At the beginning of each blink, the canaliculi and lacrimal sac are filled with the tears from the previous blink. As the blink begins, both papillae elevate and are forced into apposition at half closure of the lids. This effectively occludes the puncta and prevents regurgitation. During the rest of the blink, the contraction of the orbicularis muscle squeezes the canaliculi and lacrimal sac, forcing tears into the nose. At completion of a blink, the drainage system is compressed and for the most part empty. When the lids begin to open, the puncta are still closed, and the valves of Rosenmüller and Hasner prevent reflux of fluid or air. At this point, the orbicularis is no longer contracting, releasing compression on the drainage system. The elastic walls of the canaliculi and sac then try to re-expand, causing a vacuum in the system. When the lids are two-thirds open, the puncta pop open, allowing tears to be drawn into the canaliculi and sac.[8] The cycle, which takes 258 msec, then repeats itself.[10]

CONCLUSION

The tearing patients should be approached in a systematic manner. A complete examination of the patient, the eye, and the lacrimal system is necessary to locate the source of tearing. The ophthalmologist must remember not to focus on the first anatomic abnormality discovered without considering a multifactorial cause. A complete work-up performed prior to the initiation of treatment will ensure the correct diagnosis and greater patient satisfaction.

Key Points

1. The main lacrimal gland is thought to be responsible for reflex tear production. It is located in the lacrimal fossa of the superotemporal orbit and consists of 2 lobes.
2. The accessory lacrimal glands of Krauss and Wolfring are believed to be the main contributors to basal tear production.
3. The upper punctum is 6 mm and the lower is 6.5 mm from the medial canthus. Each is approximately 0.3 mm in diameter and sits on a papilla, an elevated ridge of tissue.
4. An opening is made in the ampullae during punctoplasty to create a larger "drain" for tears to enter.
5. Tear production occurs at approximately 0.8 to 1.2 μL/min, resulting in about 1.5 cc/day.

References

1. Hornblass A, ed. *Oculoplastic, Orbital, and Reconstructive Surgery.* Baltimore, Md: Williams & Wilkins; 1990:1331.

2. Chen WP. *Oculoplastic Surgery: The Essentials.* New York: Thieme; 2001:17, 263–288.

3. Ciftci F, Tse DT, Wesley RE, et al. Histopathologic changes in the lacrimal sac of dacryocystorhinostomy patients with and without silicone intubation. *Ophthal Plast Reconstr Surg.* 2005;21:59–64.

4. Blaylock WK, Moore CA, Lindberg JV. Anterior ethmoid anatomy facilitates dacryocystorhinostomy. *Arch Ophthalmol.* 1990;108:1774–1777.

5. Botega AA, Goldberg SH. Margins of safety in dacryocystorhinostomy. *Ophthalmic Surg.* 1993;24:320–323.

6. Plugfelder SC, Solomon A, Stern ME. The diagnosis and management of dry eye, a twenty-five-year review. *Cornea.* 2000;19:644–649.

7. Stern ME, Beuerman RW, Fox RI, et al. The pathology of dry eye: the interaction between the ocular surface and the lacrimal glands. *Cornea.* 1998;17:584–589.

8. Doane MG. Blinking and the mechanics of the lacrimal drainage system. *Ophthalmology.* 1981;88:844–851.

9. Jones LY. Anatomic approaches to problems of the eyelids and lacrimal apparatus. *Arch Ophthalmol.* 1961;66:111.

10. Doane MG. Interactions of eyelids and tears in corneal wetting and the dynamics of the normal human eyelid blink. *Am J Ophthalmol.* 1980;89:507–516.

3

Anatomy, Physiology, and Biochemistry of the Tear Film

Ashok Garg, MS, PhD, FRSM, FIAO;
Amar Agarwal, MS, FRCS, FRCOphth; and
C. Sujatha, DO

INTRODUCTION

The tear film[1-6] is not grossly visible on the surface of the eye but can be seen at the upper and lower lid margins as a 1-mm strip of tear fluid with a concave outer surface. This thin fluid film, known as preocular tear film, is a highly specialized and well-organized moist film that covers the exposed parts of the ocular globe—the cornea and the bulbar conjunctiva. It is the surface of the eye that remains most directly in contact with the environment. It is critically important for protecting the eye from external influences and for maintaining the health of the underlying cornea and conjunctiva. The optical stability and normal functions of the eye depend on an adequate supply of fluid covering its surface. It also serves a protective function for the eye. The presence of a continuous tear film over the exposed ocular surface is imperative for good visual acuity and the well-being of the epithelium and facilitates blinking.

Tear film serves the following functions:
- An optical function by maintaining an optically uniform corneal surface.
- A mechanical function by flushing cellular debris and foreign matter from the cornea and conjunctival sac and by lubricating the ocular surface.
- A corneal nutritional function.
- An antibacterial function.

ANATOMY

The tear film can be arbitrarily divided into 4 main parts:
1. The marginal tear film along the eyelid, which lies posterior to the lipid strip secreted by the tarsal glands.

2. Portion covering the palpebral conjunctiva.
3. Portion covering the bulbar conjunctiva.
4. Precorneal tear film that covers the cornea.

The volume of tear fluid is about 5 to 10 microl with a normal rate of secretion of about 1 to 2 microl/minute. About 95% of it is produced by the lacrimal gland and lesser amounts are produced by goblet cells and the accessory lacrimal glands of the conjunctiva. The total mass of the latter is about one-tenth of the mass of the main lacrimal gland.

The tear film is composed of 3 layers.

Superficial Lipid Layer

The superficial layer at the air-tear interface is formed by the oily secretions of the meibomian glands and possibly by the accessory sebaceous glands of Zeiss and Moll. The meibomian gland openings are distributed along the eyelid margin immediately behind the lash follicles.

The chemical nature of the lipid layer is essentially waxy and consists of cholesterol esters and some sterols. The thickness of this layer varies with the width of the palpebral fissure and is between 0.1 and 0.2 μm. The lipid layer thickens with a narrowed palpebral aperture.

The outer lipid layer has the following main functions:

-   It reduces the rate of evaporation of the underlying aqueous tear layer.
-   It alters surface tension so that tears do not overflow the lower lid margin.
-   It thickens and stabilizes tear film through interaction with the underlying aqueous layer.
-   It lubricates the eyelids as they pass over the surface of the globe.

Middle Aqueous Layer

The intermediate layer of tear film is the aqueous layer, which is secreted by the main lacrimal gland and the accessory glands of Krause and Wolfring. This layer constitutes almost the entire thickness of the tear film, being about 6.5 to 10 μm thick. It contains inorganic salts, water, proteins, enzymes, glucose, urea, metabolites, electrolytes, glycoproteins, and surface active biopolymers. Its main functions are:

-   It supplies atmospheric oxygen to the corneal epithelium and carries waste products away.
-   It helps prevent corneal infection because it contains antibacterial substances like lactoferrin and lysozyme.
-   It maintains the tonicity of the tear film.
-   It provides a smooth optical surface by removing any minute irregularities of the cornea.
-   It washes away debris from the cornea and conjunctiva.

Posterior Mucin Layer

The innermost layer of tear film is a thin mucoid layer secreted by the goblet cells of the conjunctiva and also by the crypts of Henle and glands of Manz. It is only 0.02 to 0.04 μm thick. This absorbs on the naturally hydrophobic epithelial surface of the cornea and conjunctiva, rendering them hydrophilic. The preocular tear film is dependent upon a constant supply of mucus to maintain corneal and conjunctival surfaces in the proper state of hydration. The mucous layer facilitates spreading of the tear film by smoothing the film over the corneal surface to form a perfect, regular refracting surface. It also provides lubrication, allowing the eyelid margin and palpebral conjunctiva to slide smoothly over one another and covers foreign bodies with a slippery coating thereby protecting the cornea and conjunctiva against their abrasive effect.

In addition to a quantitatively and qualitatively normal tear film, other important factors necessary for effective resurfacing of the cornea by the precorneal tear film are as follows:

- A normal blink reflex is essential to ensure that the mucin is brought from the inferior conjunctiva and rubbed into the corneal epithelium.
- Congruity between external ocular surface and the eyelids ensures that the precorneal tear film spreads evenly over the entire cornea.
- Normal epithelium is necessary for the adsorption of mucin onto its surface cells.

PHYSIOLOGY

Tear Film Maintenance

Maintenance of ocular surface depends on the production, secretion, distribution, and elimination of the tear film. This results in a thorough interaction between the lids, tear film, and the ocular surface.

Production of the Tear Film

LIPID SECRETION

Meibomian glands consist of globules of secretory cells emptying into a single duct. These cells disintegrate and are discharged into the duct. The movement of lipid along the duct to the surface is facilitated by contracture of orbicularis oculi muscle. Whether the gland is under sympathetic or parasympathetic control is not yet determined.

AQUEOUS PRODUCTION

The lacrimal gland consists of the main and the accessory parts. The main gland is a tubuloacinar exocrine type of gland. Paraductal acinar cells surround the central lumen, which communicates with ducts. The myoepithelial cells that surround the acini squeeze out secreted fluid.

MUCIN PRODUCTION

These glycoproteins are stored in membrane-bound secretory granules at the apical side of the goblet cells, which can be stimulated to produce mucin by parasympathetic agonists, histamine, chemical irritants, and prostaglandins. The secondary mucous secretory system is in the nongoblet cells in the conjunctival epithelium, located in the vesicles seen in apical sides of nongoblet cells of conjunctiva. These cells are responsible for increased tear secretion in allergic conditions like vernal conjunctivitis and giant papillary conjunctivitis.

Secretion of the Tear Film

The tear film is formed and maintained by an elaborate system—the lacrimal apparatus, which has secretory, distributive, and excretory parts. The secretory part includes the lacrimal gland, accessory lacrimal gland tissue, sebaceous glands of the eyelids,

Figure 3-1. Anatomy of the facial nerve (VII cranial nerve) showing the supply to the lacrimal gland.

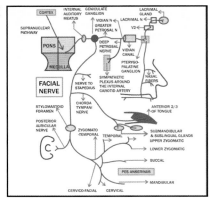

goblet cells, and other mucin-secreting elements of the conjunctiva. Basic secretion of tear fluid is made up of the secretions of the lacrimal gland and accessory lacrimal gland tissue together with the secretions of meibomian glands and the mucous glands of the conjunctiva. Reflex secretions of tears is a hundred times greater than basal or resting secretion. The stimulus to reflex secretions appear to be derived from the superficial corneal and conjunctival sensory stimulation as a result of tear breakup and dry spot formation. The secretory stimulus to the lacrimal glands is parasympathetic with reflex secretions occurring in both eyes, following superficial stimulation of one eye. The whole mass of lacrimal tissue responds as one unit to reflex tearing. Reflex secretion is reduced by topical corneal and conjunctival anesthesia.

Stimulation of the cornea gives rise to stimulation of parasympathetic VII nerve fibers via salivary nucleus through the greater petrosal nerve (Figure 3-1). The preganglionic fibers synapse in pterygopalatine ganglion from which postganglionic fibers follow zygomatic nerve via lacrimal nerve to the gland itself. Secretion of aqueous from the lacrimal and accessory glands is mediated by parasympathetic secretomotor fibers of the VII nerve. The gland also receives sympathetic inputs to the smooth muscles surrounding the arterioles. Thus these fibers have a regulatory effect on the gland's blood supply. Thus, the normal tear flow is under sympathetic control by regulating the blood supply, and reflex tear secretion is under parasympathetic control due to V nerve stimulation.

Distribution of the Tear Film

Tears forming the upper tear strip are conducted nasally from the upper temporal fornix. At the lateral canthus, the tears fall by gravity to form the lower strip, spreading medially. The upper and lower strips reach the plica and caruncle where they join together. The tear fluid does not flow over the eye by gravity, but a thin film is spread over the cornea by blinking and eye movements.

BLINK

Under normal conditions, a person blinks an average of 15 times per minute. During closure of the eyelids, the superficial lipid layer of the tear film is compressed and thickens between the eyelid edges; whereas the aqueous tear layer remains uniform under the lids and acts as a lubricant between the eyelids and the globe. When the eye-

Table 3-2 COMPOSITION OF HUMAN TEARS AND PLASMA (CONTINUED)		
7. Miscellaneous		
Citric acid	0.6 mg/100 mL	2.2 to 2.8 mg/100 mL
Ascorbic acid	0.14 mg/100 mL	0.1 to 0.7 mg/100 mL
Lysozyme	1 to 2 mg/mL	—
Amino acid	7.58 mg/100 mL	—
Lactate	1 to 5 mmol/L	0.5 to 0.8 mmol/L
Prostaglandin	75 pg PF/mL	80 to 90 pg PF/mL
	300 pg PF/mL	
	0.5 to 1.5 µg/mL	
Catecholamine	1:4 dilution	1.32 dilution

Table 3-3 AMINO ACID COMPOSITION OF HUMAN TEAR LYSOZYME	
Amino Acids	*Residues (g/100 g protein)*
Aspartic acid	13.23
Arginine	13.05
Glutamic acid	8.55
Tryptophan	6.89
Alanine	6.36
Leucine	6.11
Trypsin	5.65
Glycine	4.94
Lysine	4.92
Valine	4.62
Serine	4.02
Half-cysteine	4.01
Threonine	3.67
Isoleucine	3.59
Phenylalanine	1.97
Proline	1.72
Methionine	1.50
Histidine	1.01

Table 3-4		
RELATIVE QUANTITY OF VARIOUS PROTEIN FRACTIONS IN TEARS		
Fractions	*Normal Tears (%)*	*Stimulated Flow (Tears) (%)*
Albumin	58.2	20.2
Globulin	23.9	56.9
Lysozyme	17.9	22.9

Table 3-5			
ORIGIN OF VARIOUS TEAR PROTEIN FRACTIONS			
Protein Fraction	*Lacrimal Gland proper*	*Accessory Lacrimal gland*	*Goblet Cells*
Lysozyme	+	−	−
Component-I	−	+	±
Component-II	+	±	±
Component-III	+	±	±
Serum albumin	−	−	+
Tear albumin	+	−	−
Mucin	−	−	+

+ fraction is present.
− fraction is absent.
± fraction is indifferently present.

bacteriostatic activity in tears, making essential metal ions unavailable for microbial metabolism.

The lysozyme and beta-lysin protein fractions can be separated by filtering the tears. Beta-lysin acts primarily on cellular membrane, while lysozyme dissolves bacterial cell walls.

Transferrin

Transferrin, along with serum albumin and IgG, can be detected only after mild trauma to the mucosal surface of the conjunctiva or in tears.

Ceruloplasmin

Ceruloplasmin, a copper carrying protein, is regularly found in tears. In electrophoresis, the migration rate of tear ceruloplasmin varies from its serum counterpart.

Immunoglobulins

The details are given in Table 3-6.

Immunoglobulin A (IgA) is the major immunoglobulin present in tears, saliva, and colostrum. The possible functions of secretory IgA include prevention of viral and bacterial infections that may have an access to the external secretions (eg, tears) and participate as opsonins in the phagocytosis process.

Ig Class	Tears	Serum
Total proteins	800 mg/100 mL	6500 mg/100 mL
IgA	14 to 24 mg/100 mL	170 to 200 mg/100 mL
IgG	17 mg/100 mL	1000 mg/100 mL
IgM	5 to 7 mg/100 mL	100 mg/100 mL
IgE	26 to 250 microg/mL	2000 microg/mL

Table 3-6
IMMUNOGLOBULIN LEVELS IN TEAR AND SERUM

In the human lacrimal gland, IgA appears to be synthesized by interstitial plasma cells. After entry into the intercellular spaces, it is coupled to secretory component (SC) and secreted as secretory IgA (IgA-SC) through the blood-tear barrier involving intracellular transport by acinar epithelial cells into the lumen. In the conjunctiva, IgA and plasma cells are located in the substantia propria. Only in the acinar epithelium of the accessory lacrimal glands can SC material be present, indicating that these are the sites of synthesis of secretory IgA of the conjunctival secretions. Depending upon the method of tear collection, IgA values can vary from 10 to 100 mg%.

Immunoglobulin G (IgG) is present in very low concentrations in normal tears. However, after mild trauma to the mucosal surface of the conjunctiva, it can be easily detected. During the secondary response, IgG is the major immunoglobulin to be synthesized. Probably because of its small size, IgG diffuses more readily than other immunoglobulins into the tears; therefore, as the predominating immunoglobulin, it carries the major burden of neutralizing bacterial toxins and of binding to microorganisms (specially streptococci, pneumococci, and staphylococci) to enhance their phagocytosis. IgG is most efficient in killing and stopping the progress of microbial invasion.

Immunoglobulin M (IgM) is present in very low concentrations in normal tears. IgM is an extremely efficient agglutinating and cytolytic agent and is the first type of antibody that is formed after the initial encounter with an antigen. It appears early in the response to infection and is confined mainly to the blood stream.

Even minimum trauma to conjunctiva would cause serum proteins to leak into the tears. There is increased concentrations of IgA, IgG, and IgE in tears. Either these immunoglobulins are selectively excreted into the tears or they are locally synthesized. Increased concentrations of IgA, IgG, and IgM are reported in cases of blepharoconjunctivitis, herpes keratitis, vernal conjunctivitis, acute follicular conjunctivitis, phlyctenular conjunctivitis, keratomalacia, corneal ulcer, and acute endogenous uveitis.

Immunoglobulin E (IgE) is mostly extravascular in distribution. Normal serum contains only traces of IgE, but greatly elevated levels are seen in atopic conditions.

Immunoglobulin D (IgD) levels are quite low in tears as well as in serum. It is mostly intravascular.

Complement
Complement in tears has been shown in hemolytic assays up to dilution of 1:4, whereas serum is active in this system up to 1:32.

Table 3-7
ANTIMICROBIAL FACTORS IN TEARS

Compound	Evidence
Lysozyme	+
IgA	+
IgG	±
IgE	+
IgM	±
Complement	+
Lactoferrin	+
Tractoferrin	±
Beta-lysin	+
Antibiotic producing commensal organism	+

+ present in normal tears.
± present in tears after stimulation (mild trauma to the conjunctiva).

Glycoproteins

Glycoproteins are present in the mucoid layer as well as in the tear fluid since they are highly soluble in water. Glycoproteins contribute significantly to the stickiness of the material forming the mucoid layer. N-acetylneuraminic acid (a sialic acid) has been identified in normal tears. Glycoproteins may play a critical role in the lubrication of the corneal surface by rendering its hydrophobic surface more hydrophilic, permitting spreading and stabilization of the tear film. The glycoproteins are carbohydrate-protein complexes characterized by the presence of hexosamines, hexoses, and sialic acid. In normal tears relative hexosamine content of the protein, which is used as an indicator for glycoproteins, varies from 0.5% to 17%, the hexosamine concentration from 0.05 to 3 g/L. Sialic acid concentration of human tears has been reported to be 114 mol/100 mL.

Antiproteinases

The antimicrobial factors in tears are shown in Table 3-7.

METABOLITES

A number of metabolites have been reported to be present in normal human tears. These include organic constituents of low molecular weight like glucose, urea, and amino acids and other metabolites like lactate, histamine, prostaglandins, and catecholamines.

Glucose

Glucose is present in minimal amounts of about 0.2 mmol/L in tear fluids of normoglycemic persons. This low concentration of glucose appears to be insufficient for corneal nutrition. There is no definitive evidence that the cornea metabolizes glucose from the tears.

There is a corresponding rise in tear glucose level with elevation of plasma glucose level above 100 mg%. However, there is no significant rise in tear glucose levels in diabetics with blood glucose levels of more than 20 mmol/L, which demonstrates the barrier function of the corneal and conjunctival epithelium against loss of glucose from the tissues into the tear fluid. It is the tissue fluid that contributes to the tear glucose after mechanically stimulated methods of tear collection.

Urea
Urea concentration in tear fluid and plasma has been found to be equivalent, suggesting an unrestricted passage through the blood-tear barrier in the lacrimal gland. Urea concentration in tears decreases with increasing secretion rate.

Amino Acids
Free amino acid concentration in tears is reported to be 7.58 mg/100 mL. This value is 3 to 4 times higher than the free amino acid concentration in serum.

Lactate
Lactate levels of 1 to 5 mmol/L in tears are far higher than the normal blood levels of 0.5 to 0.8 mmol/L. Pyruvate from 0.05 to 0.35 mmol/L is about the same as is normal for blood (0.1 to 0.2 mmol/L). These levels do not show significant alterations after mechanical irritation. The epithelium does not possess a barrier function for lactate and pyruvate.

Histamine
Histamine is present in normal tears collected from the conjunctival sac at a level of about 10 mg/mL. In vernal conjunctivitis specifically a variable increase up to 125 mg/mL has been observed.

Prostaglandins
Prostaglandins are present in normal tears at a level of 75 pg prostaglandin F/mL and it is a little lower than in serum. Significantly higher values are found in inflammatory conditions of the eye, up to 300 pg/mL of tears.

Catecholamines, Dopamine, Noradrenaline, and Dopa
Catecholamines, dopamine, noradrenaline, and dopa have been found in the tear fluid. The levels vary from 0.5 to 1.5 microg/mL. Dopamine has values as high as 280 microg/mL.

In glaucoma patients, lower values have been reported for these compounds that reflect the diminished activity of the sympathetic innervation of the eye. The determination of catecholamines in tears has been advocated as a test in glaucoma diagnosis.

ELECTROLYTES AND HYDROGEN IONS
The predominant positively charged electrolytes (cation) in tears are mainly sodium and potassium, while the negative ions (anions) are chloride and bicarbonate.

Sodium
Sodium concentration in tears (120 to 170 mmol/L) is about equal to that in plasma, suggesting a passive secretion into the tears, while potassium with an average value of about 20 mmol/L is much higher than the corresponding plasma concentration of about 5 mmol/L. This indicates an active secretion of potassium into the tears. It is interesting to observe that the main cationic constituent of the aqueous and vitreous humor is sodium, while the cornea (mainly corneal epithelium) contains a much high-

er concentration of potassium than sodium. These 2 cations play an essential role in the osmotic regulation of the extracellular and intracellular spaces. In general, changes in the sodium level are the reverse of changes in the potassium level.

Calcium
Calcium is independent of tear production and is lower than the free fraction of plasma. Cystic fibrosis patients have much higher calcium values.

Magnesium
Magnesium in tears is a little lower than the corresponding serum value, possibly reflecting the free fraction of magnesium. Both calcium and magnesium play a role in controlling membrane permeability.

Chloride
Chloride, an anion essential to all tissues, also plays an important role in osmotic regulation much like sodium and potassium. The chloride concentration is slightly higher in tears than in serum.

Bicarbonate
Bicarbonate together with the carbonate ions in tears may be involved in the regulation of pH. This buffer system maintains the near neutral pH of the tear film, the surface of which is exposed to atmospheric changes.

ENZYMES

Enzymes of Energy Producing Metabolism
Glycolytic enzymes and enzymes of tricarboxylic acid cycle can be detected in high values only in human tear samples. The source of these enzymes is in the conjunctiva where they are secreted in small amounts. The lacrimal gland apparently does not secrete these enzymes. These enzymes can be obtained during mechanical irritation.

Lactate Dehydrogenase
Lactate dehydrogenase (LDH) is the enzyme in the highest concentration in tears. It can be separated electrophoretically into its 5 isoenzymes, showing a pattern with more of the slower migrating muscle type isoenzymes. This is closely related to the distribution pattern of corneal tissue in contrast to serum LDH where the faster migrating heart type isoenzymes prevail.

These findings indicate that tear LDH originates from the corneal epithelium. Therefore, in patients suffering from corneal disease, the distribution of LDH isoenzymes in tears differs from those found in healthy individuals.

Lysosomal Enzymes
Lysosomal enzymes include a number of lysosomal acid hydrolases that are present in tears in concentration of 2 to 10 times that in serum. The lacrimal gland is the main source of the lysosomal enzymes, but conjunctiva may act as a second source for lysosomal enzymes after mild trauma. Lysosomal enzyme activities in tears are used for the diagnosis and identification of carriers of several inborn errors of metabolism.

The concentration of β-hexosaminidase in tears collected on filter paper strips is an index for the development and prognosis of diabetic retinopathy. The tears would reflect the decreased enzyme activity of β-hexosaminidase and of other lysosomal glycosidases in the retina, showing a negative correlation with the increased plasma levels of these enzymes.

Amylase
Amylase is the enzyme present in tear fluid in relatively moderate levels. The origin of this enzyme is in the lacrimal gland. The reported presence of amylase in the cornea might be due to contamination by tear fluid.

Peroxidase
Peroxidase (POD) is present in human tears, originating from the lacrimal gland and not from the conjunctiva.

Plasminogen Activator
Plasminogen activator has been demonstrated in tear fluid, and corneal epithelium is suggested to be the source of this urokinase-like fibrinolytic activity.

Collagenase
Collagenase has been shown to be present in tear fluid in the presence of corneal ulceration due to infection, chemical burns, trauma, and desiccation. Corneal collagenase is present as an inactive precursor "latent collagenase" that can be activated with trypsin and *in vivo* possibly by plasmin resulting from plasminogen activator activity in tears.

Key Points

1. The tear film is formed and maintained by an elaborate system—the lacrimal apparatus, which has secretory, distributive, and excretory parts.
2. If the BUT is shorter than the average time interval between 2 consecutive blinks, premature tear film rupture can cause pathological changes in the underlying epithelium.
3. Reflex stimulation of tears in early adaptation to contact lenses results in a relative hypotonicity that may account for the corneal edema often seen in early stages of contact lens wearing.
4. HTL levels have been shown to be greatly decreased in tears of patients suffering from Sjögren's syndrome and ocular toxicity from long-term use of practolol therapy, thus making it a useful diagnostic aid. Other disease states in which HTL level is lowered include herpes simplex virus infection and malnutrition in children.
5. Normal serum contains only traces of IgE, but greatly elevated levels are seen in atopic conditions.
6. The determination of catecholamines in tears has been advocated as a test in glaucoma diagnosis.
7. Cystic fibrosis patients have much higher calcium values.
8. Lysosomal enzyme activities in tears are used for the diagnosis and identification of carriers of several inborn errors of metabolism.
9. The concentration of β-hexosaminidase in tears collected on filter paper strips is an index for the development and prognosis of diabetic retinopathy.

REFERENCES

1. Hart WM. *Eugene Wolff's Anatomy of the Eye and Orbit.* Philadelphia: WB Saunders; 1992.
2. Last RJ. *Adler's Physiology of the Eye.* 9th ed. St. Louis, Mo: Mosby Year Book, Inc; 1961.
3. Rolando M, Zierhut M. The ocular surface and tear film and their dysfunction in dry eye disease. *Surv Ophthalmol.* 2001;45:S203–S210.
4. Doane MG. Interactions of eyelids and tears in corneal wetting and the dynamics of the normal human eyeblink. *Am J Ophthalmol.* 1980;89:507–516.
5. Dilly PN. Structure and function of the tear film. *Adv Exp Med Biol.* 1994;350:239–247.
6. Tsubota K, Tseng TCG, Nordlund ML. Anatomy and physiology of the ocular surface. In: Holland EJ, Mannis MJ, eds. *Ocular Surface Disease.* New York, NY: Springer-Verlag; 2002.

4

Dry Eye Process and Ocular Surface Disorders

Soosan Jacob, MS, FRCS, Dip NB and
Amar Agarwal, MS, FRCS, FRCOphth

INTRODUCTION

The ocular surface refers to the mucosal lining of the eye bordered by the skin at the superior and inferior lid margins. This surface covers the cornea, the limbus, and the conjunctiva. The main functions of the ocular surface are to provide clear vision during open eye conditions, to maintain comfort, to prevent microbial invasion, and to protect the eye from mechanical insults. For this, the ocular surface has to be covered by a stable tear film.

The 2 components essential for maintaining ocular surface health are a healthy ocular surface epithelium and a normal, stable preocular tear film, both of which function as a unit. An alteration in the quantity or quality of any of the elements of the tear film can lead to an unstable tear film and secondary changes in the epithelium. Vice versa, primary changes of the ocular surface epithelium as part of ocular surface failure can lead to a secondary dry eye (Figure 4-1). Thus, an intimate relationship exists between the two and any change in this can lead to the occurrence of various ocular surface disorders. Because all elements of ocular surface defense are integrated and work in concert with ocular surface epithelia, the entire spectrum of ocular surface disorders are better treated as a group than isolated disease entities, no matter whether they range from ocular irritation to defective wound healing and surface destruction.

NORMAL OCULAR SURFACE DEFENSE

There are 2 factors essential for normal functioning of the ocular surface: a normal, adequate, and stable tear film and normally functioning hydrodynamic factors. The tear

Figure 4-1. Corneal epithelial defect with ocular surface disorder. Note the corneal vascularization present.

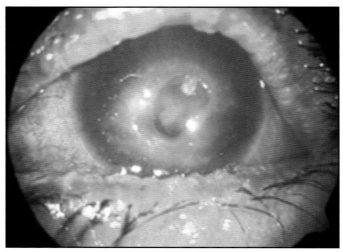

Figure 4-2. Interplay of factors essential for normal tear film and ocular surface.

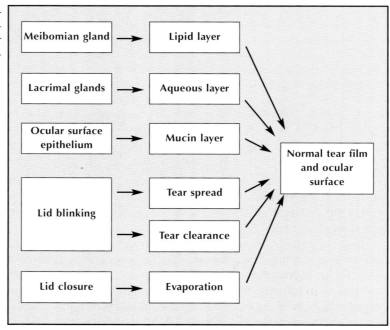

film consists of a mucin layer, an aqueous layer, and a lipid layer. Hydrodynamic factors include periodic, adequate, and complete lid blinking to distribute an even tear film over the ocular surface and proper tear clearance to ensure adequate turnover and refreshment. Thus, the eyelids, the external adnexal glands, and the ocular surface epithelia all play a major role in maintaining a normal tear film and ocular surface (Figure 4-2). Two neuronal reflex arcs function in this process. For both the arcs, the first branch of the trigeminal nerve (V1) controls the ocular sensitivity as the afferent sensory input, and the parasympathetic branch and the motor branch of the facial nerve (VII) are the afferent output.

OCULAR SURFACE FAILURE

Impression cytology has identified 2 major types of ocular surface failure based on the epithelial phenotype,[1] which will be discussed below.

With Intact Limbal Stem Cells

Here, the normal nonkeratinized ocular surface epithelium undergoes squamous metaplasia into keratinized epithelium.[1,2] This is also associated with loss of goblet cells and mucin expression, which in turn are accompanied by a switch to expression of epidermal keratins.[3] This altered epithelial differentiation renders the ocular surface epithelium nonwettable. This leads to an unstable tear film, the hallmark of various dry eye disorders.

When the nature of the primary pathology is due to poor ocular surface defense, the resulting squamous metaplasia is probably due to dryness, deficiency in factors and nutrients required for growth and differentiation, or chronic mechanical trauma by eyelid movement. This kind of squamous metaplasia is fully reversible if the ocular surface defense is restored. This indicates the stem cells of the ocular surface are not defective. Here, the dry eye may be secondary to the following:

AQUEOUS TEAR DEFICIENCY

The middle thick aqueous layer of the tear film is produced by the main lacrimal glands (reflex tearing), as well as the accessory lacrimal glands of Krause and Wolfring (basic tearing).

Aqueous tear deficiency can be idiopathic (age-related, more common in women after menopause) or due to vitamin A deficiency (xerophthalmia), sensory denervation (after surgery or severe keratitis), collagen vascular diseases (rheumatoid arthritis, Wegener granulomatosis, systemic lupus erythematosus, etc), Sjögren's syndrome and related autoimmune disorders, rheumatoid arthritis, scleroderma, polymyositis, dermatomyositis, polyarteritis nodosa, Hashimoto's thyroiditis, chronic hepatobiliary cirrhosis, lymphocytic interstitial pneumonitis, thrombocytopenic purpura, hypergammaglobulinemia, Waldenström's macroglobulinemia, interstitial nephritis, others, drugs (oral contraceptives, antidepressants, antihistamines, beta-blockers, others), lacrimal glands infiltration (amyloidosis, sarcoidosis, or tumors), fibrosis of the lacrimal glands (radiotherapy), lacrimal gland ablation, and contact lens use (impaired tear reflex).

LIPID TEAR LAYER DEFICIENCY

The superficial thin lipid layer is produced by the meibomian glands, and its principal function is to retard tear evaporation and to assist in uniform tear spreading.

A lipid tear layer deficiency may occur secondary to blepharitis, acne rosacea, contact lenses, etc.

MUCIN TEAR LAYER DEFICIENCY

The innermost hydrophilic mucin layer is produced by both the conjunctiva goblet cells and the ocular surface epithelium, and associates itself with the ocular surface via its loose attachments to the glycocalyx of the microplicae of the epithelium. It is the hydrophilic quality of the mucin that allows the aqueous to spread over the corneal epithelium.

Mucin tear layer deficiency may be due to vitamin A deficiency, trachoma, mucocutaneous disorders, topical medications, contact lenses, and conjunctival scarring

Figure 4-3. Dry eye due to ectropion. (Courtesy of Guillermo L. Simón-Castellví.)

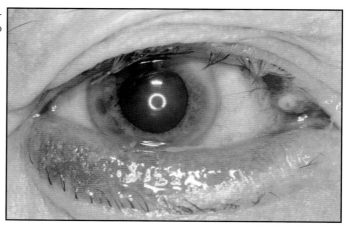

Figure 4-4. Dry eye due to thyroid eye disease. The dry eye has lead to corneal ulceration. A tarsorrhaphy has been done. (Courtesy of Guillermo L. Simón-Castellví.)

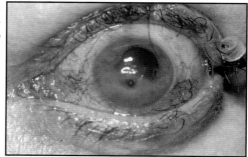

(benign ocular pemphigoid, Stevens-Johnson syndrome, atopia, trachoma, chemical/thermal/radiation burns).

Increased Tear Film Evaporation

Air conditioning, computer use (insufficient blink), blink reflex malfunction (V cranial), lid retraction, lagophthalmos, ectropion (Figure 4-3), insufficient lid closure, exophthalmos (eg, thyroid disease) (Figure 4-4), increased lid aperture, driving with the window open, etc may predispose to this.

Recently, it is thought that all tear production is controlled by sensory stimuli from different sources innervated by V1 and thus, the amount of aqueous tear formation varies according to the intensity of the total sensory drive. Defective corneal or conjunctival sensitivity may, therefore, lead to a deficiency in aqueous tear production due to a decrease in the sensory drive. It also results in inadequate blinking, resulting in increased exposure and evaporation, collectively leading to an unstable tear film. Ocular hypoesthesia is thus frequently associated with dryness-induced keratopathy.

Delayed Tear Clearance

Delayed tear clearance secondary to ineffective lacrimal pump mechanism or to obstruction in tear outflow can result in accumulation of infectious, toxic, allergic, inflammatory, or other irritant factors that can lead to ocular surface disorders by either causing an unstable tear film or by direct irritant effect on the ocular surface epithelium.

In dry eye patients, there is a disruption of the normal neuronal control of tear secretion and damage to the lacrimal glands and the ocular surface. In the healthy eye, dryness acts as a stimulus to send signals to the brain, which in turn stimulates the lacrimal gland to produce tears. In dry eye syndrome, inflammatory cells damage the lacrimal gland, causing a decreased production of tears. The little tears that are produced contain inflammatory cells that, along with the inherent dryness, damage the ocular surface and reduce corneal sensation. The corneal anesthesia decreases brainstem stimulation, which in turn reduces the firing to the lacrimal gland, causing a vicious cycle.

Histopathology of postmortem lacrimal gland tissue from dry eye patients shows a high degree of infiltration by T lymphocytes in all kinds of dry eye patients. The disease is thus autoimmune regardless of whether or not the patient has a circulating immunoglobulin. Topical therapy with cyclosporine helps in dry eye by eliminating the inflammatory component of the syndrome by causing apoptosis of T lymphocytes. This restores normal lacrimal function and corneal sensation. The quality of the tear film also improves, which provides further support to the cornea, reversing the damage to the cornea's neurological integrity.

Associated With Limbal Stem Cell Deficiency

Here, the normal corneal epithelial phenotype is replaced by conjunctival epithelium. Patients may present with severe photophobia and defective vision. The salient features seen here are conjunctivalization, vascularization, chronic inflammation, poor epithelial integrity manifested as an irregular surface, recurrent erosion and persistent ulcer, destruction of the basement membrane, and fibrous ingrowth.[4] These patients generally respond poorly to conventional corneal transplantation. Conjunctivalization is the hallmark of limbal stem cell deficiency and may be confirmed by impression cytology, which shows the presence of goblet cells.[4]

Limbal stem cell deficiency can be due to a variety of hereditary or acquired conditions.[5–12] Conditions with limbal stem cell deficiency can be classified in terms of the following.

PRIMARY LIMBAL STEM CELL DEFICIENCY

These patients exhibit a gradual loss of limbal stem cell function over time. It is generally seen in association with conditions like aniridia, congenital erythrokeratodermia, keratitis associated with multiple endocrine deficiencies, neurotrophic (neural and ischemic) keratopathy, peripheral inflammatory or ulcerative keratitis or limbitis, idiopathic keratopathy, and pterygium/pseudopterygium. It is possible that limbal stem cell function is modulated by developmental, hormonal, neuronal, vascular, and inflammatory factors in the limbal stromal microenvironment, and dysfunction of the limbal stroma can lead to limbal deficiency. It is also possible that the associated diseases alter the stroma and then indirectly affect epithelial functions.

SECONDARY LIMBAL STEM CELL DEFICIENCY

Cases with secondary limbal stem cell deficiency have a clear pathogenic cause that is responsible for destruction of the limbal stem cells. It may occur subsequent to chemical or thermal injuries, Stevens-Johnson syndrome, ocular rosacea, ocular pemphigoid, contact lens wear, severe microbial infection or "iatrogenic" causes such as multiple surgeries or cryotherapies at the limbal region, and antimetabolite (5-FU) toxicity.[13] The limbal stem cell destruction may be secondary to stromal inflammation or loss of vascular supply as a result of scarring in the stroma. The resultant squamous metaplasia leads to an unstable tear film and hence results in a dry eye even if there are adequate amounts of aqueous tear fluid. Limbal autografts[14–24] can be used for patients with focal or unilateral limbal deficiency and allograft source[21,22,25–29] of either HLA-matched living donors or nonmatched cadavers for those with bilateral and diffuse limbal deficiency.

CONCLUSION

We see that ocular surface health is maintained by a close relationship between ocular surface epithelium and the preocular tear film, the whole mechanism being under neuroanatomic control. Limbal stem cell function is supported by stromal fibroblasts and matrix, and their primary or secondary deficiency can lead to a variety of ocular surface disorders.

Key Points

1. An alteration in the quantity or quality of any of the elements of the tear film can lead to an unstable tear film and secondary changes in the epithelium. Vice versa, primary changes of the ocular surface epithelium as part of ocular surface failure can lead to a secondary dry eye.
2. There are 2 factors essential for normal functioning of the ocular surface: a normal, adequate, and stable tear film and normally functioning hydrodynamic factors. The tear film consists of a mucin layer, an aqueous layer, and a lipid layer. Hydrodynamic factors include periodic, adequate, and complete lid blinking to distribute an even tear film over the ocular surface and proper tear clearance to ensure adequate turnover and refreshment.
3. Impression cytology has identified 2 major types of ocular surface failure based on the epithelial phenotype: with intact limbal stem cells and without intact limbal stem cells.
4. In ocular surface failure with intact limbal stem cells, the normal nonkeratinized ocular surface epithelium undergoes squamous metaplasia into keratinized epithelium. This is also associated with loss of goblet cells and mucin expression, which in turn are accompanied by a switch to expression of epidermal keratins.[3]
5. Limbal stem cell deficiency can be primary or secondary.

REFERENCES

1. Tseng SCG. Staging of conjunctival squamous metaplasia by impression cytology. *Ophthalmology*. 1985;92:728–733.
2. Lemp MA. Report of the National Eye Institute/Industry Workshop on clinical trials in dry eyes. *CLAO J*. 1995;21:4–15.

3. Tseng SCG, Hatchell D, Tiemey N, Huang AJW, Sun TT. Expression of specific keratin markers by rabbit corneal, conjunctival, and esophageal epithelia during vitamin A deficiency. *J Cell Biol.* 1984;99:2.279–2.286.
4. Puangsricharern V, Tseng SCG. Cytologic evidence of corneal diseases with limbal stem cell deficiency. *Ophthalmology.* 1995;102:1.476–1.485.
5. Dua HS, Azuara Blanco A. Limbal stem cells of the corneal epithelium. *Surv Ophthalmol.* 2000;44:415–425.
6. Thoft RA, Wiley LA, Sundarraj N. The multipotential cells of the limbus. *Eye.* 1989;3:109–113.
7. Tseng SC. Concept and application of limbal stem cells. *Eye.* 1989;3:141–157.
8. Dua HS. Stem cells of the ocular surface: scientific principles and clinical applications. *Br J Ophthalmol.* 1995;79:968–969.
9. Tseng SC. Regulation and clinical implications of corneal epithelial stem cells. *Mol Biol Rep.* 1996;23:47–58.
10. Chen JJ, Tseng SC. Abnormal corneal epithelial wound healing in partial thickness removal of limbal epithelium. *Invest Ophthalmol Vis Sci.* 1991;32:2219–2233.
11. Dua HS, Saini JS, Azuara Blanco A, Gupta P. Limbal stem cell deficiency: concept, aetiology, clinical presentation, diagnosis and management. *Indian J Ophthalmol.* 2000;48:83–92.
12. Huang AJ, Tseng SC. Corneal epithelial wound healing in the absence of limbal epithelium. *Invest Ophthalmol Vis Sci.* 1991;32:96–105.
13. Schwartz GS, Holland EJ. Iatrogenic limbal stem cell deficiency. *Cornea.* 1998;7:31–37.
14. Tseng SCG, Chen JJY, Huang AJW, Kruse FE, Maskin SL, Tsai RJF. Classification of conjunctival surgeries for corneal disease based on stem cell concept. *Ophthalmol Clin North Am.* 1990;3: 595–610.
15. Holland EJ, Schwartz GS. The evolution of epithelial transplantation for severe ocular surface disease and a proposed classification system. *Cornea.* 1996;15:549–556.
16. Kenyon KR, Tseng SCG. Limbal autograft transplantation for ocular surface disorders. *Ophthalmology.* 1989;96:709–723.
17. Copeland RA, Char DH. Limbal autograft reconstruction after conjunctival squamous cell carcinoma. *Am J Ophthalmol.* 1990;110:412–415.
18. Kenyon KR. Limbal autograft transplantation for chemical and thermal bums. *Dev Ophthalmol.* 1989;18:53–58.
19. Jenkins C, Tuft S, Liu C, Buckley R. Limbal transplantation in the management of chronic contact-lens-associated epitheliopathy. *Eye.* 1993;7:629–633.
20. Ronk JF, Ruiz-Esmenjaud S, Osorio M, Bacigalupi M, Goosey JD. Limbal conjunctival autograft in a subacute alkaline corneal burn. *Cornea.* 1994;13:465–468.
21. Tan DTH, Ficker LA, Buckley RJ. Limbal transplantation. *Ophthalmology.* 1996;103:29–36.
22. Holland EJ. Epithelial transplantation for the management of severe ocular surface disease. *Trans Am Ophthalmol Soc.* 1996;94:677–743.
23. Mashima Y, Yamada M, Yamada H, Tsunoda K, Arimoto M. Limbal autograft transplantations for chronic ocular surface failure. *Jpn J Clin Ophthalmol.* 1993;47:607–610.
24. Morgan S, Murray A. Limbal autotransplantation in the acute and chronic phases of severe chemical injuries. *Eye.* 1996;10:349–354.
25. Kenyon KR, Rapoza PA. Limbal allograft transplantation for ocular surface disorders. *Ophthalmology.* 1995;102(Suppl):101–102.
26. Tsai RJF, Tseng SCG. Human allograft limbal transplantation for corneal surface reconstruction. *Cornea.* 1994;13:389–400.
27. Tsubota K, Toda I, Saito H, Shinozaki N, Shimazaki J. Reconstruction of the corneal epithelium by limbal allograft transplantation for severe ocular surface disorders. *Ophthalmology.* 1995; 102:1.486–1.496.

28. Theng JTS, Tan DTH. Combined penetrating keratoplasty and limbal allograft transplantation for severe corneal burns. *Ophthal Surg Lasers.* 1997;28:765–768.
29. Sangwan VS, Tseng SCG. New perspectives in ocular surface disorders. An integrated approach for diagnosis and management. *Indian J Ophthalmol.* 2001;49:153–168.

Section II

Clinical Assessment

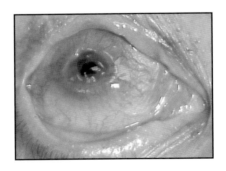

5

Evaluation of the Dry Eye Patient

Grant D. Gilliland, MD

INTRODUCTION

Patients with dry eye frequently have a long history of complaints for burning or a "sand-like" or "gritty" sensation in their eyes. Symptoms can range from mild and infrequent to severe, constant, and debilitating. Other symptoms described include dryness, grittiness, redness, and ocular fatigue. Studies have shown, however, that signs and symptoms do not always correlate and that clinical dry eye examination did not correlate with symptoms when corrected for age and artificial tear usage.[1] Furthermore, the frequency of symptoms has not been shown to correlate with clinical examination of the dry eye.[1] Other studies have examined the repeatability of dry eye examination tests and found them to be largely unrepeatable. The same study examined the repeatability of dry eye symptomatology and found moderately high repeatability there.[2]

INCIDENCE

The incidence of dry eye has been shown to be significant in several studies. The Beaver Dam study demonstrated an incidence of dry eye of 13% that was significantly correlated with patient age.[3] Dry eye symptoms are well known to be associated with middle to older aged females. It is estimated to affect 3.2 million American women and involves 5.7% of women aged 50 or less and 9.8% of women older than age 75.[4]

RISK FACTORS

Risk factors for dry eye have been studied extensively. Sjögren's syndrome is a well known cause and risk factor for dry eye. As stated above, advanced age and female race are also associated with the presence of dry eye symptoms. Other risk factors include the presence of diabetes, allergy, use of antihistamines or diuretics, premature ovarian failure, and the presence of a pterygium.[3,5,6]

DRY EYE DIAGNOSIS

Because dry eye is a significant health problem and there has been a paucity of reliable, repeatable clinical tests until recently, there is an obvious need for standardized repeatable testing to diagnose the presence and severity of dry eye pathology. Dry eye is in reality a group of diseases that adversely affect the corneal epithelium. This epithelial disease may in turn lead to tear film instability, becoming an endless vicious cycle unless treated. The clinical presentation may be so variable as to give no indication to the cause of the disease. Recent advances in dry eye disease diagnosis and treatment have been significant. Dry eye diagnosis can roughly be divided into 4 groups:

1. The first is based on clinical presentation.
2. The second relates to tear film composition, osmolality, and tear film dynamics.
3. The third is tear film related and includes tear BUT, evaporation, and lipid abnormalities. Several new assays for lipids in the tear film have been shown to be useful.
4. The fourth relates to the ocular surface and is evaluated by surface staining, impression cytology, and surface microscopy.[7]

Clinical History

For years, clinical history was regarded as the most accurate measure of whether a patient had a significant dry eye disease. It is felt that symptoms appear earlier than objective manifestation of the disease in many patients and are more consistent than many of the early objective measures of dry eye disease. A careful and thorough clinical history is extremely useful in classifying the etiology of the disease and directing potentially significant treatment modalities. Most patients can not elucidate a specific date or time that their symptoms started in that most dry eye diseases are insidious in onset. Patients that can point to a specific date as the starting point for their symptoms usually have a well-defined etiology of their dry eye disease. Certainly, an abrupt onset of an eyelid abnormality could cause dry eye disease. Examples include facial nerve palsy (posttraumatic, postsurgical, idiopathic, Ramsay-Hunt syndrome, etc), ectropion (senile, posttraumatic, neoplastic, cicatricial, etc), entropion (senile, cicatricial, neoplastic, posttraumatic, developmental), lagophthalmos (postsurgical, posttraumatic, neoplastic, etc), and lid retraction (autoimmune, cicatricial, posttraumatic, neoplastic, postsurgical, etc). A history of an insidious onset is less helpful in defining etiology and is far more common than a history of an abrupt onset.

A careful history of associated factors is also helpful in further defining the etiology and potential treatment of the dry eye disease. Certainly, all patients should be questioned regarding the use of contact lenses. How long the patient has worn contact lenses and recent changes in cleaning and wearing patterns may give a clue as to the etiology of dry eye disease. The type of contact lens—whether gas permeable, soft, or polymethylmethacrylate (PMMA)—is useful information. A recent change in cleaning practice or cleaning solutions may indicate a chemical keratitis as the cause of the dry eye symptoms. Contact lens patients should always be questioned regarding the length of time contacts are worn, whether the patient sleeps in the contact lens, and the timing of symptoms relating to contact lens usage. Certainly, a history of marginal ulcers, neovascularization, or contact lens intolerance is useful in assessing the dry eye patient.[8] Other associations may be less obvious but no less important. Consideration should be given to over-the-counter and prescription medications. It is well known that antihistamines, diuretics, and some antidepressants may exacerbate or cause a dry eye syndrome. A history of arthritis, smoking, thyroid disease, gout, HDL/cholesterol ratio, and diabetes have been associated with dry eye disease.[9] Associations that were not found to be important include history of cardiovascular disease, body mass index, blood pressure, white blood cell count, hematocrit, history of osteoporosis, stroke, history of allergies, alcohol consumption, time spent outdoors, maculopathy, cataract, and lens surgery.[9] A history of dry mouth may indicate that the patient has Sjögren's syndrome. This should lead to autoimmune testing to confirm the presence of Sjögren's syndrome and surveillance to ensure the patient does not develop lymphoproliferative neoplastic disease. Patients that have undergone head and neck irradiation for cancer are certainly prone to develop a dry eye if the periocular area was included in the field of radiation.[10] Patients should also be carefully questioned about previous eyelid surgery—either functional or aesthetic. It is not unusual for patients to be less than forthcoming regarding their history of previous aesthetic surgery. Even a remote history of blepharoplasty may be critical in evaluating the dry eye patient.[11] More recently, LASIK surgery has been associated with dry eye symptoms. This has variably been described in approximately 10% of patients undergoing LASIK surgery and is almost always transient in nature.[12]

It is important to question patients about dry eye symptoms upon waking, which implies lagophthalmos and exposure with evaporative dry eye as the etiology. Dryness late in the day may relate to evaporation and/or lipid abnormalities as the etiology. Dryness symptoms when exposed to an environment with low humidity or high winds indicates an evaporative phenomenon as the cause of symptoms.

Tear Film Composition and Dynamics

SCHIRMER 1 TEST

Since its introduction in 1903 by Schirmer, this test has been the mainstay of evaluation of the dry eye patient for decades. It is still in wide use today, although the meaning of the results is frequently misunderstood. This test is performed by placing filter paper strips in the midportion of the lower eyelid. Prior to placement of the filter strips, the patient must have his or her eyes thoroughly blotted to remove any excess tears. After 5 minutes, the wetting is assessed on the filter paper. Normal results are generally considered to be more than 10 mm of wetting in the 5 minute time period. Excessive tear formation is generally considered to be more than 25 mm of wetting in the same 5 minute time period. Moderate tear production correlates with 5 to 10 mm of wetting of the filter paper. Severe decreased tear production is less than 5 mm of wetting of the filter paper. A recent study has found a strong association between the 1-minute Schirmer test and the standard 5-minute test. A severe dry eye measures less than 2 mm of wetting of the filter paper with the 1-minute test.[13]

Repeatability of the Schirmer test and correlation with severity of patient symptoms has been shown to be poor. However, the Schirmer 1 test does give some indication of tear production—both basal and reflexive. This may be important in elucidating the nature of the dry eye symptoms when taken in conjunction with other tear tests.

SCHIRMER 2 TEST

The Schirmer 2 test is performed in the same manner as the Schirmer 1 test with the exception that the nasal mucosa is irritated with a camel's hair brush or cotton-tipped applicator to elicit reflex tear secretion.

BASIC SECRETION TEST

The basic secretion test is performed in the same manner as the Schirmer 1 test but the eye and conjunctiva are anesthetized prior to the placement of the filter paper. It is important that the eye be thoroughly blotted and the conjunctival cul-de-sac be blotted dry with a cotton-tipped applicator prior to the placement of the filter paper strips. This test measures the basal secretion of the glands of Krause and Wolfring.

Many times, all 3 tests (Schirmer 1, Schirmer 2, and basic secretion test) will need to be assessed to define tear production levels in a given patient. It is frequently necessary to do these tests on several occasions at different times of the day to get an average basal, reflex, and total tear production level.

PHENOL RED THREAD TEST

The phenol red thread test is thought to be a test of tear volume. Phenol red is pH sensitive and changes from red to yellow when exposed to tears. The crimped end of a 70-mm thread is placed in the lower conjunctival fornix and wetting measured at 15 seconds. Normal values range from 9 to 20 mm and dry eye patients typically measure less than 9 mm. However, many practitioners believe the phenol red thread test cannot reliably differentiate between a dry eye and a normal eye but has shown the ability to differentiate between an aqueous deficient dry eye and a nonaqueous deficient dry eye with 15 mm of wetting and 22 mm of wetting, respectively.[14] Most likely the phenol red thread test stimulates some reflex tear production, measures uptake by the thread, and is based upon tear film composition.[15]

MENISCOMETRY (REFRACTIVE MENISCOMETRY/VIDEOMENISCOMETRY)

The radius of curvature of the tear meniscus has been shown to be linearly related to the tear volume. A new instrument—the video meniscometer—can digitally assess the radius of curvature of the tear meniscus.[15] This device measures the specular reflex of an illuminated target from the concave mirror effect of the tear meniscus to assess the radius of curvature of the meniscus.[16] Patients with dry eye have a significantly lower radius of curvature of the tear meniscus than normal patients.

FLUORESCEIN MENISCUS TIME

Fluorescein meniscus time (FMT) is a measure of the rate at which a fluorescent tear meniscus is formed using 2% sodium fluorescein. This is a timed test performed with suitable illumination—usually at the slit lamp. It has been shown to be more sensitive and reliable in diagnosing aqueous tear deficiency.[17]

OSMOLARITY/OSMOLALITY

Tear film osmolarity and osmolality have been shown to increase in patients with dry eyes. This is due to evaporation of the aqueous component or decreased

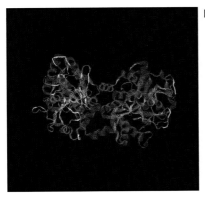

Figure 5-1. Lactoferrin molecule.

production of the aqueous component in patients with a dry eye. This test is accomplished by a nanoliter freezing point depression type osmometer. It has been shown to be variable relating to sampling errors, reflex tearing, and evaporation.[18]

TEAR FILM ENZYME ASSAY

Recently, tear film lactoferrin levels have been assayed in the assessment of dry eye states, ocular inflammatory conditions, and in the perioperative phase of refractive surgery. It is an immunoassay that has shown a high degree of sensitivity in detecting patients with Sjögren's syndrome and dry eye states (Figure 5-1).[19,20]

Tear Film Lipid Measurement

PHOSPHOLIPASE A2 MEASUREMENT

This test is done by time-resolved fluoroimmunoassay. It has been shown to be significantly decreased in patients with atopic blepharoconjunctivitis and dry eye disease.[21]

MEIBOMETRY

Meibometry can be performed via laser interferometry or absorptive spectroscopy. It is one of the few methods that directly measures the lipid content of the tear film.[22] The lipid content of the preocular tear film is delivered from the meibomian glands and is reduced in diseases associated with meibomian dysfunction, including meibomitis, blepharitis, and acne rosacea.

TEAR BREAKUP TIME

A strip of fluorescein is applied in the lower eyelid fornix and then removed. The patient is asked to stare straight ahead and not blink. The tear film is observed under cobalt-blue filtered light of the slit lamp microscope and the time that elapsed between the last blink and appearance of the first break in the tear film is recorded with a stopwatch (a break is seen as a dark spot in a sea of blue). A tear BUT of less than 10 seconds is considered abnormal. This is an important test of tear film stability induced by the lipid layer. There are important considerations when evaluating the fluorescein tear BUT. Reflex tearing and the effect of the fluorescein dye on the lipid layer can alter the results. Another method to assess tear film lipid layer stability is the noninvasive BUT. This is accomplished by viewing the tear film through a keratometer and measuring the time until the keratometer mire is distorted. This is known as the prerupture phase that

Figure 5-2. Fluorescein and rose bengal staining in a patient with dry eye. (Courtesy of Guillermo L. Simón-Castellví.)

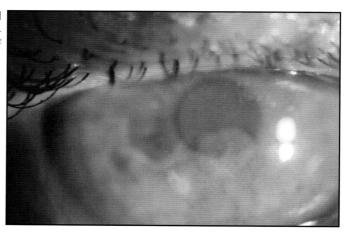

precedes the actual breakup of the tears. Normal values are considered greater than 15 seconds.

MUC5AC Assay

MUC5AC is a major secretory mucin of the conjunctival goblet cells and precorneal tear film. It is measured by quantitative immunoassay and has been shown to be significantly reduced in patients with a dry eye state.[23]

Videokeratography

Videokeratography is performed by capturing keratographic images of the cornea over time (usually every second for 10 to 15 seconds) and analyzing the images for tear BUT and tear breakup area. This has been shown to be very sensitive and specific for a dry eye state and is significantly more accurate than a slit lamp fluorescein tear BUT.[23]

Ocular Surface Evaluation

Surface Stains

A variety of vital stains have been utilized for detection of surface damage of the corneal and conjunctival epithelium due to desiccation. Each of the stains has advantages and disadvantages, but none are very sensitive.

Fluorescein

Fluorescein diffuses between corneal or conjunctival cells that have been disrupted due to dryness, degeneration, or death. This causes a greenish staining when viewed through a cobalt blue filter and is graded upon severity (Figure 5-2). The pattern of staining frequently gives clues as to the etiology of the dry eye state (ie, inferior corneal staining may indicate lagophthalmos with an evaporative dry eye). Fluorescein staining has not been shown to be very sensitive in the diagnosis of a dry eye.

Sulphorhodamine B

Sulphorhodamine B acts like fluorescein but gives an orange fluorescence, which gives greater contrast to the natural green fluorescence of the ocular tissues.

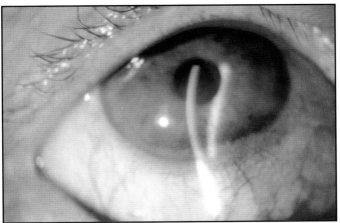

Figure 5-3. Rose bengal staining in a patient with dry eye. (Courtesy of Guillermo L. Simón-Castellví.)

Rose Bengal

Rose bengal stains dead and devitalized epithelium of the cornea and conjunctiva (Figure 5-3). Recently, it has been shown to stain cells inadequately protected by mucins and the tear film. Patients with severe rose bengal staining have been frequently shown to have lost the ability to produce tears in response to sensory stimulation.

Lissamine Green

Like rose bengal, this vital dye stains devitalized epithelium of the cornea, conjunctiva, and mucous. It is more patient friendly than rose bengal (ie, stains the eye for shorter periods of time and is less painful).

Corneal Thickness

Several studies have demonstrated a decrease in corneal thickness in patients with dry eye syndrome.[24,25] Corneal thinning is most notable in the central region and midperiphery and most likely due to desiccation and inflammation related to the dry eye state.

Impression Cytology

A nitrocellulose filter paper is applied to the eye or, frequently, a Biopore membrane device (Millicell-CM 0.4 μm PICM 012550, Millipore Corp, Bedford, Mass) is gently applied to gather surface epithelial cells from the cornea and conjunctiva. These surface cells when stained can aid in the diagnosis of a dry eye state. Specifically, the number of goblet cells are decreased and the nuclear/cytoplasmic ratio of the epithelial cells is decreased. Other findings in a dry eye patient include squamous metaplasia and hyperkeratosis (Figure 5-4).[26]

CONCLUSION

The diversity and number of tests to assess the dry eye make it apparent that dry eye symptoms in actuality represent a variety of differing disease states. As such, no one test can be used to diagnose, quantify, stratify, and assess therapy in all dry eye patients. It

Figure 5-4. Impression cytology of the cornea.

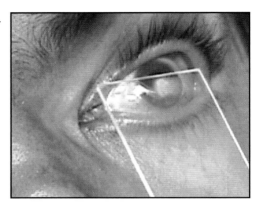

is a combination of these tests that helps the clinician diagnose and treat dry eye patients. There are a multitude of factors that affect the 3 layers of the tear film (mucous, aqueous, and lipid), and each should be assessed based on the patient's disease. Many of the methods described previously are logistically beyond the average clinician and provide significant benefit in a small number of patients that cannot be diagnosed and treated with less sophisticated methodology. Clinicians must always keep in mind the diagnosis of Sjögren's syndrome. This is important not only because of the potential beneficial effect a clinician can have in treating the dry eye as well as the dry mouth, but also because these patients need to be surveyed for lymphoproliferative disorders. In addition, a simple blood test can help confirm the diagnosis of Sjögren's syndrome—the anti-Rho/SS-A and anti-La/SS-B antibodies.[19] Most practitioners prefer the clinical history as the single most important "test" in evaluating a dry eye patient. The second most preferred test is the fluorescein tear BUT followed by fluorescein and rose bengal staining and finally Schirmer's tear test.[27]

Key Points

1. Patients with a dry eye frequently have a long history of complaints for burning or a "sand-like" or "gritty" sensation in their eyes.
2. Since its introduction in 1903 by Schirmer, Schirmer's test has been the mainstay of evaluation of the dry eye patient for decades.
3. A simple blood test can help confirm the diagnosis of Sjögren's syndrome—the anti-Rho/SS-A and anti-La/SS-B antibodies.
4. A new instrument—the video meniscometer—can digitally assess the radius of curvature of the tear meniscus.
5. A variety of vital stains have been utilized for detection of surface damage of the corneal and conjunctival epithelium due to desiccation.

REFERENCES

1. Nichols KK, Nichols JJ, Mitchell GL. The lack of association between signs and symptoms in patients with dry eye disease. *Cornea*. 2004;23(8):762–770.

2. Nichols KK, Mitchell GL, Zadnik K. The repeatability of clinical measurements of dry eye. *Cornea*. 2004;23(3):272–285.

3. Moss SE, Klein R, Klein BE. Incidence of dry eye in an older population. *Arch Ophthalmol*. 2004; 122(3):369–373.

4. Schaumberg DA, Sullivan DA, Buring JE, Dana MR. Prevalence of dry eye syndrome among US women. *Am J Ophthalmol*. 2003;136(2):318–326.

5. Smith JA, Vitale S, Reed GF, et al. Dry eye signs and symptoms in women with premature ovarian failure. *Arch Ophthalmol*. 2004;122(2):151–156.

6. Lee AJ, Lee J, Saw SM, et al. Prevalence and risk factors associated with dry eye symptoms: a population based study in Indonesia. *Br J Ophthalmol*. 2002;86(12):1347–1351.

7. Holly FJ. Diagnostic methods and treatment modalities of dry eye conditions. *Int Ophthalmol*. 1993;17(3):113–125.

8. Nomura K, Nakao M, Matsubara K. Subjective symptom of eye dryness and lifestyle factors with corneal neovascularization in contact lens wearers. *Eye Contact Lens*. 2004;30(2):95–98.

9. Moss SE, Klein R, Klein BE. Prevalence of and risk factors for dry eye syndrome. *Arch Ophthalmol*. 2000;118(9):1264–1268.

10. Parsons JT, Bova FJ, Fitzgerald CR, Mendenhall WM, Million RR. Severe dry-eye syndrome following external beam irradiation. *Int J Radiat Oncol Biol Phys*. 1994;30(4):775–780.

11. Hwang K, Lee DK, Lee EJ, Chung IH, Lee SI. Innervation of the lower eyelid in relation to blepharoplasty and midface lift: clinical observation and cadaveric study. *Ann Plast Surg*. 2001;47(1):1–5; discussion 5–7.

12. Ang RT, Dartt DA, Tsubota K. Dry eye after refractive surgery. *Curr Opin Ophthalmol*. 2001;12(4): 318–322.

13. Bawazeer AM, Hodge WG. One-minute Schirmer test with anesthesia. *Cornea*. 2003;22(4): 285–287.

14. Patel S, Farrell J, Blades KJ, Grierson DJ. The value of a phenol red impregnated thread for differentiating between the aqueous and non-aqueous deficient dry eye. *Ophthalmic Physiol Opt*. 1998;18(6):471–476.

15. Tomlinson A, Blades KJ, Pearce EI. What does the phenol red thread test actually measure? *Optom Vis Sci*. 2001;78(3):142–146.

16. Yokoi N, Bron AJ, Tiffany JM, Maruyama K, Komuro A, Kinoshita S. Relationship between tear volume and tear meniscus curvature. *Arch Ophthalmol*. 2004;122(9):1265–1269.

17. Yokoi N, Bron AJ, Tiffany JM, Kinoshita S. Reflective meniscometry: a new field of dry eye assessment. *Cornea*. 2000;19(3 Suppl):S37–S43.

18. Nelson JD, Wright JC. Tear film osmolality determination: an evaluation of potential errors in measurement. *Curr Eye Res*. 1986;5(9):677–681.

19. Da Dalt S, Moncada A, Priori R, Valesini G, Pivetti-Pezzi P. The lactoferrin tear test in the diagnosis of Sjögren's syndrome. *Eur J Ophthalmol*. 1996;6(3):284–286.

20. Danjo Y, Lee M, Horimoto K, Hamano T. Ocular surface damage and tear lactoferrin in dry eye syndrome. *Acta Ophthalmol (Copenh)*. 1994;72(4):433–437.

21. Peuravuori H, Kari O, Peltonen S, et al. Group IIA phospholipase A2 content of tears in patients with atopic blepharoconjunctivitis. *Graefes Arch Clin Exp Ophthalmol*. 2004;242(12):986–989.

22. Yokoi N, Komuro A. Non-invasive methods of assessing the tear film. *Exp Eye Res*. 2004;78(3): 399–407.

23. Zhao H, Jumblatt JE, Wood TO, Jumblatt MM. Quantification of MUC5AC protein in human tears. *Cornea*. 2001;20(8):873–877.

24. Sanchis-Gimeno JA, Lleo-Perez A, Alonso L, Rahhal MS, Martinez-Soriano F. Reduced corneal thickness values in postmenopausal women with dry eye. *Cornea*. 2005;24(1):39–44.
25. Liu Z, Pflugfelder SC. Corneal thickness is reduced in dry eye. *Cornea*. 1999;18(4):403–407.
26. McKelvie P. Ocular surface impression cytology. *Adv Anat Pathol*. 2003;10(6):328–337.
27. Korb DR. Survey of preferred tests for diagnosis of the tear film and dry eye. *Cornea*. 2000; 19(4):483–486.

6

Dry Eye Secondary to Aqueous Tear Deficiency (Sjögren's Syndrome)

Mahmoud M. Ismail, MD, PhD;
M. Alaa El Danasoury, FRCS; and
Akef El-Maghraby, MD, FRCS

INTRODUCTION

The tear film consists of 3 layers: the inner mucin layer, the middle aqueous layer, and the outer lipid layer. Dry eye can, therefore, be caused by a deficiency or defect in any of these 3 layers. The tear layer affected most frequently is the aqueous layer, resulting in aqueous tear deficiency (ATD) or lacrimal hyposecretion. Keratoconjunctivitis sicca (KCS) (dry eye syndrome) is an ocular surface disorder of the natural function and protective mechanism of the external eye, leading to an unstable tear film. This disorder affects 3% to 5% of the population in north Europe and up to 7% in north Africa. The origin of this disease is believed to be multifactorial related to the pathological conditions of the main lacrimal gland together with the accessory components of the tear film. Also, autoimmune factors are documented to contribute as an adjuvant cause of the disease.

Dry eye conditions have been classified into 2 main categories by the National Eye Institute: ATD and evaporative dry eye (EDE). Tear deficient dry eye can be further separated into Sjögren's syndrome dry eye and non-Sjögren's syndrome that entitles the range of other tear deficiency conditions, including iatrogenic local causes (Figure 6-1). In the early 20th century, a Swedish physician named Henrik Sjögren first described this disease in a group of women whose chronic arthritis was accompanied by dry eyes and dry mouth (xerostomia).

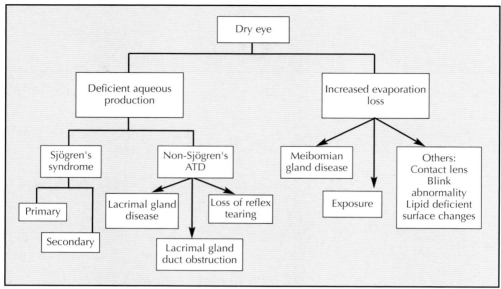

Figure 6-1. Classification scheme for dry eye proposed by NEI/Industry Workshop. (Adapted from Lemp MA. Report of the National Eye Institute/Industry Workshop on clinical trials for dry eyes. *CLAO J.* 1995;21:221–232.)

Sjögren's syndrome

Epidemiology

Sjögren's syndrome affects 1 to 4 million people in the United States. The average age group at the time of diagnosis is around 40 years. Ninety percent to 95% of the patients are females. It can affect people of all races and ethnic backgrounds. It is rare in children but may occur.

Clinical Features

Sjögren's syndrome is a chronic inflammatory connective tissue disorder that can affect many different parts of the body, but most often affects the lacrimal and salivary glands. It affects 1.2% to 1.5% of the population between 45 and 55 years of age with 10-fold prevalence in women. Patients with this condition may notice irritation, a gritty feeling, or painful burning in the eyes. Red eye and visual fatigue may follow after the initial stage of the disease (Figure 6-2). Dry mouth, difficulty in eating dry food, and swelling of the parotid glands are also common. Some patients experience dryness of other mucous membranes (nasal passages, throat, and vagina) and skin. Rarely, patients may have complications related to inflammation in other body systems, including the following:
- Joint and muscle pain with fatigue.
- Lung problems that may mimic pneumonia.
- Abnormal liver and kidney function tests.
- Skin rashes related to inflammation of small blood vessels.
- Neurologic problems causing weakness and numbness.

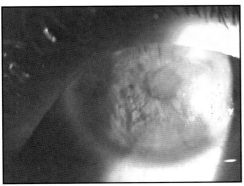

Figure 6-2. Dry eye disease with limited keratopathy.

- In about 2% of Sjögren's syndrome patients it may be associated with lymphoma.

It is an autoimmune exocrinopathy characterized by oral and ocular dryness with or without impairment of other organ systems. It can cause substantial serologic autoimmune reactivity and may be associated with other connective tissue autoimmune disorders, such as rheumatoid arthritis, scleroderma, or systemic lupus erythematosus.[1] Although the underlying immunomediated glandular destruction is thought to develop slowly over several years, a long delay from the start of the symptoms to final diagnosis has been frequently reported.[2–3] It is characterized by a combination of ATD and dry mouth (xerostomia). Immune cells attack and destroy the glands that produce tears and saliva. In addition, Sjögren's syndrome may cause skin, nose, and vaginal dryness and may affect other organs of the body, including the kidneys, blood vessels, lungs, liver, pancreas, and brain. It may cause symptoms such as dry skin, skin rashes, thyroid problems, joint and muscle pain, pneumonia, vaginal dryness, and numbness and tingling in the extremities. It also increases the risk for developing malignant non-Hodgkin's lymphoma. Ocular signs include squamous metaplasia of the ocular surface epithelium; corneal epitheliopathy; filamentary keratitis; and, in more severe cases, poor epithelial integrity, recurrent erosion, and persistent ulcer.

Classification of Sjögren's Syndrome

"Primary" Sjögren's syndrome occurs in people with no other rheumatologic or systemic disease. "Secondary" Sjögren's syndrome occurs in patients who do have another rheumatologic disease and later may develop dry eye symptoms. Most often it is seen secondary to systemic lupus erythematosus, rosacea, and rheumatoid arthritis (Table 6-1).

Complications due to progression of Sjögren's syndrome can lead to recurrent corneal ulcers and subsequent leucomas, recurrent herpetic keratitis, and infectious corneal affection. Also, stem cell failure and deep corneal vascularization with severe visual affection can occur (Figure 6-3). However, development of desmatocele and corneal melting might be an end result of a visual threatening complication of such disease (Figure 6-4).

	Primary	Secondary
	Table 6-1	
	DIFFERENCES BETWEEN PRIMARY	
	AND SECONDARY SJÖGREN'S SYNDROME	
Etiology	Lacrimal gland degeneration	Rheumatic diseases
Progression	Slow	Rapid
IgG levels	Low	High
Anti-SSA and SSB antibodies	High	Low

Figure 6-3. Stem cell failure with desmatocele.

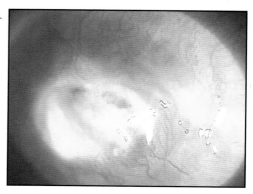

Figure 6-4. Corneal melting and perforation.

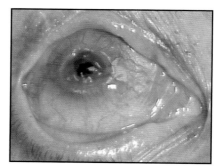

Pathogenesis of Sjögren's Syndrome

The cause of Sjögren's syndrome is not known, but it is considered to be an autoimmune disorder. The emergence and persistence of autoimmune T cells and a subsequent failure of apoptosis of these activated cells might result in a persistent stimulation of B cells. This occurs after a critical decrease in androgen level, leading to atrophy of the lacrimal glands. Resulting apoptotic fragments of the interstitial and acinar cells will act as a source of potential autoantigens. This subsequently might be presented to the CD4 cell antigen receptors and start an immune response.

In primary Sjögren's syndrome, patients with rather severe ocular surface disease were compared to initial cases with regard to severity of disease as indicated by serum IgG. No differences in serum IgG between both patient groups were found. Thus, the degree of dryness seems not to be linked directly to the severity of disease.

Key Points

1. Dry eye secondary to ATD and dry eye secondary to increased evaporation may sometimes coexist in patients with multifactorial dry eyes.
2. Sjögren's syndrome is an autoimmune exocrinopathy characterized by oral and ocular dryness with or without impairment of other organ systems. It can cause substantial serologic autoimmune reactivity and may be associated with other connective tissue autoimmune disorders, such as rheumatoid arthritis, scleroderma, or systemic lupus erythematosus
3. There is progressive lymphocytic (predominantly B and CD4 lymphocytes) infiltration of the lacrimal and salivary glands that leads to disorganization of the normal gland architecture and consequent loss of function in all cases of Sjögren's syndrome.
4. Histopathology of postmortem lacrimal gland tissue from dry eye patients shows a high degree of infiltration by T lymphocytes in all kinds of dry eye patients. The disease is thus autoimmune regardless of whether or not the patient has a circulating immunoglobulin.

REFERENCES

1. Chambers MS. Sjögren's syndrome. *ORL Head Neck Nurs.* 2004;22(4):22–30; quiz 32–33.
2. Mignogna MD, Fedele S, Russo LL, Muzio LL, Wolff A. Sjögren's syndrome: the diagnostic potential of early oral manifestations preceding hyposalivation/xerostomia. *J Oral Pathol Med.* 2005;34(1):1–6.
3. Rozman B, Novljan MP, Hocevar A, et al. Epidemiology and diagnostics of primary Sjögren's syndrome. *Reumatizam.* 2004;51(2):9–12.
4. Ono M, Takamura E, Shinozaki K, et al. Therapeutic effect of cevimeline on dry eye in patients with Sjögren's syndrome: a randomized, double-blind clinical study. *Am J Ophthalmol.* 2004;138(1):6–17.
5. Moore BD. Lacrimal system abnormalities. *Optom Vis Sci.* 1994;71:182–183.
6. Smith RS, Maddox SF, Collins BE. Congenital alacrima. *Arch Ophthalmol.* 1968;79:45–48.
7. Kroop IG. The production of tears in familial dysautonomia: preliminary report. *J Pediatr.* 1956;48:328–329.
8. Obata H, Yamamoto S, Horiuchi H, et al. Histopathologic study of human lacrimal gland. *Ophthalmology.* 1995;102:678–686.
9. Lemp MA. Report of the National Eye Institute/Industry Workshop on clinical trials for dry eyes. *CLAO J.* 1995;21:221–232.
10. Heath P. Ocular lymphomas. *Am J Ophthalmol.* 1949;32:1213–1223.
11. James DG, Anderson R, Langley D, Ainslie D. Ocular sarcoidosis. *Br J Ophthalmol.* 1964;48:461–470.
12. Fox RI. Systemic diseases associated with dry eye (review). *Int Ophthalmol Clin.* 1994;34:71–87.
13. Itescu S. Diffuse infiltrative lymphocytosis syndrome in human immunodeficiency virus infection: a Sjögren's like disease. *Rheum Dis Clin North Am.* 1991;17:99–115.
14. Pflugfelder SC, Crouse CA, Monroy D, Yen M, Rowe M, Atherton SS. Epstein-Barr virus and the lacrimal gland pathology of Sjögren's syndrome. *Am J Pathol.* 1993;143:49–64.
15. Scherz W, Dohlman CH. Is the lacrimal gland dispensable? Keratoconjunctivitis sicca after lacrimal gland removal. *Arch Ophthalmol.* 1975;93:281–283.

16. Lopez FM, Pflugfelder SC. Disorders of tear production and the lacrimal system: cornea and external disease. In: Krachmer JH, Mannis MJ, et al, eds. *Fundamentals of Corneal and External Disease.* St. Louis, Mo: Mosby Year Book; 1997:663–686.

17. Schaumberg DA, Buring JE, Sullivan DA, Dana MR. Hormone replacement therapy and the prevalence of dry eye syndrome. *JAMA.* 2001;286:2114–2119.

18. Sullivan DA, Yamagami H, Liu M, et al. Sex steroids, the meibomian gland and evaporative dry eye. *Adv Exp Med Biol.* 2002;506(Pt A):389–399.

19. Krenzer KL, Dana MR, Ullman MD, et al. Effect of androgen deficiency on the human meibomian gland and ocular surface. *J Clin Endocr Metab.* 2000;85:4874–4882.

20. Sullivan BD, Evans JE, Krenzer KL, Dana MR, Sullivan DA. Impact of anti-androgen treatment on the fatty acid profile of neutral lipids in human meibomian gland secretions. *J Clin Endocr Metab.* 2000;85:4866–4873.

21. Sullivan BD, Evans JE, Dana MR, Sullivan DA. Impact of androgen deficiency on the lipid profiles in human meibomian gland secretions. *Adv Exp Med Biol.* 2002;506(Pt A):449–458.

7

Dry Eye Secondary to Increased Evaporation

Amar Agarwal, MS, FRCS, FRCOphth and Soosan Jacob, MS, FRCS, Dip NB

INTRODUCTION

People with dry eye syndrome usually present with complaints of burning, stinging, redness of the eyes, and tearing. The tearing seems paradoxical at first but is explained by the fact that an underlying dry eye may become irritated, thus sending a signal for increased tear production to flush out the irritants. Tearing that becomes symptomatic usually occurs in conditions that result in more rapid evaporation of tears from the eye, such as being outdoors in the wind. Heat, low humidity, and the presence of smoke may compound the problem.

EPIDEMIOLOGY

Dry eye's prevalence increases with age. It is extremely common in older people of both sexes. The condition affects 2 to 3 times more women than men. About 6 million women and 3 million men in the United States have moderate or severe symptoms of the disease, and it is estimated that an additional 20 to 30 million people in this country have a mild form of dry eye. Dry eye syndrome is not a frequent cause of blindness; however, it is an important public health problem, the main reason being that it is so common. Visits for dry eye syndrome are one of the leading reasons for patients to seek eye care. This is because its symptoms are very bothersome and lead to a decreased quality of life, reduced work capacity, and poorer psychological health. Furthermore, dry eye syndrome is associated with a decreased ability to perform activities that require visual attention, such as reading and driving a car. It is estimated that meibomian gland disease, which also occurs in Sjögren's syndrome, may be a contributing factor in more than 60% of all dry eye cases.[1]

> ## Table 7-1
> ## ETIOLOGY OF EVAPORATIVE DRY EYE
>
> - Central heating (forced air dry heat), hair dryer, car windscreen demisting, air travel, dry climates, wind, air pollution (cigarette smoke), contact lens wear (reduced blinking), driving, watching TV, computer work, and reading.
> - Blepharitis, rosacea, and meibomian gland dysfunction are major causes of this form of dry eye. Ocular rosacea has been suggested to be present in up to 75% of perimenopausal women with facial rosacea.
> - Tears are not spread adequately over the eye surface due to proptosis, ectropion, entropion, nocturnal lagophthalmos, Bell's palsy, pterygium/pinguecula (Figure 7-1), and conjunctivalchalasis.

CLASSIFICATION OF DRY EYE

- Tear-deficient dry eye: Tear-deficient dry eye is the largest category of dry eye. It is due to a deficiency of the aqueous component of the tear film.
- Tear-sufficient dry eye or dry eye secondary to increased evaporation or evaporative dry eye (EDE): In EDE, there is normal composition of the tear film; however, there is an increase in tear evaporation.[2] Dry eye occurs where lacrimal function is normal and the volume and composition of the lacrimal fluid are adequate and regarded as sufficient, with the tear abnormality created by other periocular disease usually leading to increased tear evaporation.

THE NATIONAL EYE INSTITUTE/ INDUSTRY WORKSHOP REPORT

This report[3] defines dry eye as a disorder of the tear film due to tear deficiency or excessive tear evaporation that causes damage to the interpalpebral ocular surface and is associated with symptoms of ocular discomfort. Dry eye is most frequently caused by a decrease of lacrimal gland function but may also occur when lacrimal gland function is normal. The various etiologies may act independently or may interact to cause dry eye. These disorders or combinations have features in common that may be embraced by this single definition.

ETIOLOGY

A simple classification of the etiology of EDE is given in Table 7-1.

Blepharitis

Anterior blepharitis independent of other forms of lid disease may cause dry eye. It is a common inflammatory condition of the eyelids characterized by itching, burning,

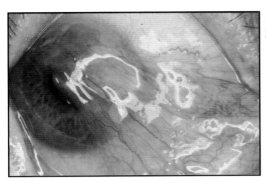

Figure 7-1. Advanced elevated fleshy pterygium affecting the visual axis. (Courtesy of Pablo Gili.)

foreign body sensation, and crusting of the eyelids especially prominent in the mornings. Microscopic examination may show crusting of the eyelashes and red, thickened eyelid margins with dilated blood vessels. Skin lipid breaks up the normal tear film.[4] Desquamated cells derived from the lid margin in squamous blepharitis may deliver such lipid to the tear film and give rise to punctate keratitis by causing tear instability and increased tear evaporation. Qualitatively altered meibomian lipid may also directly damage the ocular surface.[4–7] Many patients will also have meibomian gland dysfunction characterized by inspissation of the oils and perhaps plugging of the glands. There may also be a seborrheic (dandruff) or infectious (usually "staph") component that contributes to the disorder. Blepharitis is more common in patients with rosacea.

Meibomian Gland Disease

The oil normally produced by the meibomian glands in the eyelid coats the tear film, acting like a biological plastic wrap to retard evaporation and keep the eye moist.

Various forms of meibomian gland disease can cause dry eye. It is thought to be due to an insufficient lipid layer for resurfacing the tear film with each blink and/or a qualitative alteration of the meibomian lipid in such a way as to destabilize the tear film. The occurrence of dry eye is dependent on the severity and extent of gland dysfunction. The most common form of meibomian gland disease is obstructive. Obstructive meibomian gland disease is diagnosed on the basis of reduced expressibility of meibomian oil, qualitative abnormality of the expressed oil, and morphologic abnormality of the gland acini and ductules. Such changes can be graded by meibography[8,9] and a clinical grading approach,[10] and methods have been devised to measure the amount and quality of the lid oil more precisely using meibometry and a clinical grading scheme.[11–13] Meibomitis leads to EDE by causing meibomian gland dysfunction—oil production by the glands decreases and the oils that are produced are of altered composition. With the reduction of the quantity and quality of the oil layer, evaporation increases and these patients develop dry eye. Various lid scrubs have been marketed for this condition, but the results have not been very effective.

Altered lipid pattern in gland secretion causes decreased tear film BUT leading to functional dry eye. Congenital absence or malformation of meibomian gland occurs in ectodermal dysplasia. Acquired gland dysfunction occurs due to old age; trauma; contact lens wear; inflammatory, topical, and systemic chemical toxicity; androgen deficiency; radiation; and oral retinoids.

Figure 7-2. Dry eye due to lagophthalmos because of facial Bell's palsy. (Courtesy of Guillermo L. Simón-Castellví.)

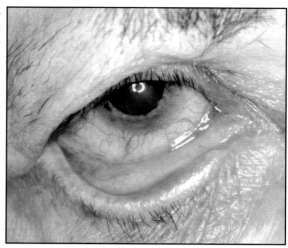

Meibomian gland disease causes dry eye by the following 2 methods:
1. Increased evaporation rates and elevated tear osmolarity.
2. Evaporation losses due to gland drop out.

Meibomian gland dysfunction is commonly associated with blepharitis. The bacteria, mostly *Staphylococcus aureus*, produces lipases that hydrolyze and produce free fatty acid, which are surface active and capable of rupturing the tear lipid layer.

Meibomian gland diseases may be secondary to a reduced number (congenital deficiency[14] or metaplastic), replacement distichiasis,[15] or hyposecretory or obstructive meibomitis[16-20] (focal or diffuse[15]). Obstructive meibomitis may be primary or secondary to local diseases such as anterior blepharitis; conjunctivitis (eg, trachoma, pemphigoid, and atopy); chemical burns; systemic diseases such as sebaceous dermatitis[20] anhydrotic ectodermal dysplasia, acne rosacea,[20] ectrodactyly syndrome,[21,22] atopy,[20] Turner syndrome, ichthyosis,[15] fungus,[23,24] or psoriasis.[20] Toxic causes such as 13-Cis ret. acid,[4,25,26] polychlorinated biphenyls,[5–7] and epinephrine[27] may also cause meibomian gland dysfunction.

Blink Disorders

Infrequent blinking such as in Parkinson's disease and seventh nerve palsy (Figure 7-2) leads to increased evaporation and drying of the ocular surface. The anticholinergic drugs used for treatment of Parkinson's diseases further precipitate dry eye. Trigeminal nerve palsy leads to decreased corneal sensation and reflex lacrimation and decreased blink rates. The dynamics of the blink can be recorded by special techniques.[28]

Disorders of Lid Aperture and Lid/Globe Congruity

Increased width of the palpebral aperture such as in thyroid exophthalmos (Figure 7-3) may be associated with ocular drying and tear hyperosmolarity.[29] Lid deformity and poor lid-globe apposition lead to inadequate resurfacing of the ocular surface with tears.[30] Wide palpebral fissures increase the exposure area, as do conditions like entropion, ectropion, symblepharon, and notched lid.

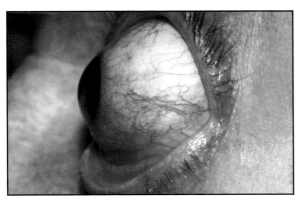

Figure 7-3. Proptosis. (Courtesy of Guillermo L. Simón-Castellví.)

Infections

Infections like rosacea cause squamous metaplasia of ductal opening. Seborrheic dermatitis causes oily scaling of epidermis and hyperkeratinization, leading to obstruction of meibomian gland orifice, leading to altered lipid layer and thus dry eye.

Ocular Surface Disorder

Any elevation of the ocular surface is associated with localized surface drying. In xerophthalmia, both aqueous-adequate and aqueous-deficient dry eye can occur. There is defective surface wetting (xerosis) associated with surface metaplasia.[18] Ocular surface changes include goblet cell loss.[31] Although the metaplasia could be due entirely to goblet cell loss, it is also possible that it is due to a more subtle abnormality of the surface glycocalyx caused by the vitamin A deficiency itself.[32]

Other Tear Film Disorders

This includes those disorders that cause ocular surface damage in the presence of normal lacrimal function and whose mechanism is as yet unclear. Ocular surface disorders due to contact lens wear and drying of the ocular surface under a high water content soft lens are included.[33] Extended wear contact lens and hard contact lens wearers are prone to decreased corneal sensitivity, decreased reflex tear production, and increased osmolarity. Meibomian gland dysfunction is also common in chronic contact lens wearers, which acts as an additive factor in producing dry eyes.

Combined Disorder

Any of the above conditions, whether aqueous deficient or aqueous adequate, may occur in conjunction with any other condition. Lacrimal gland deficiency may be accompanied by meibomian gland deficiency, cicatricial conjunctival disease may cause dry eye by a combination of occlusion of the lacrimal gland ductules as well as by causing a lid incongruity that interferes with tear resurfacing with each blink.

Environmental Factors

Dry climate, high altitudes, low humidity, and a windy environment lead to increased evaporation. Prolonged watching of television and reading for long hours are conditions in which the blink rate is decreased, leading to increased evaporation.

Hormonal Factors

Although age leads to decreased tear secretion and functioning of the meibomian gland, hormonal influence has also been one of the factors associated with high incidence of dry eye in menopausal women.

A major reason for the prevalence of dry eye syndromes in women appears to be the impact of sex steroids, or the lack thereof, on the meibomian gland. This tissue secretes the tear film's lipid layer and is very important in preventing the evaporation of the tear film and maintaining its stability.[34] Recent research indicates that androgen deficiency, as well as systemic HRT or estrogen HRT, in postmenopausal women may lead to both meibomian gland dysfunction and EDE. The rationale for why androgen insufficiency might influence the meibomian gland is that this tissue, like other sebaceous glands, is an androgen target organ. Androgens typically regulate the development, differentiation, and lipid production of sebaceous glands throughout the body.[34] Similarly, androgens appear to modulate meibomian gland function, improve the quality and/or quantity of lipids produced by this tissue, and promote the formation of the tear film's lipid layer.[34] These hormone actions seem to be mediated through androgen receptors within epithelial cell nuclei and to involve the regulation of numerous genes (including those related to lipid, sex steroid, and other cellular metabolic pathways).[35] Conversely, androgen deficiency is associated with meibomian gland dysfunction, an altered lipid profile in meibomian gland secretions, a reduced tear film BUT, and/or a significant increase in dry eye signs and symptoms.[34,36–38] This association between androgen deficiency, meibomian gland disease, and EDE might help to explain why topical or systemic androgen administration has been reported to stimulate the production and secretion of meibomian gland lipids, prolong the tear film BUT, and decrease the signs and symptoms of dry eye in women and men.[34]

A recent study suggests that estrogen HRT may promote both meibomian gland dysfunction and EDE. An epidemiological evaluation of 25,389 postmenopausal women demonstrated that those using estrogen HRT have a significantly higher prevalence of severe dry eye symptoms and clinically diagnosed dry eye syndrome as compared to women who never used HRT.[39] This hormone effect may be targeted to the meibomian gland, given that estrogens have been shown to induce a significant decrease in the size, activity, and lipid production of sebaceous glands in a variety of species. For years, estrogens were used clinically to reduce sebaceous gland function and secretion in humans.[34]

SYMPTOMS

Irritation, foreign body sensation, burning, and occasional itching may be seen amongst others. A ropelike secretion may be found in the lower fornix due to increased mucin secretion. Photophobia may also be present in some cases.

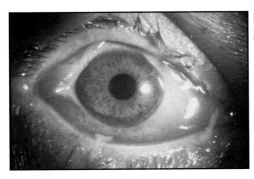

Figure 8-1. Photograph depicting marked conjunctival chemosis and injection in SAC.

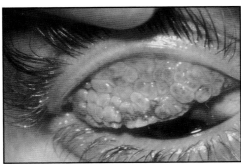

Figure 8-2. Giant papillae of the upper tarsus in VKC.

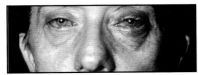

Figure 8-3. External photograph of the eyelid in AKC depicting severe periocular atopic disease along with diffuse conjunctival hyperemia.

demonstrable findings may include limbal follicles, punctate keratitis (keratitis of Tobgy), corneal scarring (shield ulcers), and corneal vascularization. AKC is a chronic, continuous conjunctivitis that typically occurs in young adults with a history of atopic disease such as eczema or asthma (Figure 8-3). Symptoms are similar to VKC but with the potential for more severe vision-threatening sequelae from abnormalities such as symblepharon, tear film destabilization, persistent epithelial defects, corneal scarring and vascularization from stem cell dysfunction, and subsequent risk of secondary bacterial or viral keratitis.[4-6] Papillary conjunctivitis is also present in the upper and lower palpebral conjunctiva. Large papillae may form, but the classic giant papillae are only seen with VKC. Limbal papillae are often seen with AKC but are not typically seen as with VKC. However, the limbal form of VKC, seen more often in sub-Saharan Africa, can have pronounced limbal lesions including giant papillae.[7]

DIFFERENTIAL DIAGNOSIS

Allergic conjunctivitis can be difficult to differentiate between primary dry eye disease (KCS) and toxic medication effects to the ocular surface (Table 8-1). Some key generalizations can be made to aid in differentiation of these ocular surface disorders. In general, allergic ocular disease can be linked to chronic symptoms in relation to

Table 8-1
DRY EYE VS. ALLERGIC CONJUNCTIVITIS

Features	*Dry Eye*	*Allergic Conjunctivitis*
Ocular Signs		
Tear BUT	Short	Normal
Lacrimal meniscus	Scarce	Normal
Conjunctival redness	Discrete	Milky or pale pink conjunctivitis with moderate vascular injection
Conjunctival morphology	Smooth	Frequent papillary conjunctivitis
Temporality	Permanent with fluctuations	Seasonal
Ocular Symptoms		
Sensation	Dryness, rubbery	Itching, burning
Occasional blurry vision	Improves on blinking	Improves when tearing resolves
Photophobia	Little	More pronounced
Circadian pattern	Worse in the evening and night	Worse in the morning and evening
Extraocular Frequent Associations		
Other dryness	Mouth, nose, vagina	None or exocrinic hypersecretion (nose, lungs)
Other inflammations	None, except with Sjögren's syndrome type 2	Atopic dermatitis or mucositis (rhinitis, pharyngitis, bronchitis)
Tests		
Tear	Hyperosmolarity	Normal osmolarity
Total IgE in blood	<70 kU/l	>70 kU/l
Specific IgE in blood	<0.35 kU/l	>0.35 kU/l
IgE in tear	<2 kU/l	>2 kU/l
Prick test to allergens	Negative	Positive
Impression cytology	Lymphocytes, macrophages	Eosinophils, lymphocytes, macrophages
Histamine	About 10 microgram/l	>50 microgram/l

Courtesy of Juan Murube.

repeated exposure to a particular allergen. A period of time must usually occur from the initial introduction of the allergen until repeat exposure occurs with activation of a subsequent hypersensitivity reaction. Ocular itching is typically a hallmark of allergic disease symptomatology. Classic teaching suggests that if an eye has itching, an allergic disorder is the cause. Conversely, a similar philosophy suggests, "no itching, no allergy."[8] While this key concept remains an important consideration with ocular disease diagnosis, allergic disease should not be the only consideration in patients reporting itching alone. In fact, itching can often be misinterpreted or improperly ascribed to other symptoms such as burning, stinging, or ocular irritation. Clinical findings in allergic disease typically include diffuse and broad conjunctival injection, chemosis, eyelid swelling, thin and clear mucoid discharge, and papillary conjunctivitis.[9,10] In contrast, dry eye disease does not typically present with mucopurulent discharge, although severe dry eye may present with long mucous threads. The palpebral conjunctiva in dry eye will exhibit a papillary response that often reflects severity. While medication toxicity may present with itching and presence of conjunctival papillae, a follicular component may also be present unlike typical allergic eye disease. In fact, a number of medications have been associated with a follicular conjunctivitis (Table 8-2).[11,12] Unfortunately, follicles may also be seen occasionally in allergic eye disease if chronic staphylococcal eyelid colonization is also present. Allergic eye disease classically creates diffuse bulbar conjunctival chemosis and hyperemia, whereas a toxic conjunctivitis is not typically diffusely distributed because the superior bulbar conjunctiva may show relative sparing. Toxic conjunctivitis may also demonstrate a more purulent discharge as opposed to the thin and clear mucous discharge present in allergic disease.

A variety of vital dyes can aid external ocular disease diagnosis by staining of the ocular surface. The staining pattern of these vital dyes not only assists with characterization of disease states, but they also allow for a method of assessing disease severity and response to treatment. While a number of dyes may be used for ocular surface staining, the most common dyes used in clinical practice include fluorescein sodium, rose bengal, and lissamine green.[13–15] Corneal surface topology may allow differentiation between ocular surface disease states based on the pattern and distribution of epitheliopathy (Figure 8-4).[16] KCS typically displays a pattern of punctate keratitis in the interpalpebral zone or middle third of the cornea, although severe disease can extend beyond these zones. Toxicity-induced punctate keratitis is commonly located in the inferior or inferonasal cornea. The inferior location of epitheliopathy relates to gravity's effect on maintaining contact between the toxic medication and the inferior cornea, while the inferonasal epitheliopathy relates to the directional flow of toxic substances toward the nasally located puncta.[16] Toxic ulcerative keratopathy can produce oval epithelial defects located in the inferonasal cornea with coarse surrounding keratitis.[17] The edges of the epithelial defect demonstrate rolled margins in the setting of iatrogenic or factitious toxic keratoconjunctivitis. The distribution of punctate corneal staining in allergic disorders such as VKC and AKC classically involves the superior cornea, possibly because of trapped antigen beneath the upper eyelid as it covers and apposes the superior cornea.[16]

Several salient points can help differentiate KCS from other ocular surface disorders. While symptoms of KCS may mimic allergic eye disease and medication toxicity, KCS patients typically report symptoms are worse at the end of the day or after performing

Table 8-2
COMMON MEDICATIONS CAUSING FOLLICULAR CONJUNCTIVITIS

- Physostigmine.
- Neostigmine.
- Echothiophate.
- Diisopropylfluorophosphate.
- Furtrethonium iodide

- Pilocarpine.
- Idoxuridine.
- Atropine.
- Apraclonidine, brimonidine.
- Dipivefrin.

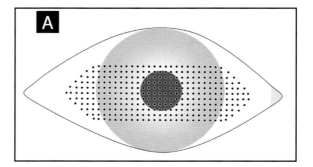

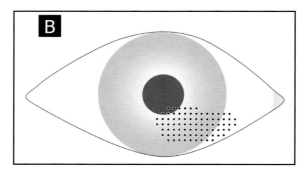

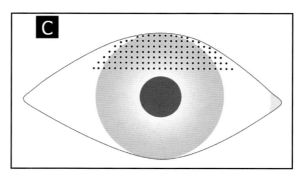

Figure 8-4. The staining pattern of vital dyes on the corneal and conjunctival surface may suggest the underlying cause of ocular surface disease. (A) Interpalpebral staining in KCS. (B) Inferonasal staining in toxic keratoconjunctivitis. (C) Superior staining in vernal and atopic keratoconjunctivitis. (Illustrations by Annette Joglar.)

extended length vision-requiring activities such as computer work, driving, or reading. Any activity in which the blink rate is decreased will tend to exacerbate KCS symptoms. Tear film abnormalities may also help identify KCS. Dry eye patients commonly have a low precorneal tear meniscus in both eyes associated with prominent bulbar conjunctival folds and redundancy. The bulbar conjunctival changes result from the constant surface friction from eyelid-ocular surface touch with each blink in the setting of a poor tear film. Additional tests for assessment of poor lacrimal gland function in KCS may include an abnormal phenol red thread test or Schirmer's test and fluorophotometric techniques to demonstrate poor tear secretion and tear volume. Laboratory testing for KCS may also include elevated tear film osmolarity, abnormal tear protein analysis, and a delay in tear clearance testing.[18] Eyelid margin disease may also contribute to KCS symptoms and findings. Meibomian gland dysfunction can represent a key component of KCS with meibomian gland orifice inspissation and ductal metaplasia, eyelid margin telangiectasias (brush marks), increased viscosity of expressed glandular material, and meibomian gland acinar dropout.[19] Different forms of anterior blepharitis such as staphylococcal disease or seborrheic disease may also contribute to KCS symptoms, thus close inspection of the eyelids can provide specific clues for accurate disease diagnosis. Additional tests may include assessment of tear BUT, the ocular ferning testing, and impression cytology for goblet cell quantification.[20]

Although a variety of diagnostic tests for allergic eye disease are available, they are rarely used in the clinical setting. The intradermal skin test is the gold standard for diagnosis of type-I hypersensitivity reactions. This test involves intradermal injection of the suspected agent to elicit a wheal and flare response on the skin within minutes of exposure. This test may also be performed on the ocular surface by instillation of the offending agent into the eye. A positive test demonstrates an analogous reaction to the wheal and flare reaction of the skin with development of eyelid edema, erythema, conjunctival chemosis, hyperemia, and itching along the ocular surface.[11] The gold standard for type-IV hypersensitivity reactions is the patch test. The suspected substance is applied to the skin and covered. A positive test demonstrates a contact dermatitis at the application site within 24 to 48 hours. Conjunctival scrapings can also assist in diagnosis of an allergic reaction. Allergic ocular disease typically demonstrates eosinophils on microscopic analysis after conjunctival scraping. Toxic reactions may reveal large basophilic granules within the cytoplasm of epithelial cells, mononuclear cells, and polymorphonuclear cells; however, these granules are not specific for toxicity.[11]

ERYTHEMA MULTIFORME, STEVENS-JOHNSON SYNDROME, AND TOXIC EPIDERMAL NECROLYSIS

Medication-related side effects can not only have serious implications for the ocular surface, but they can also create significant systemic complications throughout the body. Erythema multiforme (EM), Stevens-Johnson syndrome, and TEN represent a continuum of disorders resulting from a combination of type-III and type-IV hypersensitivity reactions secondary to complications of drug-induced reactions or systemic infectious agents. Over 50 medications have been reported to cause TEN and SJS, yet the most common offending agents represent nonsteroidal anti-inflammatory agents; salicylates; allopurinol; antibiotics such as penicillins, cephalosporins, and sulfonamides; anticonvulsants such as phenytoin and barbiturates; and antimalarial agents (Table 8-3).[21,22] Drug-

---

Table 8-3
COMMON DRUG-RELATED CAUSES OF ERYTHEMA MULTIFORME
(STEVENS-JOHNSON SYNDROME)

---

1. Antibiotics
   - Sulfonamides
   - Aminopenicillins
   - Trimethoprim-sulfamethoxazole
   - Cephalosporins
   - Fluoroquinolones
   - Antituberculous agents
2. Anticonvulsants
   - Phenobarbital
   - Phenytoin
   - Valproic acid
   - Carbamazepine
3. Anti-inflammatory agents
   - Acetaminophen
   - Nonsteroidal anti-inflammatory agents
   - Allopurinol
   - Corticosteroids
4. Others
   - Sulfa-derivative medications
   - Sulfonylureas
   - Carbonic anhydrase inhibitors
   - Chlormezanone

---

induced reactions have been reported with oral, parenteral, and topical medication administration.[23] Infectious agents commonly include herpes simplex virus, herpes zoster virus, streptococci, *Mycoplasma pneumoniae*, measles, and adenovirus.[21]

While these acute, self-limiting disorders truly represent a spectrum of acute mucocutaneous disease, a common classification system has been designated to differentiate findings and prognosis of the various diseases. This scheme includes EM minor, EM major, SJS, and TEN. The minor form of EM primarily involves the skin with no or minimal mucous membrane involvement, whereas the major form affects the skin and 2 or more mucous membranes. Some authors consider SJS and EM major as interchangeable disorders, while recent reports suggest SJS and EM major actually represent separate entities based on clinical findings, course, and prognosis.[24,25] TEN is the most severe form of this continuum, displaying sheet-like epithelial loss and raised flaccid blisters that spread with pressure, a positive Nikolsky sign. Several reports suggest an autoimmune disease origin and genetic predisposition for development of TEN and EM because several phenotypic HLA-linkages have been identified in affected individuals.

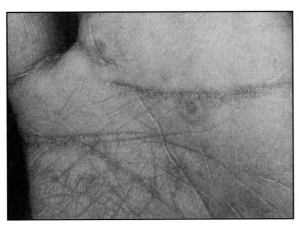

Figure 8-5. The classic "target lesion" seen on the palm of a patient with Stevens-Johnson syndrome.

Stevens-Johnson syndrome is associated with an increased incidence of HLA-Bw44 (a component of HLA B-12), HLA-DQB1, HLA-Aw33, and HLA-DRw53.[22,26,27] The HLA B-12 phenotype has also been associated with a 3-fold increase in the development of TEN.[28]

EM, originally described by Von Hebra in 1866,[29] is estimated to have an incidence of 0.1% to 1% with an estimated range of 0.5 to 5 cases per million per year.[21,23,29] The disorder begins with prodromal symptoms, including fever, chills, malaise, myalgias, headache, cough, rhinorrhea, and sore throat, and symptoms may begin as early as 1 week prior to the onset of the disease. Prodromal symptoms are followed by a symmetrical erythematous maculopapular rash with an array of lesion patterns from macules, papules, vesicles, and bullae to the classic "target lesion" (Figure 8-5). Target lesions consist of an erythematous macula or papule with a central pale or vesicular core that represents epidermal injury with necrosis or blister formation. A middle zone of pale edema may also be present. The rash begins on extensor surfaces of the extremities and spreads to the palms, soles, face, mucous membranes, and the trunk in more severe cases. Mucosal involvement occurs in 25% to 70% of EM cases, with involvement of more than one mucous membrane surface. Stevens-Johnson syndrome includes extensive vesicobullous formation involving the skin, oral mucosa, conjunctiva, pharynx, and urogenital region with a mortality rate from 5% to 15%.[21] The skin manifestations of SJS more commonly affect the trunk, palms, and soles in comparison to EM. The skin lesions of SJS and EM typically resolve in 1 to 6 weeks; however, new lesions can arise as old skin lesions heal. Some patients with EM may experience frequent episodes of recurrence over the course of several years.[30,31] The mucosal involvement in SJS includes nearly 100% of patients with stomatitis and 90% to 100% with varying degrees of conjunctivitis. Oral lesions occur with a varied incidence in 40% to 60% of cases. The skin and mucosal lesions in SJS and EM involve less than 20% of the total body surface area by definition.

TEN was first described by Lyell in 1956.[32] This disorder has an estimated incidence of 1.2 to 6 cases per million per year with a mortality rate ranging from 25% to 40%.[21,23–25] TEN results from a drug reaction or underlying infectious agent and most commonly occurs in children and people with AIDS. It includes a painful localized erythema of the skin that begins on the trunk and proximal extremities and rapidly dis-

Figure 8-6. Chronic cicatricial conjunctivitis in TEN (Lyell syndrome) with trichiasis, symblepharon, and severe corneal scarring and neovascularization from stem cell damage.

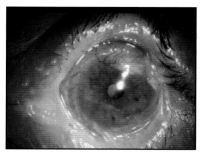

seminates to involve widespread areas forming blisters and subsequent peeling of the epidermis. This disease represents a desquamating disease that involves over 30% of the skin's epidermis with a potential for 100% of epidermal desquamation. A positive Nikolsky sign is present with epidermal detachment at the dermal-epidermal border after light pressure application. Constitutional symptoms such as fever, chills, malaise, myalgias, and arthralgias typically precede the skin and mucosal damage with widespread development of erosions that commonly affect the conjunctiva and oral mucosa in addition to the skin. The classic target lesions seen in EM and SJS are not present in TEN, and mucosal involvement in TEN is almost 100%. The alarming mortality rate of 25% to 40% results from the heightened risk of shock and multiorgan dysfunction as a result of extensive fluid and electrolyte depletion. The extremely high risk for secondary infection and subsequent septicemia as a result of the severe skin and mucosal damage also contributes to the higher risk for death.

Ocular surface findings in EM, SJS, and TEN can vary considerably depending on the type and severity of disease. Ocular complications occur in both the acute and chronic course of each of the disorders. Acute findings may include extensive periorbital edema and erythema, eyelid target lesions, severe bilateral conjunctivitis, conjunctival bullae and excoriations, subconjunctival hemorrhage, and chemosis. Eyelid edema may be one of the first ocular findings in these mucocutaneous disorders. The conjunctivitis may be mucopurulent, hemorrhagic, membranous, pseudomembranous, and/or cicatricial in nature. Associated symptoms commonly include photophobia, tearing, intense hyperemia, chemosis, and subconjunctival hemorrhage with rare instances of vesicle formation. A pseudomembranous conjunctivitis is the most common ocular manifestation of EM and SJS; however, a cicatricial conjunctivitis may also frequently occur in these disorders along with TEN (Figure 8-6). The acute complications spontaneously resolve as the skin findings disappear. Chronic ocular surface complications resulting from cicatricial changes typically create loss of goblet cell density, obliteration of accessory lacrimal glands, and lacrimal gland orifice scarring. Ocular findings from the cicatricial changes can include trichiasis, distichiasis, entropion, punctal occlusion, fornix foreshortening, symblepharon, ankyloblepharon, and KCS (Figure 8-7). Corneal complications typically develop as a result of corneal epithelial stem cell deficiency. The stem cell deficiency can potentially create findings such as punctate epithelial keratitis, corneal neovascularization, corneal scarring, nonhealing epithelial defects, corneal ulceration, keratinization, corneal melting, and subsequent perforation. Blindness can result from complete conjunctivalization and keratinization of the cornea in association with cicatricial eyelid changes and ankyloblepharon or from sequelae following ocular perforation.[21,33,34]

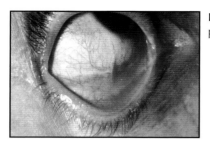

Figure 8-7. Subconjunctival fibrosis and early symblepharon formation of the inferior fornix.

The diagnosis of EM, SJS, and TEN is most often made by presentation, symptoms, and clinical observation; however, in some cases, a biopsy of a skin lesion is warranted to assist in diagnosis. The histopathology of these disorders demonstrates an immune-complex mediated vasculitis with mononuclear cell infiltration surrounding anterior dermal blood vessel wall leading to tissue-specific effects of inflammation and injury. Early lesions show a superficial lymphocytic infiltrate surrounding dermal perivascular structures with lymphocyte accumulation along the epidermal-dermal junction. Cytotoxic lymphocytes create additional tissue injury by creating epidermal keratinocyte necrosis of the basal epithelial layer with concomitant subepidermal blister formation. TEN demonstrates full thickness epidermal necrosis, subepidermal blister formation, and only minimal cellular infiltrate around dermal blood vessels. Direct immunofluorescence from a tissue biopsy demonstrates immune complex formation and deposition of C3, IgM, and fibrin around the anterior dermal blood vessels, while indirect immunofluorescence may show immune complexes from serology specimens. Immunofluorescence studies are nonspecific for differentiation between mucocutaneous disorders.

TREATMENT OF OCULAR SURFACE DISORDERS

Ocular allergy treatment requires a proper diagnosis and identification of the particular type of allergic eye disease. Treatment begins with avoidance and elimination of the offending allergen when possible. A specific allergen can be identified by history or allergy testing in some cases. Systemic and topical antihistamines and mast cell stabilizers represent the first line of medicinal therapy. These medications historically work better in SAC than PAC. AKC and VKC often require additional treatment with topical, subconjunctival, or supratarsal corticosteroids. In severe cases, systemic corticosteroids or more potent immunosuppressants, such as topical and/or oral cyclosporine or tacrolimus, may be needed for appropriate therapeutic response.

In cases of toxic ocular surface disease, the offending agent must be identified and eliminated. The diagnosis and recognition of the toxic agent is often the key to treatment in drug-related toxicity cases. Elimination of as many topical medications as possible may help to hasten return of a normal and healthy ocular surface. Use of preservative-free medications may also aid in the restoration process. In cases in which a medication is required and an oral agent of the same drug class is available, a switch from topical to oral therapy should be considered. Preservative-free lubricant drops and ointments may represent an adjunctive treatment in helping with ocular surface rehabilitation.

Medical treatment of EM, SJS, and TEN involves withdrawal of the offending medication or administration of the appropriate antibiotic/antiviral treatment directed at the underlying infectious agent. Once the offending agent has been identified, management remains supportive. Maintenance of adequate fluid and electrolyte balance and avoidance of cutaneous or mucosal infections is of utmost importance. Aggressive ocular surface lubrication with preservative-free lubricant tears and ointments along with adjunctive topical antibiotic medications may help limit long-term ocular surface complications from secondary infections. Treatment of early symblephara remains controversial. Some authors recommend daily lysis of symblephara with or without adjunctive symblephara ring placement in the fornices, while other authors feel repeated lysis exacerbates conjunctival inflammation, creating worsening of ocular surface damage long-term.[21,33] Use of systemic immunosuppression with corticosteroids also remains controversial. Some authors avoid use of systemic steroids because they are felt to delay epithelial healing and increase the risk for subsequent infection, gastrointestinal bleeding, and electrolyte imbalance.[21,31] Other studies show systemic corticosteroids at a dose of 1 mg/kg/day reduce the high mortality rate otherwise observed in severe disease states.[21,31] Additional systemic immunosuppressive agents, such as cyclosporine, tacrolimus, and cyclophosphamide, have shown benefit in promoting re-epithelialization and lowering mortality rates in SJS. More studies are needed to investigate the therapeutic response of additional immunosuppressive agents in the treatment of mucocutaneous disorders. Plasmapheresis and intravenous immunoglobulin have also shown benefit in treatment of TEN and SJS.[21,33]

In severe cases of SJS and TEN, surgical intervention is required to correct damage resulting from cicatricial effects on the eyelids and ocular surface. Eyelash abnormalities, such as trichiasis and distichiasis, should be corrected with epilation, cryotherapy, argon laser, electrolysis, or blepharotomy to destroy abnormal lash follicles.[35] Entropion repair should be performed to correct the eyelid position and prevent mechanical trauma to the cornea and conjunctiva. Oral and nasal mucosal membrane grafting and amniotic membrane have been used with success to correct severe fornix shortening and symblephara formation in association with entropion repair.[36–38] A medial or lateral tarsorrhaphy can treat an abnormal corneal surface with irregular epithelium, persistent epithelial defects, or neurotrophic corneal defects. A therapeutic bandage contact lens can be used temporarily to treat the same corneal abnormalities; however, close observation must be used to monitor for the increased risk of infection associated with bandage contact lens use in the setting of an abnormal corneal epithelial barrier to microbes. Penetrating keratoplasty, amniotic membrane grafting, cadaveric keratolimbal allografts, and combined conjunctival and keratolimbal allografting can be used to correct corneal scarring and severe corneal opacification.[39,40] These procedures carry a guarded prognosis and require systemic and topical immunosuppression for any hope of a successful outcome. The main postoperative complications of cadaveric grafts may include neurotrophic keratitis, persistent epithelial defects, infectious corneal ulcers, corneal melting, endophthalmitis, and rejection. Keratoprosthetic devices have also been used in these patients with a guarded prognosis because complications may include the same limitations of cadaveric grafts, as well as prosthetic extrusion, aqueous leaks, retroprosthetic membrane formation, and uncontrolled glaucoma.[41,42]

CLOSING CONSIDERATIONS

Allergic ocular disease and medication toxicity can affect the ocular surface with a variety of symptoms and clinical findings. Although the ocular surface manifestations of the various disease states may be similar, subtle differentiating factors can help to discern the appropriate underlying diagnosis. Once the appropriate diagnosis is confirmed, treatment strategies directed at the underlying cause for disease can be implemented. While the majority of these disorders have local ocular surface effects, certain ocular surface disorders such as EM, SJS, and TEN can also have severe systemic complications with high mortality rates and heightened risks for severe vision loss. Early recognition and appropriate differentiation between the various causes of ocular surface diseases is essential for adequate treatment and successful prognostic outcomes.

Key Points

1. Diagnosis of either ocular allergy or ocular medication toxicity can present a challenge in situations in which the signs and symptoms may be difficult to differentiate. These disorders may also mimic manifestations of KCS, thus careful scrutiny of the specific signs and symptoms typical of the various ocular disease states remains crucial for proper diagnosis and successful treatment outcomes.
2. Ocular allergy can be classified into 4 main categories including SAC, PAC, VKC, and AKC.
3. Classic teaching suggests that if an eye has itching, an allergic disorder is the cause. Conversely, a similar philosophy suggests, "no itching, no allergy." While this key concept remains an important consideration with ocular disease diagnosis, allergic disease should not be the only consideration in patients reporting itching alone. In fact, itching can often be misinterpreted or improperly ascribed to other symptoms such as burning, stinging, or ocular irritation.
4. TEN displays sheet-like epithelial loss and raised flaccid blisters that spread with pressure, a positive Nikolsky sign.
5. Ocular allergy treatment requires a proper diagnosis and identification of the particular type of allergic eye disease. Treatment begins with avoidance and elimination of the offending allergen when possible. A specific allergen can be identified by history or allergy testing in some cases. Systemic and topical antihistamines and mast cell stabilizers represent the first line of medicinal therapy.

References

1. Descotes J, Choquet-Kastylevsky G. Gell and Coombs's classification: is it still valid? *Toxicology.* 2001;158:43–49.

2. Jackson BJ. Differentiating conjunctivitis of diverse origin. *Surv Ophthalmol.* 1993;38:91–104.

3. Stahl JL, Barney NP. Ocular allergic disease. *Curr Opin Allergy Clin Immunol.* 2004;4:455–459.

4. Tanaka M, Dogru M, Takano Y, et al. The relation of conjunctival and corneal findings in severe ocular allergies. *Cornea.* 2004;23:464–467.

5. Casey R. Atopic keratoconjunctivitis. In: Abelson MB, ed. *Allergic Diseases of the Eye.* Philadelphia, Pa: WB Saunders; 2000:137.

6. Bonini S, Bonini S, Lambiase A, et al. Vernal keratoconjunctivitis revisited. A case series of 195 patients with long-term follow-up. *Ophthalmology.* 2000;107:1157–1163.

7. Tuft SJ, Cree IA, Woods M, Yorston D. Limbal vernal keratoconjunctivitis in the tropics. *Ophthalmology.* 1998;105:1489–1493.

8. Berdy GJ, Hedqvist B. Ocular allergy disorders and dry eye disease: associations, diagnostic dilemmas, and management. *Acta Ophthalmol Scand.* 2000;78:32–37.

9. Fijishima H, Toda I, Shimazaki J, Tsubota K. Allergic conjunctivitis and dry eye. *Br J Ophthalmol.* 1996;80:994–997.

10. Dart JK, Buckley RJ, Monnickendan M, Prasad J. Perennial allergic conjunctivitis: definition, clinical characteristics and prevalence. *Trans Ophthalmol Soc UK.* 1986;105:513–520.

11. Wilson FM II. Adverse external ocular effects of topical ophthalmic medications. *Surv Ophthalmol.* 1979;24:57–88.

12. Reilly CD, Mannis MJ, Chang SD. Toxic conjunctivitis. In: Krachmer JH, Mannis MJ, Holland EJ, eds. *Cornea.* 2nd ed. Vol 2. Philadelphia, Pa: Elsevier Mosby; 2005:703–711.

13. Pfluger OK. Zur ernahrung der cornea. *Klin Monatsbl Augenheilkd.* 1882;20:69–81.

14. Joyce P. Corneal vital staining. *Ir J Med Sci.* 1967;500:357–367.

15. Bron AJ, Evans VE, Smith JA. Grading of corneal and conjunctival staining in the context of other dry eye tests. *Cornea.* 2003;22:640–650.

16. Marsh PB, Schwab IR. Corneal surface disease topology. *Int Ophthalmol Clin.* 1998;38:1–13.

17. Schwab IR, Abbott RL. Toxic ulcerative keratopathy. An unrecognized problem. *Ophthalmology.* 1989;96:1187–1193.

18. De Paiva CS, Pflugfelder SC. Diagnostic approaches to lacrimal keratoconjunctivitis. In: Pflugfelder SC, Beuerman RW, Stern ME, eds. *Dry Eye and Ocular Surface Disorders.* New York, NY: Marcel Dekker, Inc; 2004:269–308.

19. Gutgesell VJ, Stern GA, Hood CI. Histopathology of meibomian gland dysfunction. *Am J Ophthalmol.* 1982;94:383–387.

20. Rolando M. Tear mucus ferning test in normal and keratoconjunctivitis sicca eyes. *Chibret Int J Ophthalmol.* 1984;2:33–41.

21. Holland EJ, Palmon FE, Webster GF. Erythema multiforme, Stevens-Johnson syndrome, and toxic epidermal necrolysis. In: Mannis MJ, Macsai MS, Huntley AC, eds. *Eye and Skin Disease.* Philadelphia, Pa: Lippincott-Raven; 1996:273–284.

22. Power WJ, Saidman SL, Zhang DS, et al. HLA typing in patients with ocular manifestations of Stevens-Johnson syndrome. *Ophthalmology.* 1996;103:1406–1409.

23. Lam N, Yang Y, Wang L, Lin Y, Chiang B. Clinical characteristics of childhood erythema multiforme, Stevens-Johnson syndrome and toxic epidermal necrolysis in Taiwanese children. *J Microbiol Immunol Infect.* 2004;37:366–370.

24. Auquier-Dunant A, Mockenhaupt M, Naldi L, et al. Correlations between clinical patterns and causes of erythema multiforme majus, Stevens-Johnson syndrome, and toxic epidermal necrolysis. *Arch Dermatol.* 2002;138:1019–1024.

25. Schofield JK, Tatnall FM, Leigh IM. Recurrent erythema multiforme: clinical features and treatment in a large series of patients. *Br J Dermatol.* 1993;128(5):542–545.

26. Mondino BJ, Brown SI, Biglan AW. HLA antigens in Stevens-Johnson syndrome with ocular involvement. *Ophthalmology.* 1982;100:1453–1454.

27. Mobini N, Ahmed AR. Immunogenetics of drug-induced bullous diseases. *Clin Dermatol.* 1993;11:449–460.

28. Roujeau JC, Huynh TN, Bracq C, et al. Genetic susceptibility to toxic epidermal necrolysis. *Arch Dermatol.* 1987;123:1171–1173.

29. von Hebra F. *On Diseases of the Skin, Including the Exanthematha.* Vol 1, translated and edited by C. H. Fagge. London: New Sydenham Society; 1866.

30. Sen P, Chua SH. A case of recurrent erythema multiforme and its therapeutic complications. *Ann Acad Med Singapore.* 2004;33:793–796.

31. Leaute-Labreze C, Lamireau T, Chawki D, Maleville J, Taieb A. Diagnosis, classification, and management of erythema multiforme and Stevens-Johnson syndrome. *Arch Dis Child.* 2000;83:347–352.

32. Lyell A. Toxic epidermal necrolysis: an eruption resembling scalding of the skin. *Br J Dermatol.* 1956;68:355–361.

33. Holland EJ, Palmon FE, Webster GF. Erythema multiforme, Stevens-Johnson syndrome, and toxic epidermal necrolysis. In: Macsai MS, Mannis MJ, Huntley AC, eds. *Eye and Skin Disease.* 1st ed. Philadelphia, Pa: Lippincott-Raven; 1996:273–284.

34. Ostler HB, Maibach HI, Hoke AW. Vasculitis and necrobiotic disorders. In: Ostler HB, Maibach HI, Hoke AW, Schwab IR, eds. *Diseases of the Eye & Skin. A Color Atlas.* Philadelphia, Pa: Lippincott Williams & Wilkins; 2003:129–144.

35. Sodhi PK, Verma L. Surgery for trichiasis. *Ophthalmology.* 2004;111:578–584.

36. McCord CD Jr, Chen WP. Tarsal polishing and mucous membrane grafting for cicatricial entropion, trichiasis and epidermalization. *Ophthalmic Surg.* 1983;14:10210–10215.

37. Tseng SC, Di Pascuale MA, Liu DT, Gao YY, Baradaran-Rafii A. Intraoperative mitomycin C and amniotic membrane transplantation for fornix reconstruction in severe cicatricial ocular surface diseases. *Ophthalmology.* 2005;112:896–903.

38. Nakamura T, Inatomi T, Sotozono C, et al. Transplantation of cultivated autologous oral mucosal epithelial cells in patients with severe ocular surface disorders. *Br J Ophthalmol.* 2004;88:1280–1284.

39. Tsubota K, Toda I, Saito H, et al. Reconstruction of the corneal epithelium by limbal allograft transplantation for severe ocular surface disorders. *Ophthalmology.* 1995;102:1486–1495.

40. Holland EJ, Schwartz GS, Nordlund ML. Surgical techniques for ocular surface reconstruction. In: Krachmer JH, Mannis MJ, Holland EJ, eds. *Cornea.* 2nd ed. Vol 2. Philadelphia, Pa: Elsevier Mosby; 2005:1799–1812.

41. Khan B, Dudenhoefer EJ, Dohlman CH. Keratoprosthesis: an update. *Curr Opin Ophthalmol.* 2001;12:282–287.

42. Hicks CR, Crawford GJ, Lou X, et al. Corneal replacement using a synthetic hydrogel cornea, AlphaCor: device, preliminary outcomes and complications. *Eye.* 2003;17:385–392.

9

Chemical Burns and the Dry Eye

Vatinee Y. Bunya, MD;
Christopher J. Rapuano, MD; and
Kristin M. Hammersmith, MD

INTRODUCTION

Ocular trauma, including chemical injury, is a leading cause of blindness. Young males are most commonly affected. These injuries occur both at home and in the workplace. In addition, chemicals have been used in assaults in urban settings. Chemical injury can cause a wide spectrum of eye problems, ranging from mild surface disease to blindness. The severity of the injury depends on several factors, including the type of chemical, time of exposure, and management after the injury. Chemical injuries can have long-term ocular morbidity, including dry eye. Dry eye in the setting of chemical burns can be challenging to manage due to the variety of complications that may occur after chemical injuries.

OCULAR EFFECTS OF CHEMICAL INJURIES

Acids tend to cause less severe ocular damage than alkalis because of their effect on the tissues that they contact. These chemicals cause precipitation and denaturation of proteins, which acts as a barrier to further penetration of acid into tissues.[1] In addition, the cornea acts as a partial buffer. However, strong acids in high concentrations can cause significant ocular injury similar to alkalis.

The most severe chemical injuries are caused by strong alkalis. These substances raise the pH of tissues and cause saponification of cell membranes, which facilitates rapid and deep chemical penetration. Alkalis can quickly penetrate through the cornea and actually enter the eye, causing intense inflammation and tissue damage.[2]

Table 9-1 CLASSIFICATION OF CHEMICAL BURNS[4]	
Grade I	Injury to epithelium; no limbal ischemia.
Grade II	Cornea hazy but iris details visible; ischemia one half or less at limbus; occasional symblepharon.
Grade III	Total corneal staining with hazy cornea and iris details obscured; ischemia up to one half at limbus.
Grade IV	Cornea opaque with iris details totally obscured; ischemia of over one half of limbus.

Table 9-2 CLASSIFICATION OF CHEMICAL BURNS[5]		
Grade	*Limbal Involvement*	*Conjunctival Involvement*
I	None	None
II	<3 clock hours	<30%
III	3 to 6 clock hours	30% to 50%
IV	6 to 9 clock hours	50% to 75%
V	>9 to <12 clock hours	>75% to <100%
VI	Total (12 clock hours)	Total (100%)

Ischemia of the anterior segment develops after severe chemical burns that extend beyond the limbus.[3] This ischemia is accompanied by an inflammatory response to the ischemic tissue. Tissues are infiltrated by leucocytes and destructive enzymes are released that can lead to corneal ulceration and perforation.

CLINICAL EXAMINATION

The initial ophthalmic examination should be performed after the eye has been copiously irrigated and the pH has normalized. In rare cases, the pH remains elevated despite copious irrigation secondary to the chemical continuing to leach out of tissues over time. Particulate matter and necrotic tissue can continue to release the toxic chemical and, therefore, should be removed under topical anesthesia. The eyelids should be flipped to search for these materials, and double eversion of the upper eyelid should be performed to check the upper fornix.

On examination, important signs to note include the size of the epithelial defect, the amount of stromal haze, and the presence of limbal blanching. The eyelids should also be examined for involvement and extent of damage. Grading chemical burns can be helpful in predicting prognosis as well as determining how aggressively to manage a particular patient (Tables 9-1 and 9-2; Figures 9-1 through 9-4).

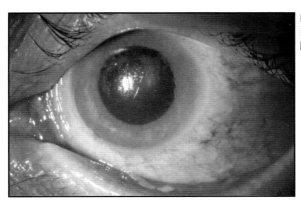

Figure 9-1. A mild to moderate alkali injury causing a large epithelial defect but minimal limbal blanching.

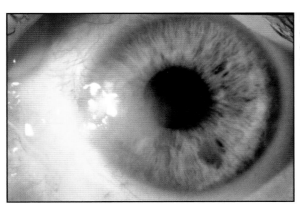

Figure 9-2. Six weeks after a moderate chemical injury causing less than 3 clock hours of limbal blanching and mild to moderate corneal haze.

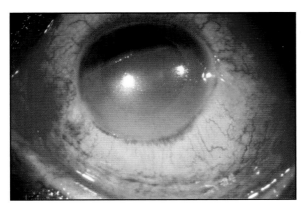

Figure 9-3. A moderate chemical injury with 6 clock hours of limbal blanching, a large epithelial defect, and stromal haze.

Figure 9-4. The sequelae of a severe chemical injury demonstrating a scarred and vascularized cornea. This eye underwent a permanent kerato-prosthesis.

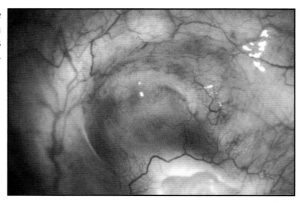

MECHANISMS OF CHEMICAL INJURIES LEADING TO DRY EYES

Chemical injury can lead to problems with dry eyes via several mechanisms, including loss of corneal innervation, damage to secondary lacrimal glands, and diffuse goblet cell loss.[6] Loss of corneal innervation disrupts the sensory, autonomic neural reflex loop between the ocular surface and lacrimal glands that is important for the maintenance of a healthy ocular surface.[7] In addition, chemical injury also leads to dry eye through disruption of the tear film at both the aqueous layer via the destruction of lacrimal glands, as well as the lipid layer through the loss of goblet cells.

Recently, attention has been focused on the important relationship between inflammation and dry eye. Inflammation of the lacrimal glands and ocular surface can lead to an abnormal tear film.[8] Changes in the tear film composition appear to promote inflammation on the ocular surface by decreasing the secretion of natural anti-inflammatory factors, increasing proinflammatory cytokines, and activating cytokines and proteases.[9] Therefore, it is important to treat ocular inflammation seen after chemical injury because it can exacerbate the dry eye changes seen in these patients.

TREATMENT OF CHEMICAL BURNS AND COMPLICATIONS

Acute Management of Chemical Injuries

The most important step for the initial management of an ocular chemical burn is immediate and copious irrigation with water or normal saline solution at the site of injury. If these liquids are not readily available, any nontoxic liquid available immediately should be used to avoid any delay in treatment. Irrigation should be started on site and ideally continued until the patient can be evaluated by a physician. Another base or acid should never be used to "neutralize" the initial agent because this may cause more injury.[1] The initial examination of the patient should be delayed until the patient has received adequate irrigation and the pH of the tears has normalized. The pH should be checked 5 to 10 minutes after stopping irrigation to allow the pH to equalize between the tear film and tissues. Irrigation should be performed for at least 30 minutes and then repeated every 30 minutes until the pH has normalized.

Long-Term Management and Complications of Chemical Injuries

After the initial management, the goals of further treatment include promoting re-epithelialization of the cornea, decreasing inflammation, monitoring intraocular pressure, and managing eyelid complications. These patients can develop many complications, including eyelid malposition, corneal scarring, symblepharon formation, limbal stem cell deficiency, cataracts, glaucoma, and dry eye.

TREATMENT OF CORNEAL EPITHELIAL DEFECTS, INFECTION, AND ULCERATION

Antibiotic Ointments and Bandage Contact Lens

Antibiotic ointments can be used to prevent superinfection after injury as well as to promote re-epithelialization of the cornea. Frequent lubrication is necessary to promote healing. A bandage soft contact lens can sometimes be useful to help the corneal epithelium heal; however, the patient should be watched closely for infection.

Tetracyclines

Oral tetracyclines, such as doxycycline, may help protect the cornea against ulceration and perforation after chemical injury. These agents inhibit matrix metalloproteinases through the suppression of the expression of neutrophil collagenase and epithelial gelatinase, inhibition of alpha-1 antitrypsin degradation, and scavenging of reactive oxygen species.[10] A typical dose is doxycycline 100 mg orally (PO) 2 times a day (BID), which can be taken with food, or tetracycline 250 mg PO once 4 times a day (QID), but tetracycline cannot be taken with food.

Ascorbic Acid

In the rabbit model, severe alkali burns result in a decrease in aqueous humor ascorbate levels. This is thought to be due to damage to the ciliary processes, which normally transfer ascorbic acid (vitamin C) from the blood into the aqueous humor.[11] In theory, the risk of corneal ulceration is increased because ascorbic acid is needed for collagen synthesis. Wishard et al showed that the systemic administration of ascorbic acid reduced the rate of corneal ulceration in acid injuries in the rabbit model.[12] Therefore, it is possible that ascorbic acid may help to promote collagen synthesis in the cornea.

Similarly in the rabbit model, systemic administration of vitamin C has been shown to raise aqueous ascorbate levels and reduce the risk of corneal perforation.[11] If these data are extrapolated to humans, then systemic administration of vitamin C may be useful in preventing corneal ulcerations after chemical injury. Of note, there have not been any randomized clinical trials demonstrating this effect in humans to date. However, Brodovsky et al found that there was a trend toward more rapid healing and better visual outcome in grade 3 burn patients treated with a standard protocol, which included intensive treatment with both topical and oral ascorbate.[13] One empiric approach is to give patients 2 g of vitamin C daily. However, this high dose of vitamin C should not be used in patients with renal disease.

In addition, topical ascorbate 10% drops may also be helpful in reducing the risk of corneal ulcerations after chemical injuries, as demonstrated in the rabbit model.[14] Topical ascorbate promotes the production of collagen by fibroblasts in the cornea, which could help healing after chemical burns.

Topical Acetylcysteine Drops

Topical acetylcysteine may be useful in the treatment of chemical burns and dry eye. Fraunfelder et al found that 24% of patients with long-term KCS had corneal mucous plaques.[15] In this study, these plaques were found to be a mixture of mucus, epithelial cells, proteins, and lipids. The authors found that these plaques were prevented by topical 10% acetylcysteine 1 to 4 times daily. In addition, the existing plaques often quickly loosened and dissolved with treatment. It is possible that treating corneal mucous plaques may alleviate the severity of dry eye. In addition, using topical acetylcysteine 10% drops QID may help control collagenase activity and corneal melting that can occur after chemical injuries.[16]

Early Amniotic Membrane Transplantation

Amniotic membrane transplantation (AMT) can be beneficial in facilitating healing and minimizing possible complications after chemical injuries.[17,18] Therefore, AMT within the first 7 to 10 days following the acute injury may be a first-line treatment for severe chemical burns along with immediate intensive medical therapy.[19]

TREATMENT OF INFLAMMATION

Topical Corticosteroids

Topical corticosteroids are extremely useful for the first 2 weeks following a chemical injury in order to limit inflammation and destruction of tissue by polymorphonuclear leucocytes. In the rabbit model, topical medroxyprogesterone may prevent or delay corneal perforation after alkali injury through decreasing collagenase activity.[20,21] Although this benefit has not been studied in a clinical trial, some physicians feel that this is a useful treatment in certain patients. However, after the acute phase, steroids should be limited because they can impede wound healing and increase the risk of infection. Donshik et al showed in the rabbit model that steroid use could increase the risk of ulceration and perforation if used after the acute phase of healing.[22]

Cycloplegia

Topical cycloplegia (eg, scopolamine 0.25% or cyclopentolate 1% to 2%, 2 to 3 times a day) is recommended if there is a significant anterior chamber reaction.

TREATMENT OF GLAUCOMA

Increased intraocular pressure after chemical injuries can be due to scleral shrinkage or decreased outflow due to damage to severe inflammation or damage to the the trabecular meshwork. Intraocular pressure can be controlled with various medications, including topical beta-blockers, alpha-blockers, and carbonic anhydrase inhibitors.

Miotics and prostaglandin analogues should be avoided because they could promote further inflammation.

TREATMENT OF SYMBLEPHARON AND EYELID MALPOSITION

Symblepharon should be broken under topical anesthesia daily or a scleral shell can be used. Patients may require surgery to correct eyelid malpositions, particularly if they are causing breakdown of the ocular surface or exposure.

TREATMENT OF DRY EYE AFTER CHEMICAL INJURY

Lubricants

Patients should be treated with frequent administration of preservative-free artificial tears and lubricants. Lubrication provides symptomatic relief as well as promotes healing of the ocular surface.

Autologous Serum

The use of autologous serum to make eye drops was first described in 1984 by Fox et al.[23] In theory, autologous serum eye drops contain growth factors and nutrients that may be useful in the treatment of severe ocular surface disorders. Serum eye drops have been used for the management of severe dry eyes, persistent epithelial defects, superior limbal keratoconjunctivitis, and as an adjunctive treatment in ocular surface reconstruction.[24] Autologous serum drops may be helpful in the treatment of severe chemical injuries. However, the difficulty in preparation and the possibility of complications such as infection and inflammation from potential immune complex deposition limit their use.[24]

Cyclosporin A

The immunomodulatory agent cyclosporin A (CsA) appears to have potentially beneficial effects on the inflammatory process underlying dry eyes. Sall et al showed that there were both objective and subjective improvements in moderate to severe dry eye disease in patients using topical CsA 0.05%.[25] This study supported previous studies that demonstrated that CsA could improve the signs and symptoms of dry eye. In addition, cyclosporine appears to be a safe medication that may treat the cause of dry eye, not just the symptoms.[7]

Punctal Occlusion

Temporary or permanent occlusion of the puncta in the upper and/or lower eyelids can be helpful in treating dry eyes by increasing tear film retention. Temporary punctal occlusion can be achieved using various types of punctal plugs,[26] while thermal or electrocautery is used to cause permanent closure of the puncta.[27]

Figure 9-5. Superior limbal stem cell abnormality after a chemical injury.

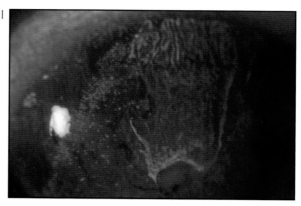

Lateral Tarsorrhaphy

Conservation of the tear film through the use of a lateral tarsorrhaphy can be very effective in alleviating dry eye signs and symptoms. A tarsorrhaphy can be temporary or permanent and works through decreasing the evaporation of the tear film.

OCULAR RECONSTRUCTION

Corneal Glue

In cases of small impending or frank corneal perforations, glue can sometimes be useful as a temporizing measure. Sharma et al showed that fibrin glue and cyanoacrylate tissue adhesive were both effective in sealing corneal perforations up to 3 mm in diameter.[28]

Amniotic Membrane Transplantation

Amniotic membrane has many qualities that make it ideal for use after chemical injury. It is known to promote ocular surface healing through various mechanisms, including inhibition of epithelial cell apoptosis and through the presence of various growth factors. In addition, AMT may help decrease inflammation and prevent scarring and symblepharon formation. AMT can serve as a temporizing measure that can be used to stabilize the ocular surface prior to a more definitive reconstructive procedure such as a penetrating keratoplasty (PK). Hick et al found that combining AMT and fibrin glue was a successful way of treating nonhealing ulcers and perforations of up to 3 mm in diameter.[29]

Limbal Stem Cell Transplantation

Patients with ocular chemical burns can have mild to severe limbal stem cell deficiency depending on the extent of the injury (Figure 9-5). Limbal stem cell deficiency can lead to persistent corneal epithelial defects, neovascularization of the cornea, and scarring.[30] Limbal stem cell transplantation may be performed as early as 2 weeks after the injury. Ideally, this surgery should be postponed until any inflammation is controlled in order to decrease the risk of stem cell failure. Stem cells can be used from the unaffected fellow eye, a living relative, or a cadaver. Kim et al have shown a higher success rate of allogeneic stem cell transplantation survival using systemic immunosuppression compared to patients treated with topical immunosuppression alone.[30] The authors recommended that patients receiving any systemic immunosuppression be followed in consultation with a transplantation medicine specialist for appropriate monitoring.

Tectonic Grafts

Tectonic (reconstructive) lamellar or PK can be used in selected patients with corneal thinning or perforation. Vanathi et al demonstrated that tectonic grafts are a useful option in certain cases of paracentral perforations or larger areas of thinning or perforation.[31] Smaller grafts can be used to stabilize the eye prior to undertaking a more definitive central PK.

Corneal Transplantation

PK has a poor prognosis in patients with ocular damage from chemical injuries. Corneal transplants have the best chance for survival when preoperative inflammation has been minimized or, ideally, eliminated. Therefore, PK is often not considered until many months to years after the initial injury. Of note, conjunctival flaps may be useful in decreasing ocular inflammation in preparation for a possible future PK.[32,33] Similarly, as described above, AMT may also be useful for quieting the eye prior to performing a PK.

Keratoprosthesis

Because PK has a poor prognosis in patients with previous or ongoing chronic inflammation, including patients after severe chemical injuries, keratoprosthesis (KPro) surgery may be indicated. However, because there is a significant rate of complications after KPro surgery, this procedure should only be reserved for those patients who are not good candidates for other reconstructive surgeries.[34]

There are 2 general types of keratoprostheses. The first type is used in patients with a good tear film and blink function, such as the Dohlman-Doane Type I (Massachusetts Eye & Ear Infirmary, Boston, Mass) and AlphaCor (CooperVision, Fairport, NY).[35,36] The second type, such as the Dohlman-Doane Type II, is placed through the eyelid in eyes with end-stage dry eye or poor blink function.[34] The Strampelli osteo-odonto-keratoprosthesis, which incorporates part of the patient's own tooth, can also be used in eyes with end-stage dry eye.[37,38] Yaghouti et al found that patients with ocular chemical injuries had an intermediate prognosis after KPro procedures when compared to graft failure-noncicatrizing disease, OCP, and Stevens-Johnson syndrome.[34]

SUMMARY

When managing dry eye in the setting of a chemical injury, it is important to be aware of the many ocular complications that can occur, including corneal scarring, symblepharon formation, eyelid malposition, limbal stem cell deficiency, cataracts, and glaucoma. In addition to treating the symptoms of dry eye, recent efforts have been focused on attempting to treat the causes of dry eye both medically and surgically. Patients with chemical injuries require long-term follow-up and may benefit from reconstructive procedures once the initial inflammation has been controlled.

Key Points

1. Acids tend to cause less severe ocular damage than alkalis. They cause precipitation and denaturation of proteins, which acts as a barrier to further penetration of acid into tissues.
2. The most severe chemical injuries are caused by strong alkalis. These substances raise the pH of tissues and cause saponification of cell membranes, which facilitates rapid and deep chemical penetration.
3. Chemical injuries to the eye require immediate and copious irrigation.
4. Chemical injury can lead to problems with dry eye via several mechanisms, including loss of corneal innervation, damage to secondary lacrimal glands, and diffuse goblet cell loss.
5. In addition to the standard treatments for dry eye, it is important to control ocular inflammation after chemical injuries because this can exacerbate dry eye symptoms.
6. Ocular inflammation should also be minimized prior to any attempts of ocular reconstruction.

REFERENCES

1. Pfister DR, Pfister RR. Acid injuries of the eye. In: Krachmer JH, Mannis MJ, Holland EJ, eds. *Cornea: Volume 1 Fundamentals, Diagnosis and Management.* Philadelphia, Pa: Elsevier Mosby; 2005:1277–1283.
2. Pfister RR, Pfister DR. Alkali injuries of the eye. In: Krachmer JH, Mannis MJ, Holland EJ, eds. *Cornea: Volume 1 Fundamentals, Diagnosis and Management.* Philadelphia, Pa: Elsevier Mosby; 2005:1285–1293.
3. Reim M. The results of ischaemia in chemical injuries. *Eye.* 1992;6:376–380.
4. Roper-Hall MJ. Thermal and chemical burns. *Trans Ophthalmol Soc UK.* 1965;85:631–653.
5. Dua HS, King AJ. A new classification of ocular surface burns. *Br J Ophthalmol.* 2001;85:1379–1383.
6. Djalian AR, Hamrah P, Pflugfelder SC. Dry eye. In: Krachmer JH, Mannis MJ, Holland EJ, eds. *Cornea: Volume 1 Fundamentals, Diagnosis and Management.* Philadelphia, Pa: Elsevier Mosby; 2005:521–540.
7. Perry HD, Donnenfeld ED. Dry eye diagnosis and management in 2004. *Curr Opin Ophthalmol.* 2004;15:299–304.
8. Stern ME, Beuerman RW, Fox RI, Gao J, Mircheff AK, Pflugfelder SC. The pathology of dry eye: the interaction between the ocular surface and the lacrimal glands. *Cornea.* 1998;17:584–589.
9. Pflugfelder SC. Antiinflammatory therapy for dry eye. *Am J Ophthalmol.* 2004;137:337–342.
10. Ralph RA. Tetracyclines and the treatment of corneal stromal ulceration. *Cornea.* 2000;19:274–277.

11. Pfister RR, Paterson CA. Ascorbic acid in the treatment of alkali burns of the eye. *Ophthalmology.* 1980;87:1050–1057.

12. Wishard P, Paterson CA. The effect of ascorbic acid on experimental acid injuries of the rabbit cornea. *Invest Ophthalmol Vis Sci.* 1980;19:564–566.

13. Brodovsky SC, McCarty CA, Snibson G, et al. Management of alkali burns: an 11-year retrospective review. *Ophthalmology.* 2000;107:1829–1835.

14. Pfister RR, Haddox JL, Yuille-Barr D. The combined effect of citrate/ascorbate treatment in alkali-injured rabbit eyes. *Cornea.* 1991;10:100–104.

15. Fraunfelder FT, Wright P, Tripathi RC. Corneal mucus plaques. *Am J Ophthalmol.* 1977;83: 191–197.

16. Rapuano CJ, Heng W. *Color Atlas & Synopsis of Clinical Ophthalmology: Cornea.* New York, NY: McGraw-Hill; 2003:282–287.

17. Ucakhan OO, Koklu G, Firat E. Nonpreserved human amniotic membrane transplantation in acute and chronic chemical eye injuries. *Cornea.* 2002;21:169–172.

18. Meller D, Pires RTF, Mack RJS, et al. Amniotic membrane transplantation for acute chemical or thermal burns. *Ophthalmology.* 2000;107:980–990.

19. John T. Human amniotic membrane transplantation: past, present, and future. *Ophthalmol Clin N Am.* 2003;16:43–65.

20. Huang Y, Meek KM, Ho MW, Paterson CA. Analysis of birefringence during would healing and remodeling following alkali burns in rabbit cornea. *Exp Eye Res.* 2001;73:521–532.

21. Newsome NA, Gross J. Prevention by medroxyprogesterone of perforation in the alkali-burned rabbit cornea: inhibition of collagenolytic activity. *Invest Ophthalmol Vis Sci.* 1977;16:21–31.

22. Donshik PC, Berman MB, Dohlman CH, Gage J, Rose J. Effect of topical corticosteroids on ulceration in alkali-burned corneas. *Arch Ophthalmol.* 1978;96:2117–2120.

23. Fox RI, Chan R, Michelson JB, et al. Beneficial effect of artificial tears made with autologous serum in patients with keratoconjunctivitis sicca. *Arthritis Rheum.* 1984;27:459–461.

24. Geerling G, MacLennan S, Hartwig D. Autologous serum eye drops for ocular surface disorders. *Br J Ophthalmol.* 2004;88:1467–1474.

25. Sall K, Stevenson OD, Mundorf TK, Reis BL, CsA Phase 3 Study Group. Two multicenter, randomized studies of the efficacy and safety of cyclosporine ophthalmic emulsion in moderate to severe dry eye disease. *Ophthalmology.* 2000;107:631–639.

26. Tai MC, Cosar CB, Cohen EJ, Rapuano CJ, Laibson PR. The clinical efficacy of silicone punctal plug therapy. *Cornea.* 2002;21:135–139.

27. Foulks GN. The evolving treatment of dry eye. *Ophthalmol Clin N Am.* 2003;16:29–35.

28. Sharma A, Kaur R, Kumar S, et al. Fibrin glue versus N-butyl-2-cyanoacrylate in corneal perforations. *Ophthalmology.* 2003;110:291–298.

29. Hick S, Demers PE, Brunette I, La C, Mabon M, Duchesne B. Amniotic membrane transplantation and fibrin glue in the management of corneal ulcers and perforations. *Cornea.* 2005;24: 369–377.

30. Kim JY, Djalilian AR, Schwartz GS, Holland EJ. Ocular surface reconstruction: limbal stem cell transplantation. *Ophthalmol Clin N Am.* 2003;16:67–77.

31. Vanathi M, Sharma N, Titiyal JS, Tandon R, Vajpayee RB. Tectonic grafts for corneal thinning and perforations. *Cornea.* 2002;21:792–797.

32. Laibson PR. Current concepts and techniques in corneal transplantation. *Curr Opin Ophthalmol.* 2002;13:220–223.

33. Geria RC, Zarate J, Geria MA. Penetrating keratoplasty in eyes treated with conjunctival flaps. *Cornea.* 2001;20:345–349.

34. Yaghouti F, Nouri M, Abad JC, Power WJ, Doane MG, Dohlman CH. Keratoprosthesis: preoperative prognostic categories. *Cornea.* 2001;20:19–23.

35. Yaghouti F, Dohlman CH. Innovations in keratoprosthesis: proved and unproved. *Int Ophthalmol Clin.* 1999;39:27–36.

36. Hicks CR, Crawford GJ, Lou X, et al. Corneal replacement using a synthetic hydrogel cornea, AlphaCor: device, preliminary outcomes and complications. *Eye*. 2003;17:385–392.
37. Hicks CR, Fitton JH, Chirila TV, Crawford GJ, Constable IJ. Keratoprostheses: advancing toward a true artificial cornea. *Surv Ophthalmol*. 1997;42:175–189.
38. Falcinelli G, Falsini B, Taloni M, Colliardo P, Falcinelli G. Modified osteo-odonto-keratoprosthesis for treatment of corneal blindness: Long-term anatomical and functional outcomes in 181 cases. *Arch Ophthalmol*. 2005;123:1319–1329.

10

Ocular Cicatricial Pemphigoid and Dry Eye Syndrome

Vasudha A. Panday, MD;
Kristin M. Hammersmith, MD; and
Christopher J. Rapuano, MD

INTRODUCTION

Bullous diseases of the skin and mucous membranes can be associated with ocular involvement, usually seen with pemphigus, bullous pemphigoid, and cicatricial pemphigoid. Of these, cicatricial pemphigoid most commonly affects the eyes and causes the most severe ocular manifestations. Ocular cicatricial pemphigoid (OCP) is characterized by progressive conjunctival scarring and shrinkage, and can eventually lead to blindness if left untreated. OCP has no specific race or geographic distribution, and more often affects people in their 60s to 70s.[1] However, there have been case reports of OCP affecting children as young as 12.[2] The incidence ranges from 1 in 15,000 to 1 in 40,000, with an average of approximately 1 in 20,000 patients affected.[3] Women seem to be affected more commonly than men, with a ratio of approximately 1.6:1.[1] These patients also have a 4-fold increase in the prevalence of other autoimmune diseases such as systemic lupus erythematosus, polyarteritis nodosa, and rheumatoid arthritis.[4]

CLINICAL PRESENTATION

Chronic papillary conjunctivitis is the most common manifestation early in the disease course. OCP can present as a unilateral process, but typically involves the other eye in less than 2 years.[4,5] Patients usually complain of dryness, burning, tearing, foreign body sensation, and other nonspecific ocular irritation. As the disease progresses, conjunctival vesicles appear that break down and form ulcers that are covered by a gray exudate.[6] Conjunctival fibrosis begins and leads to scarring. Early in the course of the disease, this finding may only be seen on the upper or lower tarsal conjunctiva as fine white fibrous scars. This fibrosis leads to conjunctival shrinkage and changes in the normal architecture of the superior and inferior fornix. With progression, fibrous tracts that fuse the bulbar conjunctiva to the palpebral conjunctiva (symblepharon formation) may be seen (Figure 10-1). This phenomenon is best seen by pulling the lower eyelid down while having the patient look up. Conjunctival shrinkage and fornix foreshortening generally continues if left untreated and can lead to complete fusion of the upper and lower lid to the palpebral conjunctiva (ankyloblepharon) with restriction of ocular motility (Figure 10-2).

The fibrotic process can also cause entropion, distichiasis, trichiasis, and lagophthalmos (Figure 10-3). Corneal damage can occur due to a combination of exposure and mechanical trauma from trichiasis. Corneal neovascularization, pannus formation, superficial erosions, persistent epithelial defects, bacterial superinfection, and stromal ulceration are also seen. Severe cases can lead to corneal perforation.

Extraocular manifestations of cicatricial pemphigoid include skin, scalp, oral and nasal mucosa, esophagus, larynx, pharynx, anus, vagina, and urethra.[7]

Dry Eye in Ocular Cicatricial Pemphigoid

OCP patients exhibit severe dry eye that results from an eventual change in all 3 of the tear film components: aqueous and mucin insufficiency and meibomian gland dysfunction. Early in the course of the disease, patients have an overproduction of mucin that mixes with proteins and nucleic acids from damaged cells and adheres to the epithelium.[7] The tear film breaks up more rapidly over these areas, leading to instability.[4] Because progressive conjunctival fibrosis and forniceal foreshortening causes occlusion of the ducts of the lacrimal and accessory lacrimal glands, there is a decrease in the aqueous component. Alteration in the lid margin from scarring leads to occlusion of the meibomian gland orifices, decreasing the lipid component and causing rapid break up of the tear film. Lastly, as the disease progresses, extensive conjunctival scarring destroys mucus-producing goblet cells in the conjunctiva, causing decreased mucus production and, therefore, more rapid tear film breakup. A deficient and unstable tear film, in combination with exposure due to lagophthalmos and abnormal blinking, leads to progressive corneal epithelial breakdown and eventual keratinization.

Pathogenesis

The initiating event in OCP is thought to be the binding of circulating antibodies, most commonly IgG and IgA,[8] to an antigen or antigens of the basement membrane zone. This activates the complement cascade and attracts plasma cells, polymorphonuclear leucocytes, macrophages, lymphocytes, and mast cells into subepithelial tissues. The inflammatory reaction not only releases hydrolytic enzymes that digest the lamina lucida and lead to subepithelial blister formation but also activates fibroblasts, thus leading to scar formation.[9]

Several antigens have recently been identified that may be potential targets for circulating antibodies, including IgG autoantibodies to the alpha-subunit of laminin 5 and the 180-kd bullous pemphigoid antigen BPAg2, as well as IgA autoantibodies to a

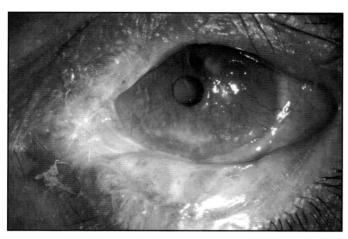

Figure 10-1. OCP with conjunctival scarring, loss of normal lid architecture, and corneal scarring. (Courtesy of Dr. Irving Raber.)

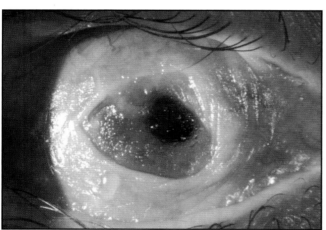

Figure 10-2. Advanced OCP with almost complete ocular surface keratinization. (Courtesy of Dr. Irving Raber.)

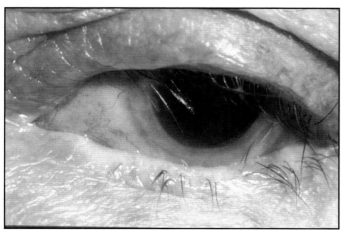

Figure 10-3. Lid and lash changes observed in OCP. Note the upper lid cicatricial entropion and lower lid distichiasis. (Courtesy of Dr. Irving Raber.)

45-kd antigen.[10–14] In addition, there has been an association of OCP with HLA-DQw7[15] and HLA B-12,[16] suggesting a genetic susceptibility to the development of the disease. High levels of tumor necrosis factor-alpha (TNF-α), interleukin-1 alpha, and interleukin beta with low levels of interleukin-1 receptor antagonist have been found in active OCP.[9] These abnormal levels can return to baseline once the active disease process has been controlled.[17]

Histologically, conjunctival specimens show infiltration with macrophages, neutrophils, plasma cells, lymphocytes, eosinophils, and Langerhans' cells. There is an increase in the number of mast cells and a decrease in the population of goblet cells. These changes may reverse after remission has been achieved. Electron microscopy of conjunctival specimens shows thinning of the surface epithelium with thickened lamina propria infiltrated with inflammatory cells. Areas of discontinuity, duplication, and focal thickening, with prominent tonofilaments and tonofibrils, are also seen.[7]

OCP can be idiopathic, medication induced, or of an infectious etiology, more appropriately termed *pseudopemphigoid*. Medications known to cause pseudopemphigoid include pilocarpine, epinephrine, echothiophate iodide, and practolol. The disease process is identical to idiopathic OCP, except for manifestation of symptoms only in the eye receiving the medication, and cessation of progression and potential reversal after discontinuation of the drug. Adenovirus, diphtheria, trachoma, primary HSV keratoconjunctivitis, and beta-hemolytic streptococcus are among the infections known to cause an OCP-like disease.

DIAGNOSIS

The diagnosis of OCP is based on conjunctival biopsy demonstrating linear deposition of immunoglobulin or complement at the epithelial basement membrane zone. Immunofluorescent techniques, or the more sensitive and equally specific immunoperoxidase techniques, should be used. The diagnostic sensitivity of immunofluorescence alone is thought to be between 50% to 52%, increasing to 83% with immunoperoxidase.[18] Serologic indirect immunofluorescent (IIF) evaluation, looking for circulatory autoantibodies to the basement membrane zone, may help to confirm the diagnosis. A negative biopsy does not rule out the presence of the disease, but a positive biopsy does confirm the diagnosis.

SYSTEMIC TREATMENT

Treatment of OCP revolves around immunosuppression. To that end, chemotherapeutic medications are used. The choice of a specific medication depends on the patient's other medical problems and overall health, as well as the amount of inflammation and rate of disease progression. Oral corticosteroids alone are ineffective in reducing conjunctival inflammation and preventing progressive scarring.[4] They are useful when used in combination with other immunosuppressive agents to treat patients with severe inflammation to quiet the inflammatory activity.

Dapsone is still considered by most to be the first-line agent for mild to moderate inflammation. It cannot be used in patients with a sulfa allergy or G6PD deficiency and can cause hemolytic anemia, agranulocytosis, and aplastic anemia. A baseline CBC and liver function tests (LFTs) should be performed on every patient prior to starting this medication. Blood work must be monitored regularly. If dapsone is not tolerated, aza-thioprine (Imuran) can be substituted. Cyclophosphamide (Cytoxan) is the drug of choice to treat moderate to severe inflammation or rapidly progressive conjunctival scarring. Side effects include anemia, alopecia, hemorrhagic cystitis, bladder carcinoma, anovulation, azoospermia, and bone marrow suppression. A CBC and urine analysis should be performed prior to initiation and regularly after initiation.

Other immunomodulating agents that are increasingly being utilized are methotrexate and mycophenolate mofetil (MMF) (Cellcept, Roche Laboratories, Inc, Nutley, NJ). MMF exerts anti-inflammatory activity via MPA, the active metabolite. MPA inhibits inosine monophosphate dehydrogenase (IMPDH), preventing guanosine nucleotide synthesis and thereby blocking T and B lymphocyte proliferation.[19] This suppresses the cell mediated immune response and antibody formation. MPA also inhibits the recruitment of monocytes and lymphocytes to the site of inflammation. MMF is not nephrotoxic or fibrogenic and has a low systemic side effect profile. Therefore, it can potentially be used as a first line of treatment. Zierhut et al[20] recently reported an analysis of the effect of MMF in 10 eyes of 5 patients with biopsy-proven OCP. All patients in this series showed subjective improvement and regression of conjunctival changes after treatment with MMF.

DRY EYE TREATMENT

Treating dry eyes in OCP patients is exceedingly difficult. Not only do OCP patients suffer from an unstable tear film due to meibomian gland dysfunction as well as aqueous and mucin insufficiency, but trichiasis and distichiasis can lead to extreme foreign body sensation and discomfort. Alterations in the lid margin due to cicatrization and scarring can cause entropion and trichiasis. Distichiasis can also occur, leading to constant mechanical trauma to the cornea. These eyelid and eyelash abnormalities can cause severe foreign body sensation and discomfort. Chronic epilation of these misdirected lashes offers a short-term solution but does not solve the problem. In fact, epilation may make things worse because the new lash stump that grows is shorter and thicker, leading to further discomfort. Cryotherapy or electrolysis should be attempted when epilation is either impractical or no longer relieves the discomfort.

For treatment of dryness, the first line of therapy in these patients is the judicious use of artificial tears. These need to be preservative free since hourly use may be necessary and preservatives can cause further irritation. A thicker tear formulation should be considered because frequency of tear usage increases. Punctal occlusion or cautery should be performed when Schirmer's testing without anesthetic measures 2 mm or less.[4] Due to scarring and changes in lid architecture caused by OCP, some patients may auto-occlude their puncta. As these changes progress and lead to lagophthalmos, lubricating ointments should be added.

Meibomian gland dysfunction can be a significant problem, leading to tear film instability. This should be treated aggressively with lid hygiene, antibiotic ointment, and oral doxycycline, if necessary. Areas of keratinized conjunctiva may respond to topical tretinoin (Retin-A [OrthoMcNeil Pharmaceuticals, Inc, Los Angeles, Calif], similar to vitamin A) ointment with potential reversal of keratinization.[21] Side effects of topical tretinoin include erythema, burning of the lid margin, and conjunctival redness. These side effects decrease with time and a lower concentration of tretinoin.

The use of oral cholinergic agents such as pilocarpine (Salagen, MGI Pharma, Inc, Bloomington, Minn) and cevimeline (Evoxac) has been studied in patients with Sjögren's syndrome and xerostomia.[22] Both of these medications are muscarinic agonists that can increase secretion by exocrine glands and have shown promising results in Sjögren's patients.[22,23] Although not studied specifically in OCP, it may have similar results and increase lacrimal gland secretion. Other oral medications such as Mucomyst (N-acetyl-cysteine) (Bristol-Myers Squibb, Princeton, NJ), usually used as a mucolytic agent in chronic respiratory illness, have shown positive results in Sjögren's patients[24] and may be beneficial as well in treating OCP patients. Lastly, topical cyclosporine 0.05% (Restasis), an immunomodulator with anti-inflammatory effects, is currently used to treat inflammation associated with KCS. Restasis has been shown to decrease the inflammatory mediators and increase goblet cell density in patients with dry eyes.[25] Many patients using Restasis noted a significant improvement in tear production and a reduction in dry eye symptoms. In 1993, Neumann et al[26] found that treatment with 2% cyclosporine eye drops controlled inflammation and stopped cicatrization in 2 patients with lichen planes. It may be beneficial in patients with OCP as well.

The treatment of dry eyes in OCP patients can be very challenging. Although various treatment options are available, not all may be successful in an individual patient. Using a stepwise approach to treatment is advisable.

11

Tear Supplements—Artificial Tears

Guillermo L. Simón-Castellví, MD;
Sarabel Simón-Castellví, MD;
José María Simón-Castellví, MD;
Cristina Simón-Castellví, MD;
José María Simón-Tor, MD; and
Demetrio Pita-Salorio, MD

INTRODUCTION

True dry eye cannot be cured, but the eyes' sensitivity can be lessened and measures taken so the eyes remain healthy by means of the use of artificial tears or tear substitutes. Topical artificial tears, gels, and ointments replace missing tears but are no definite cure to the illness.[1] When treating ocular surface disease, it is essential to address all layers of the tear film and not forget the lipid layer because a compromised lipid layer results in up to a 4-fold increase in tear evaporation.

There is not any one drop that has been proven clearly superior to all others. Most artificial tears replace the volume of tears that are missing; however, no artificial tear has all the ingredients that natural tears have (water, salts, hydrocarbons, proteins, enzymes, and lipids). A number of artificial tears try to approximate the constituents of natural tears and some have more ingredients than others, but they do not reproduce the integrity of the 3-layered lipid, aqueous, and mucin structure vital to the effective functioning of the tear film. The question of which artificial tear preparations are preferable is only answered by the patient itself; there is not one artificial tear that works well for every person. Indeed, lubrication alone is insufficient to resolve the ocular surface disorder experienced by most dry eyes sufferers.

Tear substitutes also have thickening agents in them to make them last longer. In general, we now recommend people who are using eye drops more than 3 or 4 times a day to use drops that do not contain a preservative (preservative-free)[2] because preservatives can be irritating to the eye. The best solutions are those that stay on the eye as long as possible; they are generally viscid and contain mucomimetic ingredients.

RAPID GUIDE TO DRY EYE MANAGEMENT

Various modalities of treating dry eye are shown in Tables 11-1 and 11-2.

THE PRESERVATIVE DILEMMA

Traditionally, there have been 2 types of artificial tears: multidose bottles that contain a preservative (Table 11-3) and tears packaged in individual preservative-free droppers that must be discarded immediately after one use (single-dose units).

When considering a tear substitute, close attention must be paid to the composition of the formulation. Some artificial tears contain preservatives that are toxic, in various degrees, to corneal epithelial cells.

Preservatives are responsible—in the long term—for increased immune reaction[3] against artificial tear components, increased epithelial metaplasia and subepithelial fibrosis, and tear film physiology rupture. Preservatives act like soap, breaking tear film and thus increasing the degree of dry eye. Cytotoxicity has been widely described in vivo and vitro in animals in a great number of publications[3-5]: mucin cells are destroyed most by preservatives. Increased immune reaction against artificial tear components can be responsible for glaucoma surgery failure (bleb encapsulation, early closure of trabeculectomy). Recently, a relation between cystic macular edema after cataract surgery and preservatives of antiglaucoma eye drops (dipivefrin, latanoprost, timolol, etc) has been advocated, but not yet clearly proven.

Classic signs of preservative-induced toxic conjunctivitis include conjunctival hyperemia, hyperemic lid margins, follicular conjunctivitis (inferior conjunctiva), chemosis, absence of preauricular lymphadenopathy, and superficial punctate keratopathy (corneal and conjunctival scarring in intense prolonged cases).

Symptoms of preservative-induced toxic conjunctivitis include red eye, burning, itching, increased sensation of dryness, photophobia, watery lachrymation (with mucus), and foreign body sensation while vision is unaffected.

To effectively manage preservative-induced toxic conjunctivitis, stop the application of the offending drug, solution, make-up, etc, add artificial preservative-free tear substitutes 2 to 6 times daily (eg, balanced salt solution [BSS] [sterile], sodium chloride 0.64%, sodium acetate 0.39%, sodium citrate 0.17%, calcium chloride 0.048%, magnesium chloride 0.03%, potassium chloride 0.075%. Available from Alcon in 15-ml bottles). Artificial lubricant gels (eg, Viscotears liquid eye gel carbomer 980 0.2%, Novartis Ophthalmics, East Hanover, NJ) and ointments may be of great help, especially at night. In moderate to severe reactions, topical 1% fluorometholone (2 to 4 times daily), topical antihistamine (eg, levocabastine, every 8 to 12 hours), and vaso-constricting drops provide immediate relief. We have never seen rebounding of symptoms, local toxicity, or hypersensitivity. They are not recommended for prolonged use. Oral antihistamines may help in severe reactions.

Based on clinical evidence and our own experience, it is our strong belief that preservatives should be avoided whenever possible (*"primum non nocere"*).

Affordability may become an issue because preservative-free artificial tears are more expensive. A recent study suggests that storage of open preservative-free artificial tears for 12 hours in a plastic bag inside a refrigerator does not have a significant effect on the solution.[6] This is not valid for bicarbonate-containing solutions (eg, TheraTears, Advanced Vision Research, Woburn, Mass and BION Tears, Alcon Inc, Fort Worth, Tex).

Table 11-1
RAPID GUIDE TO DRY EYE MANAGEMENT

No contact lens patient should be without extra artificial tear lubrication.

Similarly, no glaucoma trabeculectomized patient should be out of preservative-free tear substitutes.[7]

First Step

- Mild cases: Supplemental lubrication (mild and moderate keratitis sicca). Artificial tears: preferably preservative-free artificial tears (drops 4 to 14 times a day, depending on the severity of the case), viscous artificial tear drops, or gels (may blur the vision). Increase frequency of artificial tear application.
- For more severe cases: Lubricating ointments (generally reserved to bedtime because vision blur lasts minutes or hours). Not to be used with contact lenses.
- In severe cases: Patch with lubricating ointment at night.

10% N-acetylcysteine (Mucomyst), a mucolytic, 3 to 4 times daily is used in case of abundant mucus (strands or filaments).

Artificial tear insert (Lacrisert, Merck & Co, Inc, Whitehouse Station, NJ) in the inferior cul-de-sac every morning can be used, in conjunction with artificial tears. Special goggles and moist chamber glasses are used to reduce evaporation and retain humidity around the globe. In case of suspected inflammation or in case of insatisfaction, try topical steroids (CsA is only used as a last resource).

Any associated abnormalities should be treated (eg, in blepharitis, suppress inflammation with topical steroids and local antibiotics, and/or systemic tetracyclines).

Intermediate Step

- Temporary punctal occlusion with collagen (dissolvable) or silicone (permanent) plugs in case of severe aqueous tear deficiency (to preserve endogenous water). Indicated if the patient is satisfied with a previous temporal occlusion results and in-office cauterization of inferior lachrymal puncti.
- In order to minimize exposure, consider external tarsorrhaphy (first try a temporary adhesive tape tarsorrhaphy) or botulinum toxin-induced ptosis.

Last Step

In addition to previously suggested topical treatment, extremely severe cases may need one of the following:

- Surgical treatment (only for very severe cases, with ulceration or corneal perforation).
- Cyanoacrylate tissue adhesive for closure of perforation or descemetocele.
- Corneal or corneoscleral patch or conjunctival flap for an impending or frank perforation (amniotic membrane, fascia lata).
- Lateral temporary tarsorrhaphy (eg, after facial nerve paralysis, trigeminal nerve lesions, or severe exophthalmos secondary to thyroid disease).
- Amniotic membrane graft: Amniotic membrane has a naturally thick basement membrane, which makes it ideal for graft tissue. It has proven useful in treatment of ocular surface disorders.
- Limbal stem cell transplantation: The limbus contains stem cells that are capable of regeneration of corneal and conjunctival tissue. The ocular surface can be restored by limbal stem cell transplantation, either autologous or—more commonly—from a close relative.

Table 11-2
DRY EYE TREATMENT ARMAMENTARIUM*

- Artificial tear solutions (preserved and preservative-free).
- Gels and ointments.
- Sold devices (Lacrisert).
- Punctual plugs (collagen or silicone).
- Anti-inflammatory therapy (cyclosporine 0.05%).
- P2Y2 receptor agonists (Diquafosol INS365, in development by Inspire Pharmaceuticals, Inc, Durham, NC).
- Oral therapy (oral pilocarpine).
- Contact lenses (Proclear lens, CooperVision, Fairport, NY).
- Surgery (salivary gland transplantation).[4]

*Includes different therapies listed. Nevertheless, the mainstay of dry eye treatment is the use of topical artificial tears, gels, and ointments to replace missing tears.

Table 11-3
COMMON PRESERVATIVES FOUND IN TOPICAL OPHTHALMIC DRUGS*

- Benzalkonium chloride (BAC).
- Benzethonium chloride.
- Cetylpyridinum chloride.
- Chlorobutanol.
- Ethylenediaminetetraacetic acid (EDTA).
- Mercurial preservatives (phenylmercuric nitrate, phenylmercuric acetate, thimerosal).
- Methyl/propylparaben.
- Phenylethyl alcohol
- Sodium benzoate
- Sodium propionate
- Sorbic acid

Less Toxic Newer Preservatives

- Purite (stabilized oxy-chloro complex) (Allergan Pharmaceuticals, Irvine, Calif).
- Sodium perborate (decomposes to water and oxygen upon contact with the tear fluid).

*Preservatives destroy or inhibit accidental proliferation of microorganisms. Each can produce epithelial toxicity with excessive or prolonged use. Products listed are used as preservatives, either in tear substitutes or topical ophthalmic drugs. Patients with dry eyes that need to administer any topical ocular medication more often than 3 to 4 times a day should only use preservative-free eye drops.

When in contact with air, bicarbonate converts to carbon dioxide, which can diffuse trough plastic unidose vials. Once open, vials of bicarbonate-containing solutions must be discarded immediately after use.

Most available artificial tears are single-use preservative-free, fit easily into pocket or purse, and can be used quickly and conveniently, any time and anywhere. To reduce costs, a new patented bottle for eye medications called ABAK has been designed in Europe by Thea España, Barcelona, Spain. Preservative is present inside the bottle but never reaches the eye at the instillation since the preservative is retained at instillation by a special filter located inside the bottle. Therefore, tear substitutes in the ABAK system can be considered preservative-free; however, once open, the bottle can be used for 8 weeks. The third generation of the ABAK system is much easy to use than previous generations. A similar dropper is ready for launch in the United States.

Third generation multidose artificial tears contain disappearing preservatives, such as sodium perborate, that decompose to water and oxygen upon contact with the tear fluid (eg, Vistil and Oxyal [Laboratories Llorens, Barcelona, Spain]).

PHARMACOLOGY BASICS

Artificial tears contain the following:
- Viscosity-increasing agents (Table 11-4).
- Electrolytes (Table 11-5).
- Balanced amount of salts to maintain ocular tonicity (eg, NaCl, KCl).
- Buffers to adjust the pH of the formulation (eg, boric acid). The ideal pH of a tear substitute is 7.3.
- Agents to prolong eye contact time (eg, povidone).
- Preservatives to maintain sterility or avoid contamination (the ideal tear substitute is preservative-free) (see Table 11-3).

Table 11-6 shows currently marketed tear substitutes. Table 11-7 shows currently marketed artificial lubricant ointment and gels.

SODIUM HYALURONATE

The least toxic products are preferred to keep the corneal epithelium in the best condition. A revolutionary advance in the dry eye treatment has been the introduction in Europe of a 0.18% sodium hyaluronate solution (Vismed, Lab Chemedica AG, Munich, Germany). Its patented preservative-free hypotonic formula contains sodium citrate and all the ions contained in the tear film. It has an analgesic, anti-inflammatory effect that is really appreciated by the patients. Most severe dry eye patients refer a high degree of satisfaction and comfort and feel very improved with the use of this viscoelastic sodium hyaluronate solution.

The ocular surface residence time of 0.2% hyaluronic acid is significantly longer than that of 0.3% hydroxymethylcellulose or 1.4% polyvinyl alcohol. Sodium hyaluronate is not available as tear substitute in the United States but has been used for years in Europe with great success in reducing patients complaints and bengal rose corneal straining. Sodium hyaluronate is also very effective in promoting corneal re-epithelialization and has become our preferred ocular lubricant after refractive surgery. It is gaining acceptance as the first choice in dry eye patient's therapy.

Table 11-4
MAJOR CONSTITUENTS OF ARTIFICIAL TEARS ARE VISCOSITY-INCREASING AGENTS*

- Carbopol gels.
- Carboxymethylcellulose sodium (CMC).
- Dextran 70.
- Gelatin.
- Glycerin.
- Hydroxyethylcellulose.
- Hydroxypropyl methylcellulose (HPMC).
- Methylcellulose.
- Polyethylene glycol PEG.
- Poloxamer 407.
- Polysorbate 80 (also a wetting agent).
- Propylene glycol.
- Polyvinyl alcohol (PVA).
- Polyvinylpyrrolidone (povidone).
- Sodium hyaluronate.

*These are most often hydrogels: polymers that are endowed with the properties of swelling in water and retaining the moisture. Some may not be available in the United States.

Table 11-5
PHYSIOLOGICAL EFFECTS OF MOST COMMONLY FOUND ELECTROLYTES*

Electrolyte	Physiological Effect
Electrolyte-containing solutions	Increase conjunctival goblet cell density Increase corneal glycogen contents Decrease elevated tear osmolarity
Potassium	Maintains corneal thickness
Bicarbonate	Promotes recovery of damaged corneal epithelium (barrier function and ultrastructure) Helps to maintain mucin layer of tear film (protective layer)

*Electrolyte-containing solutions have proven beneficial in treating ocular surface damage in dry eye syndrome.

Table 11-6
CURRENTLY MARKETED TEAR SUBSTITUTES†

Company	Product	Active Ingredients Viscosity Agents(*)	Preservatives	Sizes	Comments
Advanced Vision Research Woburn, Mass *www.theratears.com*	TheraTears preservative free lubricant eye drops	0.25% sodium carboxymethylcellulose	None	0.6 ml 32 single-use container pack	Hypotonic Studies suggest that TheraTears restore goblet cells after LASIK. Contains NaCl, KCl, sodium bicarbonate, calcium chloride, sodium phosphate, magnesium chloride, borate buffers, and purified water. Single-use containers must be discarded after each use.
				15 ml	
Accutome Malvern, Penn *www.accutome.com*	Accu-Tears PVA Accu-Tears HPMC	Polyvinyl alcohol 1.4% and hydroxypropyl methylcellulose—dextran		15 ml 15 ml	
Akorn, Inc Buffalo Grove, Ill *www.akorn.com*	AKWA TEARS	Polyvinyl alcohol 1.4%	Benzalkonium chloride 0.001%/EDTA	15 ml	Hypotonic. Contains NaCl and sodium phosphate.
	TEARS RENEWED	0.1% dextran-70	Benzalkonium chloride 0.001%/EDTA 0.05%	15 ml	Contains hydrochloric acid, KCl, NaCl, sodium bicarbonate, and sodium hydroxide.
		0.3% hydroxypropyl methylcellulose 2906			
Alcon Laboratories Fort Worth, Tex *www.alconlabs.com*	Adsorbotear	Povidone 1.67% and water-soluble polymers, hydroxyethylcellulose Dextran-70 0.1% and 2910 hydroxypropyl methylcellulose 0.3%	Thimerosal 0.004%/EDTA 0.1%		
	Bion Tears		None	28 single use containers (0.4 ml)	Contains carbon dioxide, hydrochloric acid, and sodium hydroxide. Bicarbonate and zinc may help mucous and surface cells. Single-use containers must be discarded after each use.

(continued)

Table 11-6
CURRENTLY MARKETED TEAR SUBSTITUTES[†] (CONTINUED)

Company	Product	Active Ingredients Viscosity Agents[(*)]	Preservatives	Sizes	Comments
	Isopto Plain—Isopto Tears	2910 hydroxypropyl methylcellulose 0.5%	0.01% benzalkonium chloride	15 and 30 ml	
	Tears Naturale	0.1% dextran-70	0.01% benzalkonium chloride/EDTA		Contains NaCl, sodium citrate, and sodium phosphate.
		0.3% hydroxypropyl methylcellulose	POLYQUAD (Polyquaternium-1 0.001%)		
	Tears Naturale II	0.3% hydroxypropyl methylcellulose 2910 and 0.1% dextran-70	None (preservative free)	15- and 30-ml bottle	Contains NaCl, sodium citrate, sodium hydroxide, KCL, and NaCl.
	Tears Naturale Free	0.1% dextran-70 and 3% hydroxypropyl methylcellulose 2910	POLYQUAD (Polyquaternium-1 0.001%)	36 reclosable vial pack	Contains sodium borate, KCL, and NaCl.
	Systane	0.4% polyethylene glycol 400 and 0.3% propylene glycol	0.01% benzalkonium chloride		Contains boric acid, KCL, and NaCl.
		Hydroxypropyl guar (gel-forming matrix)		15 ml	Contains NaCl, sodium citrate, and sodium phosphate.
	Ultra Tears	1% hydroxypropyl methylcellulose 2910			
Allergan Pharmaceuticals Irvine, Calif www.allergan.com	Celluvisc Lubricant Ophthalmic Solution	Carboxymethylcellulose 1%	None (preservative free)	0.04-ml single use cartons (30 or 50 units)	Contains calcium chloride, KCL, NaCl, and sodium lactate.
	Refresh Tears	0.5% carboxymethylcellulose	Purite	15 ml	Contains boric acid, calcium chloride, magnesium chloride, KCL, NaCl, and stabilized oxy-chloro complex.
	Lacril Lubricant	Hydroxypropyl methylcellulose 0.5%	Chlorobutanol 0.5%	15 ml	
	Liquifilm Forte	Polyvinyl alcohol 3%	Thimerosal 0.002%/EDTA	15 and 30 ml	Contains NaCl.

(continued)

Table 11-6

CURRENTLY MARKETED TEAR SUBSTITUTES[†] (CONTINUED)

Company	Product	Active ingredients Viscosity agents(*)	Preservatives	Sizes	Comments
	Liquifilm Tears	Polyvinyl alcohol 1.4%	Chlorobutanol 0.5%	15 and 30 ml	Contains NaCl.
	Refresh lubricant Ophthalmic Solution	Polyvinyl alcohol 1.4% and povidone 0.6%	None	0.3-ml single use cartons (30 or 50 units)	Contains NaCl.
	Refresh Plus ophthalmic solution	0.5% carboxymethylcellulose	None	0.3-ml single use cartons (30 or 50 units)	Contains calcium chloride, magnesium chloride, KCl, NaCl, and sodium lactate.
	Tears Plus Lubricant Ophthalmic Solution	1.4% polyvinyl alcohol and 0.6% povidone	0.5% chlorobutanol	15 and 30 ml	Contains NaCl.
	Cellufresh	0.5% carboxymethylcellulose	None	30-ml bottles	
	Refresh Liquigel	1% carboxymethylcellulose sodium	Purite	0.4-ml single-use containers (20 units)	
	Refresh Endura	Castor oil, 1% glycerin, 1% polysorbate 80, and carbomer 1342	None		
Bausch & Lomb Pharmaceuticals Rochester, NY *www.bausch.com*	Murocel	1% methylcellulose and 1% propylene glycol	0.028% methylparaben 0.01% propylparaben	15 ml	Contains NaCl, boric acid, and sodium borate.
	Dry Eye Therapy	0.3% glycerin	None	30 ml	Contains KCl, NaCl, sodium citrate, and sodium phosphate.
	Moisture Eyes	1% propylene glycol and 0.3% glycerin	0.01% benzalkonium chloride	15 and 30 ml	Contains KCl, NaCl, boric acid, sodium borate, and edetate disodium.
	Moisture Eyes PF	0.95% propylene glycol	None	In 0.6 ml (single-use 32s)	
	Moisture Eyes Liquid Gel	0.1% dextran-70 and 0.8% hydroxpropylmethylcellulose	None	15 and 30 ml 15 ml	Contains KCl, NaCl, boric acid, sodium borate, and EDTA.

(continued)

Table 11-6
CURRENTLY MARKETED TEAR SUBSTITUTES[†] (CONTINUED)

Company	Product	Active Ingredients Viscosity Agents(*)	Preservatives	Sizes	Comments
	OcuCoat	0.1% dextran-70 and 0.8% hydroxypropyl methylcellulose	0.01% benzalkonium chloride	0.5 ml (UD 28s)	Contains dextrose, KCl, NaCl, and sodium phosphate.
	OcuCoat PF	0.1% dextran-70 and 0.8% hydroxypropyl methylcellulose	None		Contains dextrose, KCl, NaCl, and sodium phosphate.
Bio-Logic Aqua Technologies Grants Pass, Ore www.naturestears.com	Nature's Tears Eye Mist	Tissue-culture grade pure sterile water	None	30-ml "spray" bottle	Not eye drops. It is a propellant-free atomizer to mist the face and the eyes.
Blairex Labs, Inc Columbus, Ind www.blairex.com	Just Tears	1.4% polyvinyl alcohol	Benzalkonium chloride/EDTA	15 ml	Contains KCl and NaCl.
Fougera Melville, NY www.fougera.com	Paralube Tears	1.4% polyvinyl alcohol, 1% polyethylene glycol 400, and dextrose	Benzalkonium chloride/EDTA	15 ml	
Novartis Ophthalmics Duluth, Ga www.novartisophthalmics.com	Aquasite Drops/Drops PF	Polyethylene glycol 400 0.2%, dextran-70 0.1%, and polycarbophil	EDTA. No other preservatives.	In 6-ml single-use 24s	
	Genteal Lubricating Eye Drops	Hydroxypropyl methylcellulose 0.3% and calcium chloride	Sodium perborate (GenAqua)	15- and 25-ml bottle	Contains boric acid, NaCl, magnesium chloride, KCl, and zinc sulfate.
	Genteal Mild	Hydroxypropyl methylcellulose 0.2%	Sodium perborate (GenAqua)	15- and 25-ml bottle	Contains boric acid, NaCl, KCl, phosphoric acid, and calcium chloride dithdrate.
	Genteal PF Lubricating Eye Drops	Hydroxpropylmethylcellulose 3.3%	Preservative free	Single use vials 36s	Hypotonic.
	Hypotears Lubricating Eye Drops	Polyvinyl alcohol 1%, 1% polyethylene glycol 400, and dextrose	Benzalkonium chloride/EDTA	15- and 30-ml bottle	

(continued)

Table 11-6
CURRENTLY MARKETED TEAR SUBSTITUTES[†] (CONTINUED)

Company	Product	Active Ingredients Viscosity Agents[*]	Preservatives	Sizes	Comments
CYNACON/OCuSOFT Richmond, Tex www.ocusoft.com	Hypotears PF Eye Drops		Preservative free	0.5-ml single-use vials (30 units)	
	Tears Again Eye Drops	Polyvinyl alcohol 1.4%	0.01% benzalkonium chloride	15 ml	Contains sodium phosphate, edetate disodium, sodium phosphate, NaCl, and phosphoric acid.
	Tears Again Gel Drops	0.7% carboxymethylcellulose and carbopol 940	Dissipate preservative (stabilized peroxicomplex)	15 ml	Contains boric acid, phosphoric acid, sodium chloride, and potassium chloride.
	Tears Again MC	0.3% hydroxypropyl methylcellulose	None	15 ml	Contains boric acid, phosphoric acid, sodium chloride, and potassium chloride.
Ocumed Roseland, NJ	Ocutears PF Ocu-Tears	Polyvinyl alcohol Polyvinyl alcohol	None Unknown		
MIZA Pharmaceuticals USA, Inc (formerly Optoptics) Fairton, NJ	Nu-Tears	1.4% polyvinyl alcohol	Benzalkonium chloride/EDTA	15 ml	Contains NaCl and KCl.
	Nu-Tears II	1% polyvinyl alcohol, 1% polyethylene glycol 400, and dextrose	Benzalkonium chloride/EDTA		
Pfizer, Inc New York, NY www.pfizer.com	Visine Tears	Glycerin 0.2%, hydroxypropyl methylcellulose 0.2%, and 1% polyethylene glycol 400	Benzalkonium chloride (0.01%) and boric acid	15 and 30 ml	Within viscosity range of natural tears (contains ingredients found in natural tears: ascorbic acid, disodium phosphate, glycine, magnesium chloride, potassium chloride, sodium chloride, sodium citrate, sodium lactate, sodium phosphate, and purified water).
	Visine Tears Preservative Free	0.2% glycerin, 0.2% hydroxypropyl methylcellulose, and 1% polyethylene glycol 400	Preservative free	Free single use vials	

(continued)

Table 11-6

CURRENTLY MARKETED TEAR SUBSTITUTES[+] (CONTINUED)

Company	Product	Active Ingredients Viscosity Agents[*]	Preservatives	Sizes	Comments
Pharmafair—Bausch and Lomb Pharmaceuticals Tampa, FL *www.bausch.com*	Lubrifair Solution Tearfair Solution	Dextran-70, hydroxypropyl methyl-cellulose, and polyvinyl alcohol	None None		
Ross Laboratories Columbus, Ohio *www.ross.com*	Murine Tears	0.5% polyvinyl alcohol and 0.6% povidone	Benzalkonium chloride/EDTA	15 and 30 ml	Contains dextrose, KCl, NaCl, sodium bicarbonate, sodium citrate, and sodium phosphate.
	Clear Eyes	Hydroxypropyl methylcellulose and glycerin	Ascorbic acid/EDTA		
Rohto Orchard Park, NY *www.rohtoeyedrops.com*	Rohto Zi	1.8% povidone, poloxamer 407, and polysorbate 80	Benzalkonium chloride	12 ml	Contains 0.1% alcohol, boric acid, NaCl, KCl, and sodium borate.
S.S.S. Company Atlanta, Ga *www.sspharmaceuticals.com*	20/20 Tears	1.4% polyvinyl alcohol	Benzalkonium chloride/EDTA	15 ml	Contains KCl and NaCl. Thimerosal free.

(continued)

Table 11-6
CURRENTLY MARKETED TEAR SUBSTITUTES† (CONTINUED)

Company	Product	Active Ingredients Viscosity Agents(*)	Preservatives	Sizes	Comments
VISION Pharmaceuticals Mitchell, SD *www.visionpharm.com*	Viva-Drops	Polysorbate 80	EDTA	10 and 15 ml	Contains citric acid, mannitol, NaCl, pyruvate, retinyl palmitate, and sodium citrate.
IVAX Pharmaceuticals Miami, Fla *www.ivaxpharmaceuticals. com*	Teargen	1.4% polyvinyl alcohol	0.01% benzalkonium chloride/EDTA	15 ml	Contains NaCl and sodium phosphate.
	Teargen II	0.4% hydroxypropyl methylcellulose 2910 chloride/EDTA	0.01% benzalkonium	15 ml	Contains KCl, NaCl, and sodium phosphate.

†Listed in alphabetical order; not all inclusive.

(*) Concentrations of the listed components are identified when possible.
Ethylenediaminetetraacetic acid (EDTA) is listed as a preservative in some product descriptions and as an inactive ingredient in others.
Most of the products listed are protected by letters of patent, and their names are trademarked and registered by the firm whose name appears as *"Company."*
Distribution status of the products is OTC (over-the-counter).

NOTICE: Authors have made every effort to ensure that the products recommended herein, including brand names, composition, and presentation, are in accord with what can be found over the counters at the time of publication. The reader is invited to check the product information sheet included with any artificial tear, since changes in the formulations and clinical standards are constant. Despite this effort, some products may no longer be available at the moment you read this table or may be available under different brand names in different countries.

Table 11-7

CURRENTLY MARKETED ARTIFICIAL LUBRICANT OINTMENTS AND GELS[†]

Company	Product	Active Ingredients Viscosity Agents(*)	Preservatives	Sizes	Comments
Allergan Pharmaceuticals Irvine, Calif www.allergan.com	Lacri-Lube NP	57.3% white petrolatum, 42.5% mineral oil, and lanolin	None	0.7-g to 3.5-g tube	Ointment.
	Lacri-Lube S.O.P.	56.8% white petrolatum, 42.5% mineral oil, and lanolin alcohols,	Chlorobutanol 0.5%	0.7- to 3.5- and 7-g tubes	Ointment.
	Refresh PM	56.8% white petrolatum 41.5% mineral oil, and lanolin alcohols	None	3.5-g tube	Ointment. Contains NaCl.
	Refresh Liquigel	1% carboxymethylcellulose		15 and 30 ml	Gel. Contains KCl, NaCl, and boric acid.
Altaire Pharmaceuticals, Inc Aquebogue, NJ	Tears Again Night & Day 0.1% povidone	1.5% carboxymethylcellulose sodium	Unknown	3.5 g	Gel.
	Tears Again Preservative Free	1.5% carboxymethylcellulose sodium	None	3.5 g	Gel.
	Tears Again Ointment	White petrolatum and mineral oil		3.5 g	Ointment.
AKORN Pharmaceuticals Buffalo Grove, Ill www.akorn.com	AKWA Tears Ointment	White petrolatum, mineral oil, and lanolin	None	3.5-g tube	Ointment.
	Tears Renewed Ointment	White petrolatum, light mineral oil, and lanolin oil	None	3.5-g tube	Ointment.
Alcon Laboratories Fort Worth, Tex www.alconlabs.com	Duratears Naturale Lubricant Eye Ointment	56.8% white petrolatum, 42.5% mineral oil, and anhydrous liquid lanolin	None	3.5-g tube	Ointment.
	Tears Naturale PM Ointment	White petrolatum, mineral oil, and anhydrous liquid lanolin	None	3.5-g tube	Ointment.
Bausch and Lomb Pharmaceuticals Rochester, NY www.bausch.com	Dry Eyes	White petrolatum, mineral oil, and lanolin	None	3.5-g tube	Ointment.
	Moisture Eyes	80% white petrolatum and 20% mineral oil	None	3.5-g tube	Ointment

(continued)

Table 11-7

CURRENTLY MARKETED ARTIFICIAL LUBRICANT OINTMENTS AND GELS[†] (CONTINUED)

Company	Product	Active Ingredients Viscosity Agents(*)	Preservatives	Sizes	Comments
Chauvin Bausch & Lomb Montpellier, France	Lacrinorm 0.2%	Carbomer 980 NF		10 g	Gel.
Fougera Melville, NY *www.fougera.com*	Paralube Ointment	White petrolatum and light mineral oil	Unknown	3.5-g tube	Ointment.
Del Laboratories Uniondale, NY *www.dellabs.com*	Stye	57.7% white petrolatum, 31.9% mineral oil, and wheat germen oil	Unknown	3.5-g tube	Ointment. Contains stearic acid and microcrystalline wax.
Novartis Ophthalmics Duluth, Ga *www.novartisophthalmics.com*	Hypotears Ointment	85% white petrolatum and 15% light mineral oil	None	3.5-g tube	Preservative and lanolin free.
	Genteal Gel	0.3% hydroxypropyl methylcellulose carbopol 980	0.028% sodium perborate (GenAqua)	10-ml bottle	Gel. Contains phosphoric acid and sorbitol.
Ocumed Roseland, NJ	Ocutube	White petrolatum	Unknown		
CYNACON/OCuSOFT Richmond, Tex *www.ocusoft.com*	Tears Again Liposome Spray	Purified water and lecithin		10 ml	Spray. Contains ethanol 1%, vitamin A, vitamin E, NaCl, and 0.5% phenoxyethanol.
Pharmafair- Bausch and Lomb Pharmaceuticals Tampa, Fla *www.bausch.com*	Lubrifair Ointment	White petrolatum, mineral oil, and lanolin liquid	None		
	Petrolatum Ointment-Sterile	White petrolatum	None		
	TearFair Ointment	White petrolatum, mineral oil, and lanolin derivatives	None		

(continued)

Table 11-7

CURRENTLY MARKETED ARTIFICIAL LUBRICANT OINTMENTS AND GELS[†] (CONTINUED)

Company	Product	Active Ingredients Viscosity Agents(*)	Preservatives	Sizes	Comments
Watson Pharmaceuticals Corona, Calif www.watsonpharm.com	Artificial tears	83% white petrolatum, 1% mineral oil, and lanolin oil	Unknown	3.5 g	Ointment.

[†]Listed in alphabetical order by manufacturer; not all inclusive.

(*) Concentrations of the listed components are identified when possible.

Ethylenediaminetetraacetic acid (EDTA) is listed as a preservative in some product descriptions and as an inactive ingredient in others.

If it is not specified that an ointment contains a preservative, it is listed as "unknown."

Most of the products listed are protected by letters of patent, and their names are trade marked and registered by the firm whose name appears as "Company."

Distribution status of the products is OTC (over-the-counter).

NOTICE: Authors have made every effort to ensure that the products recommended herein, including brand names, composition, and presentation, are in accord with what can be found over the counters at the time of publication. The reader is invited to check the product information sheet included with any artificial tear, since changes in the formulations and clinical standards are constant. Despite this effort, some products may no longer be available at the moment you read this table or may be available under different brand names in different countries.

Table 11-8
STORAGE OF TEAR SUBSTITUTES

- Keep out of the reach of children.
- Store away from heat and direct light.
- Keep them from freezing.
- Do not keep outdated drops that are no longer needed.
- Remember that single-dose drops have to be discarded after use.

es alone have no place in the treatment of dry eyes. Concomitant use of artificial teardrops (and periodic check-up) is essential. Storage of tear substitutes is important and shown in Table 11-8.

Salivary gland transplantation into the inferior tarsal conjunctiva has been reported to be useful in dry eye conditions with severe permanent lacrimal gland dysfunction (not useful in Sjögren's syndrome). It is a technically complex procedure.

A new product is on the way for dry eye: diquafosol tetrasodium ophthalmic solution (INS365). It is an ophthalmic preparation under development by Inspire Pharmaceuticals, Inc, Durham, NC, aiming to stimulate the P2Y2 receptors present in the eyes and obtain a better mucosal hydration. It should increase secretion of mucin, lipids, water, and salts. At the time of this writing, it has not been proven effective enough in clinical trials.

Key Points

1. The use of topical artificial tears, gels, and ointments replaces missing tears, but is not a definite cure to the illness. When treating ocular surface disease, it is essential to address all layers of the tear film and not forget the lipid layer because a compromised lipid layer results in up to a 4-fold increase in tear evaporation.
2. Classic signs of preservative-induced toxic conjunctivitis include conjunctival hyperemia, hyperemic lid margins, follicular conjunctivitis (inferior conjunctiva), chemosis, absence of preauricular lymphadenopathy, and superficial punctate keratopathy (corneal and conjunctival scarring in intense prolonged cases).
3. A revolutionary advance in the dry eye treatment has been the introduction in Europe of a 0.18% sodium hyaluronate solution (Vismed). Also available in 0.15% concentration (Hyabak) and 0.1% concentration (Hyluprotect).
4. In addition to gel polymers, lipids and vitamins have been recently incorporated to ocular lubricants.
5. A new product is on the way for dry eye: diquafosol tetrasodium ophthalmic solution (INS365).

REFERENCES

1. Simón-Castellví JM. *Los Ojos Del Ciudadano.* Barcelona, Spain: Club de Autores Ediciones; 2000.

2. Simón-Castellví GL, Simón-Castellví S, Simón-Castellví JM, Simón-Tor JM. Tips and tricks for successful refractive surgery. In: Agarwal S, ed. *Refractive Surgery.* New Delhi, India: Jaypee Brothers Medical Publishers; 1998.

3. Badouin C, Garcher C, Haouat N, Bron A, Gastaud P. Expression of inflammatory membrane makers by conjunctival cells in chronically treated patients with glaucoma. *Ophthalmology.* 1994;101(3):454–460.

4. Friedlander M. Contact allergy and toxicity in the eye. *Int Ophthalmol Clin.* 1988;29:317–332.

5. Wilson FM II. Adverse external ocular effects of topical ophthalmic medications. *Surv Ophthalmol.* 1979;24:57.

6. Karkkainen TR. The effect of refrigeration on the osmolality and pH of nonpreserved artificial tears containing carboxymethylcellulose. *Optom Vis Sci.* 2001;78:37–39.

7. Simón-Castellví GL, Simón-Castellví S, Simón-Castellví JM, Simón-Tor JM. Assessment and management of filtering blebs. In: Agarwal S, ed. *Textbook of Ophthalmology.* Vol 3. New Delhi, India: Jaypee Brothers Medical Publishers; 2000.

8. Bury T, Bourcier T, Debbasch C, Laroche L. L'association des substitutes lacrymaux est-elle toujours synergique? *J Fr Ophtalmol.* 2003;26(4):396–399.

9. Johnson JT, Ferretti GA, Nethery WJ, et al. Oral pilocarpine for post-radiation xerostomia in patients with head and neck cancer. *N Engl J Med.* 1993;329(6):390–395.

12

Autologous Serum Drops

Kazuo Tsubota, MD and Murat Dogru, MD

INTRODUCTION

Dry eye is a chronic and unremitting disorder associated with ocular surface desiccation leading to squamous metaplasia, a pathologic transition of a nonkeratinized squamous epithelium to keratinized squamous epithelium.[1,2] Squamous metaplasia accounts for most of the ocular symptomatology in dry eye patients such as irritation, grittiness, and photophobia and is often the basis of clinical morbidity of corneal complications such as neovascularization, recurrent erosion, ulceration, scarring, and perforation.[2] Conventional therapies, including frequent application of tears, lubricants, therapeutic soft contact lenses, as well as surgical procedures such as punctal occlusion and tarsorrhaphy are not directed toward reversing the process of squamous metaplasia but rather toward alleviating the symptoms and decreasing ocular surface dye staining.[3] Traditional therapies for dry eye are palliative and their purpose is to replace or conserve the patient's tears without correcting the underlying disease process. The use of topical artificial tears and lubricants is currently the most widely preferred therapy for dry eye syndromes, and a variety of components are used to formulate a considerable number of commercially available preparations.[4–9] The goal of using tear substitutes is to increase humidity at the ocular surface and to improve lubrication while decreasing evaporation. One of the most important disadvantages of many of the commercially available artificial tear substitutes and lubricants is that they contain preservatives, stabilizers, and other additives that have been reported to be associated with ocular surface epithelial toxicity. The risk may be increased in patients with therapeutically blocked tear ducts, since the agent persists longer in the tear sac, relatively undiluted by lacrimal fluid.[10,11] Patients who require the application of tear substitutes more than 4 times daily on a long-term basis to maintain comfort may be at more risk of such toxicity and may be better off with unpreserved (usually unit-dose) formulations.[11]

Indeed, the introduction of preservative-free solutions can be considered the single most important contribution in the formulation of tear substitutes in recent years. Two drawbacks of such formulations are that they are more expensive than preserved preparations and they can induce lack of compliance because patients must carry numerous vials to maintain adequate dosage over 24 hours or more.[11] Artificial tear preparations have been reported to improve symptoms of irritation and to decrease the ocular surface vital dye staining in patients with KCS, but their use may not improve ocular surface keratinization because they lack most of the essential tear components, which led to the quest for the discovery of treatment modalities including autologous serum eye drops providing these components.[11]

Autologous Serum Eye Drops in the Treatment of Dry Eyes: The Concept

Ocular surface changes associated with Sjögren's syndrome are often more severe than non-Sjögren's dry eye, owing to a lack of both basic and reflex tearing due to lacrimal gland destruction by infiltrating lymphocytes.[12–14] Particular substances that may be lacking in dry eye patients play an important role in the regulation and maturation of the ocular surface epithelium. Accumulated knowledge in the past decade showed that the composition of tears resembled that of serum (Table 12-1) and that tear components such as EGF and vitamin A were important for the health of the ocular surface epithelium.[15–18] In addition, TGF-β concentration in human serum, which is 5 times higher than in tears, is believed to control epithelial proliferation and to maintain cells in an undifferentiated state such as the induction of basic keratins in epidermal cells.[19] Serum also contains fibronectin, substance P, and insulin-like growth factors, which are reported to be essential for wound healing in patients with dry eye-associated epithelial problems.[20–22] To date, no ideal artificial tear containing all aforementioned tear components has been developed. The concept of using autologous serum seems desirable because many essential components of tears are abundant in serum. In 1984, Fox et al reported the beneficial effects of autologous serum application to dry eye patients with Sjögren's syndrome for the first time.[23] The rationale for his observations was based upon the fact that vitamins or growth factors present in tears are also present in serum. The application of autologous serum offered an advantage over the simple use of artificial tears, which lacks such essential components.[24] The Fox report was followed by numerous studies reporting the efficacy of autologous serum eye drops in a variety of dry eye and ocular surface disorders (Table 12-2).

Our Initial Experience and Research with Autologous Serum Eye Drops

We also demonstrated a clear benefit of using autologous serum for the treatment of dry eye associated with Sjögren's syndrome. We measured EGF, vitamin A, and TGF-β concentrations in serum and tears and found that these components can be supplied to the ocular surface by this method.[25] Furthermore, we confirmed that the autologous serum samples can be preserved for more than 1 month in the refrigerator and more than 3 months in the freezer without significant changes of the concentration of the

Table 12-1
COMPOSITIONAL COMPARISON OF
TEAR FLUID AND AUTOLOGOUS SERUM

Content	Tears	Serum
Electrolytes		
Na^+	145 mEq/L	135 to 146 mEq/L
K^+	24 mEq/L	3.5 to 5 mEq/L
Cl^-	128 mEq/L	96 to 108 mEq/L
HCO_3^-	26 mEq/L	21 to 29 mEq/L
Ca_2^+	1.5 mEq/L	5 mEq/L
Proteins		
Total protein	0.74 g/dL	6.8 to 8.2 g/dL
Lysosome	0.24 g/dL	0.4 to 1.5 mg/dL
Lactoferrin	0.15 g/dL	—
Albumin	5.4 mg/dL	3.5 to 5.5 g/dL
IgA	41.1 mg/dL	90 to 450 mg/dL
Vitamins		
Vitamin A	16 ng/mL	883 ng/mL
Vitamin C	117 μg/mL	7 to 20 μg/mL
Growth Factors		
EGF	1.66 ng/mL	0.72 ng/mL
TGF-α	180 to 247 pg/mL	147 pg/mL
TGF-β	2.32 ng/mL	140.3 ng/mL

Table 12-2
THE APPLICATIONS AND INDICATIONS
OF AUTOLOGOUS SERUM EYE DROPS

- Dry eye syndromes:
  * Sjögren's and non-Sjögren's dry eyes.
  * Severe dry eyes associated with Stevens-Johnson syndrome, OCP.
  * Ocular surface keratinization with extensive meibomian gland loss associated with lid tattooing.
  * GVHD.
- Superior limbic keratoconjunctivitis.
- Persistent epithelial defects, recurrent corneal erosions.
- Neurotrophic corneal ulcers.
- Epithelial maintenance and as an adjunct in dry eyes after refractive surgery or ocular surface reconstruction procedures.

essential serum components. It was interesting to note that the components in serum were stable in the refrigerator for 1 month and in the freezer for 3 months. In serum, there are many proteins, such as albumin or globulin, that can protect the degradation of important cytokines. Although the mechanism is unknown, the prolonged preservation of these components in serum makes autologous application clinically possible. We also noted that the concentration of EGF was 0.7~8.1 ng/mL in reflex tears and 1.9~9.7 ng/mL in nonreflex tears, which is higher than EGF in serum that ranges around 0.5 ng/mL.[25] In contrast, the amounts of retinol in human tears has been reported by Speek et al to be 0.4~10.6 ng/mL.[26] Since the concentration of retinol in serum is around 55 mg/mL, serum contains more than 1000 times the amount available in tears. When vitamin A is lacking, the epithelium tends to undergo squamous metaplasia.[25,27] Application of serum may provide higher levels of retinol necessary in pathological conditions.

The TGF-β concentration in human serum is 5 times higher than in tears. TGF-β is believed to control epithelial proliferation and to maintain cells in an undifferentiated state such as the induction of the basic keratins in epidermal cells. TGF-β, for example, is known to have antiproliferative effects, and high concentrations of TGF-β may suppress wound healing of the ocular surface epithelium.[25] This was one of the reasons for using a diluted solution of serum in order to maintain TGF-β levels comparable with tears. Dilution also has the benefit of obtaining larger amounts of serum eyedrops from one sample.

PREPARATION OF AUTOLOGOUS SERUM EYE DROPS

A comprehensive explanation of the effects and drawbacks of the treatment should be provided to the patient and an informed consent should be obtained. Confirmation of the absence of HIV and hepatitis B and C infections in the subject must also be carried out.

In our experience, a 40-mL sample of venous blood from the patient is enough to last for at least 3 months. Twenty mL of serum can be obtained from 40 mL of whole blood, while diluting 1:5 with saline provides 100-mL serum solution. If each eye drop is 50 mL, 2000 drops can be obtained from 100 mL. Sjögren's syndrome dry eye patients use a maximum of 20 drops a day (10 times for each eye), thus 2000 drops are enough for more than 100 days. Patients are supplied with 20 5-mL bottles of 20% autologous serum and are advised to store bottles in the freezer until use.[25] The patients are advised to keep bottles in current use in the refrigerator. The preparation of autologous serum eye drops is summarized in Figure 12-1.

DRY EYE SYNDROMES

Our initial observations with autologous serum drops showed dramatic improvement of rose bengal and fluorescein scores in our Sjögren's syndrome and non-Sjögren's syndrome dry eye patients. The beneficial effect of autologous serum may be multifactorial. Our concomitant observations of the increased MUC-1 expression of cultured conjunctival epithelium suggested a direct effect of the serum on the ocular surface epithelium.[25]

A recent study sought to evaluate the efficacy of autologous serum for the treatment of severe ocular surface disorders using a prospective randomized controlled crossover

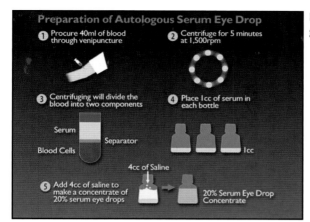

Figure 12-1. Preparation of autologous serum eye drops.

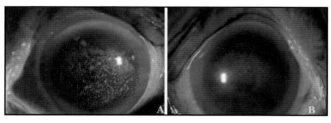

Figure 12-2. Anterior segment photographs of a representative case with severe Sjögren's syndrome treated with topical autologous serum eye drops 5 times a day for 2 weeks. Note complete resolution of corneal fluorescein staining.

study comparing 50% autologous serum eye drops with conventional therapy utilizing artificial tear solutions. The crossover design of that study confirmed that ocular surface vital staining score and cytological improvements were due to serum drops because the effects were reversed when treatment reverted to conventional therapy. This indirectly indicates that active components present in serum are required for the maintenance of a healthy ocular surface.[28]

Tananuvat et al reported that there was a nonstatistically significant trend toward improvement of vital staining scores and tear stability in both eyes in a controlled trial comparing autologous serum eye drops in one eye with the use of artificial tears in the fellow eye as a control. However, most eyes in that study had received punctal occlusion, which might have interfered with the evaluation of the solitary effects of autologous serum eye drops and artificial tear eye drops and might have caused a bias toward overevaluation of the effects of solitary artificial tears.[29]

We recently performed a randomized prospective controlled clinical trial by carrying out a wash-out for 2 weeks and assigned patients into 2 groups using only autologous serum or artificial tears, which we think allowed us to evaluate the solitary effects of these eye drops. We found significant improvements in tear stability, ocular surface vital staining scores, and pain symptom scores in patients treated with autologous serum eye drops compared to those assigned to nonpreserved artificial tears.[30] Anterior segment photographs of a representative case with severe Sjögren's syndrome treated with topical autologous serum eye drops are shown in Figure 12-2.

Another promising evidence on the efficacy and safety of autologous serum eye drops was our investigation and observations on the treatment of severe dry eyes occurring after allogeneic hematopoietic stem cell transplantation (SCT) (ie, GVHD). A total of 14 patients (4 males and 10 females; median age 31.0 years) with severe dry eye associated with chronic graft-versus-host disease (cGVHD) were enrolled in that study. All patients were refractory to treatment with conventional artificial tears. Autologous serum eye drops, a solution made of 20% autologous serum in sterile saline, were applied 10 times per eye per day. The patients were evaluated every 4 weeks according to visual acuity, corneal sensitivity, vital staining of the ocular surface, tear dynamics, and subjective assessments of symptoms. The median follow-up period was 19.4 months (range: 4 to 41 months). After 4 weeks of treatment, significant improvement was observed in both symptom scores and fluorescein staining scores (from 5.8 ± 2.0 to 2.4 ± 0.9 points). Significant improvements were observed also in rose bengal staining and tear BUT. In 7 of the 14 patients, the responses were maintained for 6 to 41 months (median: 19.4 ± 8.3 months), while 6 of the other 7 patients required treatment with punctal plugs in addition to autologous serum eye drops. One of these other 7 patients developed eczema around the eyelids, after which the treatment was discontinued. No serious adverse events were observed. We concluded that autologous serum eye drops were safe and effective for treating severe dry eye associated with cGVHD and that more efficient control of dry eye may be achieved by the combined use of autologous serum eye drops with punctal plugs.[31]

Another recent humble observation on the efficacy of autologous serum drops made by us was in a 45-year-old woman who underwent eyelid tattooing 20 years earlier that resulted in tear instability with increased ocular surface staining scores and advanced tear film lipid layer abnormality due to tattoo-related bilateral total meibomian gland dropout. Treatment with autologous serum eye drops resulted in full epithelialization in the patient in which meibomian gland disease-specific therapy did not result in any change in BUT, vital staining scores, tear film lipid layer interferometry grades, or glandular dropout state.[32]

Superior Limbic Keratoconjunctivitis

We determined the efficacy of autologous serum drops in the treatment of superior limbic keratoconjunctivitis (SLK) in 22 eyes of 11 patients who were treated with 20% diluted autologous serum eye drops 10 times a day in addition to ongoing treatment of the SLK with artificial tear drops. Fluorescein and rose bengal staining scores, as well as subjective symptom gradings, were performed before and after 4 weeks of therapy. Nine of the 11 patients (82%) responded well to treatment with complete resolution of the process. The average rose bengal and fluorescein scores improved, and there was also subjective improvement in patient symptoms. The study concluded that autologous serum application can be used as an alternative mode of therapy in SLK.[33] Anterior segment photographs of a representative case with severe SLK treated with topical autologous serum eye drops 10 times a day for 4 weeks are shown in Figure 12-3.

Recurrent Corneal Erosions and Persistent Epithelial Defects

A recent study on 11 eyes of 11 consecutive patients with acute macroform corneal erosions who had suffered several relapses despite receiving different types of treatment analyzed the outcome of treatment with autologous serum drops for 3 months.

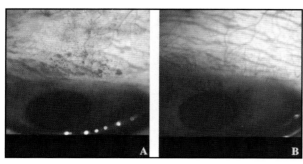

Figure 12-3. Anterior segment photographs of a representative case with severe SLK treated with topical autologous serum eye drops 10 times a day for 4 weeks. Note the resolution of rose bengal staining with treatment. (Reprinted with permission from Goto E, Shimmura S, Shimazaki J, Tsubota K. Treatment of superior limbic keratoconjunctivitis by application of autologous serum. *Cornea.* 2001;20:807–810.)

The mean follow-up time was 9.4 ± 3.7 months (range: 4 to 16). No side effects were noted in any of the treated patients. In that study, treatments prior to the use of autologous serum had failed to avoid recurrences in all patients, with the mean recurrence rate being 2.2 recurrences per month of follow-up. After the onset of serum treatment, only a single recurrence was recorded in 3 of the patients (0.028 recurrences per month of follow-up). The study concluded that the use of autologous serum for the treatment of patients with recurrent corneal erosion is effective and safe in reducing the number of recurrences experienced by patients.[34]

We also evaluated the efficacy of autologous serum application 6 to 10 times a day for the treatment of persistent epithelial defects in a prospective, clinical, noncomparative case series study that comprised 16 eyes. Among 16 persistent epithelial defects, 7 (43.8%) healed within 2 weeks, 3 (18.8%) healed within 1 month, and the remaining 6 (37.5%) did not respond within 1 month. No apparent side effect of autologous serum application was observed in our study, which confirmed the efficacy and safety of autologous serum eye drops in the treatment of persistent corneal epithelial defects.[35]

NEUROTROPHIC CORNEAL ULCERS

We evaluated the effect of autologous serum application for epithelial disorders in neurotrophic keratopathy in a recent noncomparative interventional case series that consisted of 12 eyes of 10 patients with neurotrophic keratopathy. Twenty percent topical autologous serum eye drops were applied 5 to 10 times daily until the neurotrophic ulcers healed. Patients underwent routine ophthalmic examinations, including slit lamp examination, corneal fluorescein dye testing, Cochet-Bonnet corneal sensitivity, and best-corrected visual acuity (BCVA) measurements before and at the end of the treatment. Moreover, serum samples from 10 healthy volunteers were studied for the levels of substance P (SP), insulin-like growth factor (IGF-1, and nerve growth factor (NGF) by using radioimmunoassay (RIA) and enzyme-linked immunosorbent assay (ELISA) techniques. Tear samples from 3 healthy subjects were also analyzed for NGF and IGF-1 levels by the same techniques. The changes in corneal disease state, corneal sensitivity, and BCVA with treatment were also evaluated in that study. The levels of neural healing factors like SP, IGF-1, and NGF in serum as well as NGF and IGF-1 in tears of healthy subjects were investigated in addition. We found that the epithelial disorders healed completely in all eyes within 6 to 32 days (mean: 17.1 ± 8.6 days) with a decrease in corneal

Figures 12-4. Anterior segment photographs of a representative case with severe neurotrophic ulcer treated with topical autologous serum eye drops. Note the complete epithelialization and decrease in corneal haze intensity and area with treatment. (Reprinted with permission from Matsumoto Y, Dogru M, Goto E, et al. Autologous serum application in the treatment of neurotrophic keratopathy. *Ophthalmology.* 2004;111:1115–1120.)

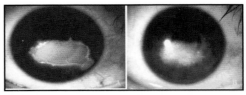

scarring and no corneal neovascularization. The mean pretreatment corneal sensitivity was 15.0±14.2 mm, which increased to 30.8±25.3 mm after treatment at the last follow-up. Five eyes attained normal corneal sensitivity with treatment. The BCVA improved by more than 2 Landolt lines in 66.7% of the eyes. The mean concentrations of SP in diluted and undiluted serum were 31.4±8.4 pg/mL and 157.0±42.1 pg/mL, respectively. The mean respective concentrations of IGF-1 in diluted and undiluted serum were 31.4±14.8 ng/mL and 157.0±73.9 ng/mL. The mean concentrations for NGF were 93.6±63.5 pg/mL and 468.3±317.4 pg/mL in serum samples with and without dilution. The mean concentration of NGF in tears was found to be 54 pg/mL. We concluded that autologous serum harbored "neurotrophic factors" and autologous serum treatment might provide "neural healers" to a compromised ocular surface and seemed promising for the restoration of the ocular surface epithelial integrity in patients with neurotrophic keratopathy.[36] Anterior segment photographs of a representative case with severe neurotrophic ulcer treated with topical autologous serum eye drops are shown in Figure 12-4.

Autologous Serum Eye Drops in Sjögren's Syndrome Patients Undergoing Refractive Surgery

We recently evaluated the efficacy and safety of LASIK in 6 eyes of 3 patients with severe dry eye associated with Sjögren's syndrome who had negative reflex tearing and were treated with topical autologous serum and/or punctal occlusion prior to LASIK to improve the ocular surface with treatment being continued postoperatively. One year after LASIK, mean uncorrected visual acuity was 1.07 (range 0.7 to 1.5), and the mean best spectacle-corrected visual acuity was 1.29 (range 1.2 to 1.5). Tear production, rose bengal and fluorescein staining, and dry eye symptoms were not exacerbated after LASIK. No complications, such as intraoperative epithelial defect, diffuse lamellar keratitis, epithelial ingrowth, or recurrent erosion occurred. In addition, all 3 patients were satisfied with the outcome of their surgery. We concluded that LASIK can be safely and effectively managed in patients with severe dry eye with reduced reflex tearing by preoperative and postoperative treatments consisting of a combination of artificial tears, topical autologous serum, and punctal occlusion.[37]

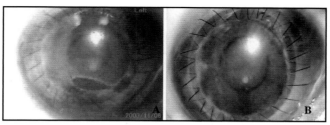

Figure 12-5. Inferior epithelial defect measuring 532 mm with surrounding edema and sterile infiltration in the corneal graft in the left eye. Nine months post deep lamellar keratoplasty (DLKP). Anterior segment photograph of the corneal graft with complete epithelialization at the final examination after treatment with autologous serum and nonpreserved artificial tears. (Reprinted with permission from Kojima T, Dogru M, Matsumoto Y, Goto E, Tsubota K. Tear film and ocular surface abnormalities after eyelid tattooing. *Ophthal Plast Reconstr Surg.* 2005;21:69–71.)

USE OF AUTOLOGOUS SERUM EYE DROPS IN CONJUNCTION WITH OCULAR SURFACE RECONSTRUCTION PROCEDURES

In our experience, autologous serum drops are also helpful in the management of epithelial problems in ocular surface reconstruction procedures when used in conjunction with tarsorrhaphy, AMT, or in the management of epithelial problems occurring after keratoplasty procedures (Figure 12-5).[38–40] In one recent study by us, a total of 11 patients were recruited. Four patients (4 eyes) had corneal perforation, 5 patients (5 eyes) had deep corneal ulcer and descemetocele, and 2 patients (2 eyes) had scleral ulcers. The ulcers were treated by AMT. Separate amniotic membranes were transplanted as material to fill the stromal layer (amniotic membrane filling), as a basement membrane (amniotic membrane graft), and as a wound cover (amniotic membrane patch). After surgery, all cases were treated with artificial tears, autologous serum drops, antibiotic eyedrops, topical corticosteroids, and sodium hyaluronate eyedrops. Eight eyes (72.7%) healed with epithelialization in 16.5 ± 8.0 days (range: 7 to 29 days), with 5 and 3 eyes showing corneal epithelialization and conjunctival epithelialization, respectively.[40]

ALBUMIN AS A TEAR SUPPLEMENT IN THE TREATMENT OF SEVERE DRY EYES

The use of serum as a tear replacement is not without problems, especially when handling serum from patients with transmissible disease such as HIV, hepatitis B, hepatitis C, and prion disease. The logical solution to this would be to develop artificial tear solutions that contain some of the key components of tear, including tear proteins. Although tears contain proteins with specific functions such as lactoferrin and immunoglobulins, a substantial quantity of other nondefined proteins in the prealbumin and albumin fractions

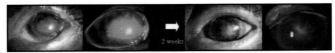

Figure 12-6. Anterior segment and cobalt blue filter photographs of a representative postkeratoplasty case with corneal ulceration and dry eye treated with topical albumin eye drops.

are also found.[41,42] Human albumin was chosen as a protein source since it is widely used in infusion therapy. We have shown in vitro that the addition of albumin can compensate for some of the cell viability lost through the process of apoptosis. Although caspase-3 activity was the only object parameter measured, cells incubated with albumin showed less degree of cell detachment than serum-deprived cells.[43]

Results of our clinical pilot study showed that staining scores significantly improved over the 4-week study period. Of special interest was rose bengal, which was said to stain areas with poor protection by the preocular tear film. The staining pattern can be blocked by the addition of lactoferrin, transferrin, as well as albumin.[44,45] Topical albumin may, therefore, compensate for the lack of soluble mucin in patients with Sjögren's syndrome. Our data also showed that fluorescein staining also improved with topical albumin. We also revealed accelerated wound healing in experimental animal model eyes receiving albumin drops. Anterior segment and cobalt blue filter photographs of a representative postkeratoplasty case with corneal ulceration and dry eye treated with topical albumin eye drops are shown in Figure 12-6. Although no adverse effects were observed during the clinical study, a minute risk of transmissible viral and prion disease still cannot be ruled out.

CONTROVERSIES AND FUTURE PROSPECTS OF AUTOLOGOUS SERUM TREATMENT

The precise mechanism of the serum on the ocular surface epithelium is unknown. Since many of the essential components in tears are also present in the serum, the use of serum as a tear substitute for the maintenance of the ocular surface remains feasible. Increased MUC-1 expression in cultured conjunctival cells by autologous serum suggested a direct effect of the serum on the ocular surface epitheliae. Whether serum upregulates other ocular surface mucins or not is still unknown. Further study is also necessary to determine the most effective concentration of serum. In addition, further experimental work remains to be carried out to delineate the cytokine specific effects of serum on corneal wound healing in dry eye patients. The major drawback of autologous serum treatment is the necessity to obtain blood from the patients. The development of an artificial tear substitute containing all essential tear components would be ideal. Comparative prospective studies on the additive effects of sodium hyaluronate eye drops and other conventional treatment modalities combined with autologous serum eye drops are essential and would provide very interesting information. The viscoelastic properties of hyaluronate might result in a longer exposure of the ocular surface to the essential autologous serum components like growth factors and retinoids. Studies clarifying the effects and risk of prolonged application of autologous serum drops or autologous serum drops of different concentrations to the ocular surface should be the subjects of future investigations. It is our belief that autologous serum eye drops may be replaced with commercially available artificial serum drops harboring essential ocular surface healers in the near future.

Key Points

1. Dry eye is a chronic and unremitting disorder associated with ocular surface desiccation, leading to squamous metaplasia, a pathologic transition of a nonkeratinized squamous epithelium to keratinized squamous epithelium.
2. One of the most important disadvantages of many of the commercially available artificial tear substitutes and lubricants is that they contain preservatives, stabilizers, and other additives that have been reported to be associated with ocular surface epithelial toxicity. The risk may be increased in patients with therapeutically blocked tear ducts, since the agent persists longer in the tear sac, relatively undiluted by lacrimal fluid.
3. Two drawbacks of preservative-free formulations are that they are more expensive than preserved preparations and they can induce lack of compliance because patients must carry numerous vials to maintain adequate dosage over 24 hours or more.
4. TGF-β concentration in human serum, which is 5 times higher than in tears, is believed to control epithelial proliferation and to maintain cells in an undifferentiated state such as the induction of basic keratins in epidermal cells. Serum also contains fibronectin, substance P, and insulin-like growth factors, which are reported to be essential for wound healing in patients with dry eye-associated epithelial problems.
5. Since the concentration of retinol in serum is around 55 mg/mL, serum contains more than 1000 times the amount available in tears. When vitamin A is lacking, the epithelium tends to undergo squamous metaplasia. Application of serum may provide higher levels of retinol necessary in pathological conditions.
6. The TGF-β concentration in human serum is 5 times higher than in tears. TGF-β is believed to control epithelial proliferation and to maintain cells in an undifferentiated state such as the induction of the basic keratins in epidermal cells.
7. Twenty mL of serum can be obtained from 40 mL of whole blood, while diluting 1:5 with saline provides 100 mL serum solution. If each eye drop is 50 mL, 2000 drops can be obtained from 100 mL. Sjögren's syndrome dry eye patients use a maximum of 20 drops a day (10 times for each eye), thus 2000 drops are enough for more than 100 days.

REFERENCES

1. Nelson JD, Havener VR, Cameron JD. Cellulose acetate impressions of the ocular surface: dry eye states. *Arch Ophthalmol.* 1983;101:1869–1872.

2. Tseng SCG. Staging of conjunctival squamous metaplasia by impression cytology. *Ophthalmology.* 1985;92:728–733.

3. Nelson JD, Farris RL. Sodium hyaluronate and polyvinyl alcohol artificial tear preparation. A comparison in patients with KCS. *Arch Ophthalmol.* 1988;106:484–487.

4. Foulks GN. The now and future therapy of the non-Sjögren's dry eye. *Adv Exp Med Biol.* 1998;438:959–964.

5. Lemp MA. The 1998 Castroviejo Lecture. New strategies in the treatment of dry-eye states. *Cornea.* 1999;18:625–632.

6. Lemp MA. Management of the dry-eye patient. *Int Ophthalmol Clin.* 1994;34:101–113.

7. Murube J, Murube A, Zhuo C. Classification of artificial tears. II: additives and commercial formulas. *Adv Exp Med Biol.* 1998;438:705–715.

8. Murube J, Paterson A, Murube E. Classification of artificial tears. I: composition and properties. *Adv Exp Med Biol.* 1998;438:693–704.

9. Pflugfelder SC. Advances in the diagnosis and management of keratoconjunctivitis sicca. *Curr Opin Ophthalmol.* 1998;9:50–53.

10. Macri A, Rolando M, Pflugfelder S. A standardized visual scale for evaluation of tear fluorescein clearance. *Ophthalmology.* 2000;107:1338–1343.

11. Berdy GJ, Abelson MB, Smith LM, George MA. Preservative-free artificial tear preparations. Assessment of corneal epithelial toxic effects. *Arch Ophthalmol.* 1992;110:528–532.

12. Tsubota K, Kaido M, Yagi Y, et al. Diseases associated with ocular surface abnormalities: the importance of reflex tearing. *Br J Ophthalmol.* 1999;83:89.

13. Tsubota K. Reflex tearing in dry eye not associated with Sjögren's syndrome. In: Sullivan D, et al, eds. *Lacrimal Gland, Tear Film and Dry Eye Syndromes.* 2nd ed. New York: Plenum Press; 1998:903–907.

14. Tsubota K, Toda I, Yagi Y, et al. Three different types of dry eye syndrome. *Cornea.* 1994; 13:202–208.

15. Ubels J, Lolay K, Rismondo V. Retinol secretion by the lacrimal gland. *Invest Ophthalmol Vis Sci.* 1986;27:1261–1269.

16. Ohashi Y, Motokura M, Kinoshita Y, et al. Presence of EGF in human tears. *Invest Ophthalmol Vis Sci.* 1989;30:1879–1887.

17. Van Setten G, Viinikka L, Tervo T. EGF is a constant component of normal human tear fluid. *Graefes Arch Clin Exp Ophthalmol.* 1989;22:184–187.

18. Van Setten, Tervo T, Tervo K, et al. EGF in ocular fluids: presence, origin and therapeutical considerations. *Acta Ophthalmol.* 1992;202:54–59.

19. Gupta A, Monroy D, Ji I, et al. TGF beta 1 and beta 2 in human tear fluid. *Curr Eye Res.* 1996; 15:605–614.

20. Nishida T, Ohashi Y, Awata T, Manabe R. Fibronectin. A new therapy for corneal trophic ulcer. *Arch Ophthalmol.* 1983;101:1046–1048.

21. Nishida T, Nakamura M, Ofuji K, et al. Synergistic effects of substance P with insulin like growth factor-1 on epithelial migration of the cornea. *J Cell Physiol.* 1996;169:159–166.

22. Nishida T, Nakagawa S, Awata T, et al. Fibronectin eye drops for traumatic recurrent corneal erosion. *Lancet.* 1983;2:521–522.

23. Fox R, Chan R, Michelson J, et al. Beneficial effect of artificial tears made with autologous serum in patients with keratoconjunctivitis sicca. *Arthritis Rheum.* 1984;27:459–461.

24. Tsubota K. *New Approaches in Dry Eye Management: Supplying Missing Tear Components to the Ocular Surface Epithelium. 1st Annual Meeting of the Kyoto Cornea Club.* Amsterdam: Kugler; 1997:27–32.

25. Tsubota K, Goto E, Fujita H, et al. Treatment of dry eye by autologous serum application in Sjögren's syndrome. *Br J Ophthalmol.* 1999;83:390–395.

26. Speek AJ, van Agtmaal EG, Saowakontha S, et al. Fluorometric determination of retinol of human tear fluid using high-performance liquid chromatography. *Curr Eye Res.* 1986;5:841–845.

27. El-Ghorab M, Capone A, Underwood B, et al. Response of ocular surface epithelium to corneal wounding ion retinol-deficient rabbits. *Invest Ophthalmol Vis Sci.* 1988;29:1671–1676.

28. Noble BA, Loh RS, MacLennan S, et al. Comparison of autologous serum eye drops with conventional therapy in a randomised controlled crossover trial for ocular surface disease. *Br J Ophthalmol.* 2004;88:647–652.

29. Tananuvat N, Daniell M, Sullivan LJ, et al. Controlled study of the use of autologous serum in dry eye patients. *Cornea.* 2001;20:802–806.

30. Kojima T, Ishida R, Dogru M, et al. The effect of autologous serum eye drops in the treatment of severe dry eye disease: a prospective randomized case-control study. *AJO.* 2005;139:242–246.

31. Ogawa Y, Okamoto S, Mori T, et al. Autologous serum eye drops for the treatment of severe dry eye in patients with chronic graft-versus-host disease. *Bone Marrow Transplant.* 2003;31:579–583.

32. Kojima T, Dogru M, Matsumoto Y, Goto E, Tsubota K. Tear film and ocular surface abnormalities after eyelid tattooing. *Ophthal Plast Reconstr Surg.* 2005;21:69–71.

33. Goto E, Shimmura S, Shimazaki J, Tsubota K. Treatment of superior limbic keratoconjunctivitis by application of autologous serum. *Cornea.* 2001;20:807–810.

34. del Castillo JM, de la Casa JM, Sardina RC, et al. Treatment of recurrent corneal erosions using autologous serum. *Cornea.* 2002;21:781–783.

35. Tsubota K, Goto E, Shimmura S, Shimazaki J. Treatment of persistent corneal epithelial defect by autologous serum application. *Ophthalmology.* 1999;106:1984–1989.

36. Matsumoto Y, Dogru M, Goto E, et al. Autologous serum application in the treatment of neurotrophic keratopathy. *Ophthalmology.* 2004;111:1115–1120.

37. Toda I, Asano-Kato N, Hori-Komai Y, Tsubota K. Ocular surface treatment before laser in situ keratomileusis in patients with severe dry eye. *J Refract Surg.* 2004;20:270–275.

38. Tsubota K, Higuchi A. Serum application for the treatment of ocular surface disorders. *Int Ophthalmol Clin.* 1999;12:113–122.

39. Tsubota K, Satake Y, Ohyama M, et al. Surgical reconstruction of the ocular surface in advanced ocular cicatricial pemphigoid and Stevens-Johnson Syndrome. *Am J Ophthalmol.* 1996;122:38–52.

40. Hanada K, Shimazaki J, Shimmura S, Tsubota K. Multilayered amniotic membrane transplantation for severe ulceration of the cornea and sclera. *AJO.* 2001;131:324–331.

41. Kijlstra A, Jeurissen SH, Koning KM. Lactoferrin levels in normal human tears. *Br J Ophthalmol.* 1983;67:199–202.

42. Sen DK, Sarin GS. Immunoglobulin concentrations in human tears in ocular diseases. *Br J Ophthalmol.* 1979;63:297–300.

43. Shimmura S, Ueno R, Matsumoto Y, et al. Albumin as a tear supplement in the treatment of severe dry eye. *Br J Ophthalmol.* 2003;87:1279–1283.

44. Feenstra RP, Tseng SC. Comparison of fluorescein and rose bengal staining. *Ophthalmology.* 1992;99:605–617.

45. Tseng SC, Zhang SH. Interaction between rose bengal and different protein components. *Cornea.* 1995;14:427–435.

13

Restasis—Topical Cyclosporin A

Renée Solomon, MD;
Henry D. Perry, MD;
John R. Wittpenn, MD; and
Eric D. Donnenfeld, MD

INTRODUCTION

Dry eye syndrome, or dysfunctional tear syndrome, is believed to be one of the most common ophthalmic problems in the United States and is found with increased prevalence in older patients, in postmenopausal women, and in patients with autoimmune disease.[1,2] In a population-based prevalence study, 14.6% of 2482 patients of subjects aged 65 years or older reported symptoms suggestive of dry eye.[2,3] Based on this study, it is estimated that 4.3 million Americans experience symptoms of dry eye syndrome. In another population-based study, 7.8% of 39,876 US women reported a prevalence of dry eye syndrome, which would extrapolate to approximately 3.2 million cases of dry eye in females aged 50 years or older.[4] Remarkably, despite these large numbers of cases, dry eye syndrome remains an underdiagnosed problem.[3–5]

The difficulty in diagnosing dry eye syndrome is partly due to the understanding of its controversies, which is undergoing revision, and partly due to the absence of one specific diagnostic test.[6] There are 2 distinct categories of dry eye syndrome; one related to insufficient production of tears and the other, more common, to increased evaporation of tears. Tests for one category may be positive and for another category negative; yet both may lead to dry eye syndrome. To compound the confusion, there is often a crossover of conditions between the 2 groups. An example of this is meibomian gland dysfunction, which is the leading cause of evaporative dry eye syndrome and may also occur in a large number of patients with aqueous deficiency.

DIAGNOSIS OF DRY EYE SYNDROME

Diagnosing dry eye syndrome begins with the patient history, including type and duration of symptoms, and any exacerbating conditions (eg, wind, prolonged computer work, air travel). Ocular history includes contact lens wear, eyelid surgery, allergic conjunctivitis, ocular surface inflammatory disease (eg, OCP, Stevens-Johnson syndrome), and topical medications (eg, antihistamines, vasoconstrictors, corticosteroids, glaucoma medications, artificial tears). Systemic history should include details about dermatological diseases (eg, rosacea), atopy, menopause, autoimmune disease (eg, Sjögren's syndrome, rheumatoid arthritis, systemic lupus erythematosus), and systemic medications (eg, diuretics, hormones, antihistamines, antidepressants).

A variety of symptoms have been associated with dry eye syndrome. These symptoms have been quantified by a questionnaire titled the Ocular Surface Disease Index (OSDI). This questionnaire (Figure 13-1) lists 12 common symptoms of dry eye patients and scores each from 1 to 4 in terms of severity. This survey permits quantification of symptoms and allows for a categorization in terms of grading for mild, moderate, or severe dry eye syndrome. Not only is there a plethora of symptoms, but also numerous diagnostic tests are available.

Examination with slit lamp biomicroscopy should particularly focus attention on the tear film, eye lashes, anterior and posterior lid margins, puncta, inferior fornix, tarsal and bulbar conjunctiva, cornea, height of tear meniscus (marginal tear strip) (Figure 13-2), and the presence or absence of tear film debris. The clinician generally relies on the history, examination with slit lamp biomicroscopy, in conjunction with Schirmer's testing (with or without anesthesia), supravital conjunctival staining, tear film BUT, and tear fluorescein clearance. Delayed tear fluorescein clearance is reported to show better correlation with the severity of ocular irritation symptoms and KCS than the Schirmer's 1 test.[6,7]

The tear BUT is the best screening test for dry eye syndrome. If the result of this test is abnormal (ie, under 5 seconds), there is usually some form of ocular surface disease; most commonly dry eye syndrome. At this point, the clinician can help confirm the diagnosis of dry eye with the use of supravital staining. Lissamine green (Figure 13-3) is a new supravital stain that combines the diagnostic advantages of fluorescein and rose bengal. Lissamine green stains healthy epithelial cells when they are not protected by a mucin layer in a manner similar to rose bengal (Figure 13-4). Lissamine green also stains dead or degenerated cells as fluorescein does.[8-10] The main advantage of lissamine green is that it avoids the ocular discomfort associated with the use of rose bengal, which can be very troublesome for patients with KCS, and is extremely helpful in diagnosing dry eye.[8,11,12] The main disadvantage of lissamine green lies in its being a little less sensitive than rose bengal, more transient, and somewhat more difficult to see on slit lamp examination. In the evaluation of refractive surgery candidates, supravital staining can reduce the risk of complications and wound healing problems related to poor outcomes by identifying high-risk patients before surgery.[13] Tear film osmolarity, tear lysozyme and tear lactoferrin concentrations, and conjunctival impression cytology are helpful tests that are rarely used outside of a research setting.

Severe untreated chronic dry eye syndrome can result in poor lubrication, altered barrier function, sterile melting, and even bacterial keratitis (Figure 13-5). Therefore, to prevent these potentially serious complications, it is extremely important to understand and treat dry eye syndrome.

Ocular Surface Disease Index^c (OSDI^c)[2]

Ask your patient the following 12 questions, and circle the number in the box that best represents each answer. Then, fill in boxes A, B, C, D, and E according to the instructions beside each.

HAVE YOU EXPERIENCED ANY OF THE FOLLOWING *DURING THE LAST WEEK*:

	All of the time	Most of the time	Half of the time	Some of the time	None of the time
1. Eyes that are sensitive to light?	4	3	2	1	0
2. Eyes that feel gritty?	4	3	2	1	0
3. Painful or sore eyes?	4	3	2	1	0
4. Blurred vision?	4	3	2	1	0
5. Poor vision?	4	3	2	1	0

Subtotal score for answers 1 to 5   (A)

HAVE PROBLEMS WITH YOUR EYES LIMITED YOU IN PERFORMING ANY OF THE FOLLOWING *DURING THE LAST WEEK*:

	All of the time	Most of the time	Half of the time	Some of the time	None of the time	
6. Reading?	4	3	2	1	0	N/A
7. Driving at night?	4	3	2	1	0	N/A
8. Working with a computer or bank machine (ATM)?	4	3	2	1	0	N/A
9. Watching TV?	4	3	2	1	0	N/A

Subtotal score for answers 6 to 9   (B)

HAVE YOUR EYES FELT UNCOMFORTABLE IN ANY OF THE FOLLOWING SITUATIONS *DURING THE LAST WEEK*:

	All of the time	Most of the time	Half of the time	Some of the time	None of the time	
10. Windy conditions?	4	3	2	1	0	N/A
11. Places or areas with low humidity (very dry)?	4	3	2	1	0	N/A
12. Areas that are air conditioned?	4	3	2	1	0	N/A

Subtotal score for answers 10 to 12   (C)

ADD SUBTOTALS A, B, AND C TO OBTAIN D (D = SUM OF SCORES FOR ALL QUESTIONS ANSWERED)   (D)

TOTAL NUMBER OF QUESTIONS ANSWERED (DO NOT INCLUDE QUESTIONS ANSWERED N/A)   (E)

Please turn over the questionnaire to calculate the patient's final OSDI^c score.

Figure 13-1. Ocular Surface Disease Index (OSDI) for evaluation of dry eye patients. (Please note that this is not the complete questionnaire.)

Figure 13-2. Clinical photograph of marginal tear strip.

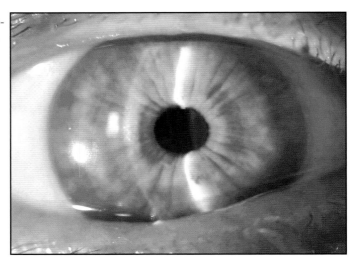

Figure 13-3. Clinical photograph demonstrating lissamine green staining pattern of the interpalpebral conjunctiva and cornea in a patient with severe dry eye syndrome.

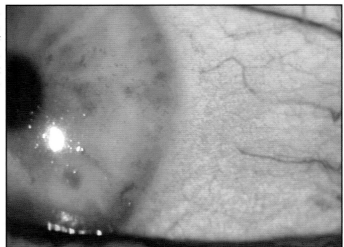

Figure 13-4. Clinical photograph demonstrating rose bengal staining pattern of the interpalpebral conjunctiva and cornea in a patient with severe dry eye syndrome.

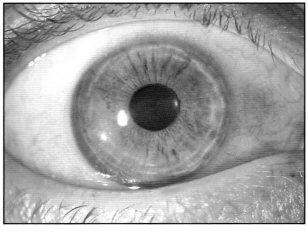

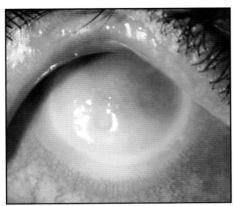

Figure 13-5. Bacterial keratitis.

CLASSIFICATION SYSTEMS: DRY EYE SYNDROME VERSUS DYSFUNCTIONAL TEAR SYNDROME

In the early 1990s, NEI had proposed a classification system for dry eye based on the differentiation between deficient aqueous production and evaporative tear loss. There are multiple subgroups in each of the categories, and there is often significant crossover between the 2 groups. Traditional therapy has included the use of artificial tears to supplement the patient's own tear production. For mild dry eye, preserved artificial tears have been effective, while for severe dry eye, nonpreserved unit dose packs have gained widespread acceptance. Recently, transiently preserved artificial tears have been developed in which the preservative is dissipated upon exposure to air. For patients in whom artificial tears are not sufficient, punctal occlusion, either temporary or permanent with plugs or cautery may be effective for both preserving the patient's own natural tears and prolonging the effect of artificial tears that have been instilled.[14]

The NEI classification does not address the inflammatory component of dry eye syndrome. An international panel of experts on dry eye syndrome, who employed the Delphi consensus approach to develop current treatment recommendations for dry eye syndrome, created a practical treatment algorithm in an attempt to cover gaps in the available literature. A new term for the disease was proposed, dysfunctional tear syndrome, which may be diagnosed as 1 of 4 severity levels with treatment recommendations for each (Tables 13-1 and 13-2). Treatment recommendations were primarily based on patient symptoms and specific clinical signs. Diagnostic tests were deemed secondary in the election of therapy. Algorithms were developed depending on the presence or absence of lid margin disease, and disease severity (mild 1 to 2, moderate 3 to 4, and severe ≥4) was assessed according to use of tear substitutes, ocular fatigue and discomfort, and visual disturbances.[15,16]

Because the abstracts reclassifying dry eye syndrome as dysfunctional tear syndrome have not yet been published and because the entity is still more commonly referred to as dry eye syndrome, for the remainder of this chapter we will refer to the entity according to the NEI classification.

Table 13-1
DYSFUNCTIONAL TEAR SYNDROME—PROGRESSION OF SEVERITY[16]

Level 1	Mild to moderate symptoms, no corneal signs Mild to moderate conjunctival signs
	⇩
Level 2	Moderate to severe symptoms Tear film signs, visual signs Mild corneal punctuate staining Conjunctival staining
	⇩
Level 3	Severe symptoms Marked corneal punctate staining Central corneal staining Filamentary keratitis
	⇩
Level 4	Extremely severe symptoms/altered lifestyle Severe corneal staining, erosions Conjunctival scarring

COMMUNICATION BETWEEN THE OCULAR SURFACE AND THE LACRIMAL GLANDS IN THE PATHOGENESIS OF DRY EYE SYNDROME

One major advance in dry eye over the past decade is the understanding that the ocular surface and lacrimal glands function as an integrated unit (Figure 13-6). A sensory/autonomic neural reflex loop facilitates communication between the lacrimal glands (Figure 13-7) and the ocular surface. The sensory nerves innervate the ocular surface and nasal mucosa synapse with efferent autonomic nerves in the brainstem that stimulate secretion of tear fluid and proteins by the lacrimal glands. Ocular surface sensitivity has been found to decrease as aqueous tear production and clearance of tears from the ocular surface decrease. This decrease in surface sensation in turn exacerbates dry eye because of a decrease in sensory-stimulated reflex tearing and decreased ability of the lacrimal glands to respond to ocular surface injury. This creates a self-perpetuating cycle of continuing inflammation mediated by tears produced by lacrimal gland tissue heavily infiltrated with T cell lymphocytes constantly secreting inflammatory mediators and cytokines that bathe the ocular surface.[17–19]

The importance of inflammation in the pathogenesis of dry eye of people 65 years of age or older has also been elucidated over the past decade (Figure 13-8) and is now being taken into account in the classification of dry eye disorder.[20] It has been found that decreased tear production and tear clearance lead to chronic inflammation on the ocular surface. This inflammatory response consists of inflammatory cell infiltration of the ocular surface, activation of the ocular surface epithelium with increased expres-

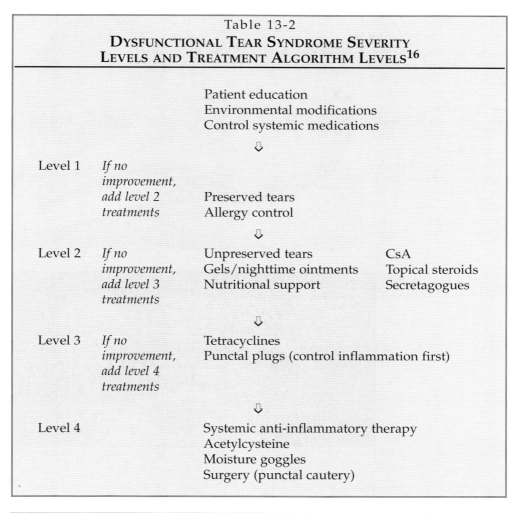

Table 13-2
**DYSFUNCTIONAL TEAR SYNDROME SEVERITY
LEVELS AND TREATMENT ALGORITHM LEVELS[16]**

		Patient education	
		Environmental modifications	
		Control systemic medications	
		⇩	
Level 1	*If no improvement, add level 2 treatments*	Preserved tears Allergy control	
		⇩	
Level 2	*If no improvement, add level 3 treatments*	Unpreserved tears Gels/nighttime ointments Nutritional support	CsA Topical steroids Secretagogues
		⇩	
Level 3	*If no improvement, add level 4 treatments*	Tetracyclines Punctal plugs (control inflammation first)	
		⇩	
Level 4		Systemic anti-inflammatory therapy Acetylcysteine Moisture goggles Surgery (punctal cautery)	

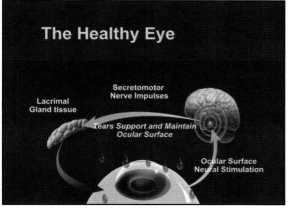

Figure 13-6. Diagram showing normal homeostasis mechanism for the ocular surface in a healthy eye.

Figure 13-7. Illustra-tion of lacrimal glands, which secrete aqueous compo-nent of tear film, mostly tear proteins including andro-gens important for glandu-lar homeostasis and pro-teins important to maintain healthy ocular surface. (Reprinted with permission from Pflugfelder SC, Beuer-man RW, Stern ME. *Dry Eye and Ocular Surface Dis-orders.* New York: Marcel Dekker; 2004:19.)

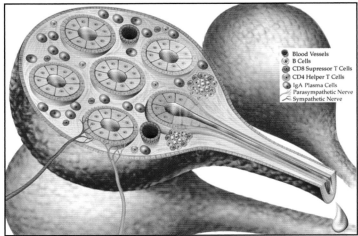

Figure 13-8. Diagram showing inflammation interrupting normal homeostasis and lead-ing to ocular surface disease and dry eye syndrome.

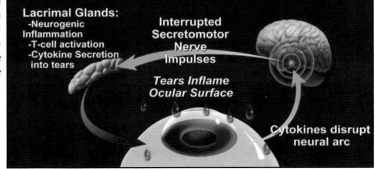

sion of adhesion molecules and inflammatory cytokines, increased concentrations of inflammatory cytokines in the tear fluid, and increased activity of matrix degrading enzymes such as matrix metalloproteinase-9 in the tear fluid (Figure 13-9).[21] A signif-icant, positive correlation has been observed between the levels of inflammatory cytokines in the conjunctival epithelium and the severity of ocular irritation symptoms and corneal fluorescein staining. The inflammatory cytokines and other inflammatory mediators also correlate positively to the severity of conjunctival squamous metaplasia in patients with Sjögren's syndrome keratoconjunctivitis.[17,18]

RESTASIS—TOPICAL CYCLOSPORIN A

For years, dry eye patients have had their symptoms treated with artificial tears, gels, ointments, steroids, punctual plugs, nonsteroidal anti-inflammatory agents, etc, but nothing provided anything beyond symptomatic relief until the breakthrough develop-ment of the pharmacologic agent, Restasis. Restasis is a 0.05% emulsion of the active ingredient cyclosporin A formulated in a castor oil-based topical emulsion vehicle con-taining glycerin, polysorbate 80, carbomer 1342, purified water, and sodium hydrox-

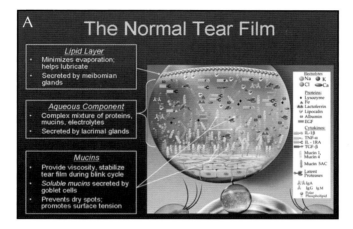

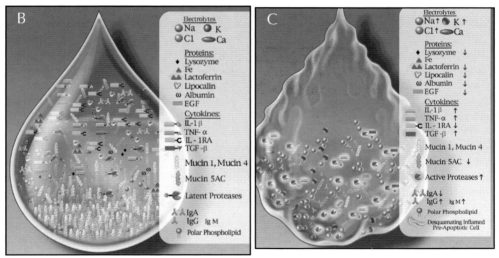

Figure 13-9. (A and B) Illustration of normal tear film, which is a complex mixture of proteins, mucins, and electrolytes coated by a lipid layer. The normal tear film contains antimicrobial proteins, growth factors and suppressors of inflammation, soluble mucin that helps stabilize tear film, and electrolytes for proper osmolarity (295 to 300) in a slightly alkaline pH (7.4). (C) Illustration of unhealthy tears in chronic dry eye, which contain decreased concentrations of many proteins (eg, antimicrobial proteins), decreased growth factors, a shift in cytokine and protease balance, loss of goblet cells resulting in a decreased soluble mucin, activated proteases that degrade extracellular matrix and tight junctions, and increased osmolarity. (Figure 13-9A reprinted with permission from Pflugfelder SC, Beuerman RW, Stern ME. *Dry Eye and Ocular Surface Disorders.* New York: Marcel Dekker; 2004:50. Figures 13-9B and 13-9C courtesy of Allergan.)

Figure 13–10. Schematic diagram of cyclic polypeptide of topical cyclosporin A.

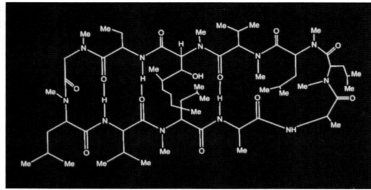

ide.[22] Topical CsA (TCSA) is the first FDA-approved medication indicated to increase tear production in patients who do not produce sufficient tears due to ocular inflammation associated with chronic dry eye syndrome.

CsA is a cyclic polypeptide (Figure 13-10) produced as a metabolite by the fungus *Beauveria nivea*, which is well known for its anti-inflammatory and immunomodulatory properties. It is most commonly used systemically to prevent rejection of transplanted tissues.[23] In addition, it is used systemically to treat psoriasis[24] and rheumatoid arthritis.[25] The mechanism of action of cyclosporine on inflammatory disease processes arises from its ability to inhibit T cell activation and thus T cell-mediated inflammation. TCSA is advantageous in blocking T cell activation because activated T cells produce cytokines that may result in recruitment of additional T cells, increased cytokine production, neural signal to the lacrimal gland that disrupts production of natural tears, which leads to a decrease in quality and quantity of tears, and damage in lacrimal gland tissue and the ocular surface.

TCSA prevents activation of T cells by cytokines and other agents of inflammation and normalizes effects of chronic dry eye syndrome processes of T cells and lacrimal gland acinar cells. Activated T cells are responsible for the production of inflammatory cytokines and other inflammatory mediators. These mediators lead to tissue damage, activation of more T cells, and the production of more inflammatory mediators.

It is important to note that TCSA has no effect on intraocular pressure (IOP) and does not inhibit the phagocytic system as greatly as do corticosteroids, allowing the antimicrobial arm of the immune system to fight infection. Furthermore, TCSA does not inhibit wound healing or produce lens changes. This creates a wide safety profile for this drug.[26] FDA guidelines indicated 2 contraindications for the use of TCSA, which are active ocular infection and any previously demonstrated hypersensitivity to the active molecule or any of the ingredients in the formulation.

COMPOSITION AND APPEARANCE OF RESTASIS WITH SLIT LAMP BIOMICROSCOPY

Restasis appears as a white to slightly translucent oil slick or micellar aggregate (Figure 13-11).[22] The micellar aggregate phenomena observed under the slit lamp in the

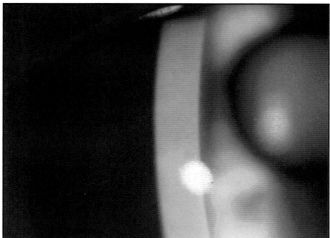

Figure 13-11. Slit lamp examination of the tear film demonstrating an accumulation of tiny droplet material with lucent centers and white looking surrounds. (Reproduced with permission from Solomon R, Perry HD, Donnenfeld ED, Greenman HE. Slit lamp biomicroscopy of the tear film of patients using topical Restasis and Refresh Endura. *J Cataract Refract Surg.* 2005;31:661–663.)

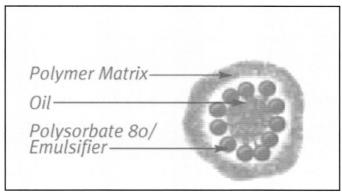

Polymer Matrix

Oil

Polysorbate 80/ Emulsifier

Figure 13-12. Illustration of a micelle. (Reproduced with permission from Solomon R, Perry HD, Donnenfeld ED, Greenman HE. Slit lamp biomicroscopy of the tear film of patients using topical Restasis and Refresh Endura. *J Cataract Refract Surg.* 2005; 31:661–663.)

tear film of patients using TCSA may be seen because TCSA is formulated as an emulsion (Figure 13-12) (ie, a medication containing 2 immiscible liquids in which one is dispersed, in the form of very small globules or droplets [internal phase], throughout the other [external phase] [eg, oil in water {milk} or water in oil {mayonnaise}]).[27,28]

The size of a micelle in TCSA is about 1 or 2 μm in diameter. When first applied, the initial micelles are too small to be seen even under the magnification of the slit lamp, but what can be appreciated is a general hazy texture to the tear film. If the emulsions in either formulation were examined with a slit lamp at highest magnification, one would appreciate the uniform hazy fluid, or oil slick due to light scatter, with no visible structure except occasional air bubbles floating at the top.

The microscopic micelles of the emulsion change over time and break apart as micelles are destabilized. The micelles are destabilized as the emulsion is diluted by tears and the viscosity of the emulsion drops. Salts enhance this destabilization process and the sodium in the fluorescein may speed the pace of the micellar destabilization. After the micelles are destabilized, they release oil and polymeric emulsifying agents into the tear film, and a portion of these may reform and coalesce into the visible aggregates described previously.[22] Tear components may participate in the formation of this aggregate and may add bulk, increasing visibility. In general, when emulsions begin to break up, it is possible for larger temporary features to form. These features might look like oil droplets or may have a creamy or foamy whitish appearance if many were trapped together. The micellar aggregates also appear white because the light shown on the tear film (the "blue" cobalt light) contains sufficient other wavelengths to appear white when reflected. Enough blue is absorbed by the miceller aggregate so that the reflected mix appears white, at least by contrast with the surrounding much bluer tissue.

Emulsifying agents are added to stabilize the emulsion and prevent coalescence of the dispersed drops.[27] The findings of micellar aggregates are specific for topical ophthalmic emulsion agents. Emulsions are advantageous as a drug delivery system because they offer the ability to deliver lipid-soluble drugs in a liquid aqueous-like form. This produces enhanced bioavailability, protection of drugs susceptible to oxidation or hydrolysis, and patient acceptability in instances in which the free drug is irritating.[27]

Careful examination under the slit lamp of patients applying Restasis can help to confirm patient compliance with the drug. We estimate the duration of time the micellar aggregates are visible to be hours based on what we have observed in patients using these emulsion agents. Break up of the micelles is necessary to release the suspended cyclosporin A to the ocular surface. This technique may help quantitate the stability of this agent on the ocular surface and help determine whether an increase or decrease in dosing is required.

INDICATIONS AND USES OF TOPICAL CYCLOSPORIN A

TCSA has been successfully used or has shown promise in the management of many other ophthalmologic conditions[29-35] (Table 13-3). These off-label uses for TCSA, some of which were tried prior to the release of commercially available Restasis, include vernal keratoconjunctivitis,[36] Thygeson's superficial punctate keratitis,[37,38] superior limbic keratoconjunctivitis,[39] improvement of LASIK outcomes in patients with dry eye,[40] postkeratoplasty glaucoma,[26] postkeratoplasty glaucoma with corticosteroid-induced ocular hypertension,[26,41] HSV stromal keratitis,[42] steroid-resistant atopic keratoconjunctivitis,[43] KCS in secondary Sjögren's syndrome,[44] as an adjunct to antifungal treatment in nonresolving severe keratomycosis,[45] inhibition of fungal growth,[46] synergistically with punctual plugs in the treatment of dry eye syndrome,[47] prevention of corneal graft rejection,[37,48-50] dysthyroid ophthalmopathy,[51] allergic conjunctivitis,[52] severe allergic keratoconjunctivitis,[53] phlyctenular keratoconjunctivitis,[54] GVHD,[55] treatment of necrotizing scleritis and corneal melting in patients with rheumatoid arthritis,[56] prevention of pterygium recurrence along with thiotepa,[57] the prevention of limbal allograft rejection,[58] in the management of therapeutic keratoplasty for mycotic keratitis,[59] treatment of contact lens intolerance,[60] stimulation of neovascularization in sterile rheumatoid central corneal ulcers as the first sign of a favorable clinical response,[61] and Mooren's ulcer.[62]

Table 13-3

ADDITIONAL POTENTIAL OFF LABEL USES FOR TOPICAL CYCLOSPORIN A, SOME OF WHICH WERE TRIED PRIOR TO THE RELEASE OF COMMERCIALLY AVAILABLE RESTASIS

- Allergic keratoconjunctivitis.
- Atopic keratoconjunctivitis (steroid-resistant).
- Contact lens intolerance.
- Corneal graft rejection.
- Dry eye syndrome.
- Dysthyroid ophthalmopathy.
- Glaucoma—postkeratoplasty glaucoma.
- Glaucoma—postkeratoplasty glaucoma with corticosteroid-induced ocular hypertension.
- GVHD.
- HSV stromal keratitis
- Keratomycosis (useful as an adjunct to antifungal treatment in severe cases).
- Limbal allograft rejection.
- LASIK—improves LASIK outcomes in patients with dry eye.
- Mooren's ulcer.
- Posterior blepharitis—meibomian gland dysfunction.
- Phlyctenular keratoconjunctivitis.
- Pterygium (prevention of pterygium recurrence when used with thiotepa).
- Rosacea (ocular rosacea).
- Scleritis (necrotizing scleritis and corneal melting in patients with rheumatoid arthritis).
- Sjögren's syndrome (KCS in secondary Sjögren's syndrome).
- Superior limbic keratoconjunctivitis.
- Therapeutic keratoplasty for mycotic keratitis.
- Thygeson's superficial punctate keratitis.
- Vernal keratoconjunctivitis.

RESTASIS AND DRY EYE SYNDROME—PHASE III STUDIES AND OTHER DRY EYE INVESTIGATIONS

Early studies suggesting Restasis's utility in dry eye syndrome came from dog studies in which topical application of cyclosporine ophthalmic emulsion twice daily reduced lymphocyte infiltration in the lacrimal glands and conjunctiva.[63–65] CsA also was associated with reduced apoptosis of lacrimal glands and conjunctival epithelial cells in dogs, effects that contribute to reduced inflammation and clinical improvement of dry eye.[64] The earliest human studies in KCS revealed that topical eye treatment with cyclosporin A relieved the signs and symptoms of the disease.[44,66,67]

Table 13-4
KEY INCLUSION AND EXCLUSION CRITERIA[29]

Inclusion	*Exclusion*
• Symptomatic dry eye disease despite conventional management.	• Severe lacrimal dysfunction —nasal-stimulated Schirmer's <3 mm.
• Schirmer's ≤5 mm/5 min.	• Permanent goblet cell loss/scarring.
• Corneal and interpalpebral conjunctival staining.	• Active ocular infection.
• OSDI score.	• Ocular rosacea.
• Normal lid anatomy/blinking function.	• Severe blepharitis/lid margin inflammation.
• BCVA Snellen ≥20/100.	• Punctal occlusion within 3 months.
	• Contact lens wear during study.

More recent data from a large, multicenter, double-masked, parallel, randomized 6-month trial evaluating 3 treatment groups: 0.05% cyclosporine in vehicle, 0.1% cyclosporine in vehicle, and vehicle all given 1 drop twice daily involving 877 patients, was the basis for approval of Restasis.[29] This study established the efficacy, safety, and anti-inflammatory activity of cyclosporin A ophthalmic emulsion compared with castor oil-based topical emulsion vehicle alone in patients with moderate to severe dry eye syndrome.[29]

Patient demographics in each group were as follows: 82%, 84%, and 31% were female, Caucasian, and Sjögren's syndrome patients, respectively. The age range was 22 to 90 years (mean: 60 years). There were no statistically significant differences between treatment groups in any demographic variable. No statistically significant differences in prior therapy or types of concomitant medications used during study for other conditions were observed. At baseline, patients were using artificial tears as required. In the 0.05% cyclosporine group, the average baseline use was 6.25 times daily. In the 0.1% cyclosporine group, the average baseline use was 5.56 times daily. These patients had been previously treated unsuccessfully—sometimes for decades—with multiple products and practices. Key exclusion and inclusion criteria are listed in Table 13-4.

The study evaluated several primary and secondary variables. The 4 primary efficacy variables included 2 objective (corneal staining and Schirmer's test with anesthesia) and 2 subjective (reliance on artificial tears and blurred vision). Six secondary efficacy variables included photophobia, sandy/gritty feeling, burning or stinging, itching, feeling of dryness, and pain. Several tertiary laboratory variables to assess immune involvement included the following: presence of inflammatory markers, goblet cell density, and status of pathological apoptosis. These were performed on conjunctival biopsy tissue obtained before and after treatment.

The rationale behind this study was the theory that insufficient ocular lubrication increases corneal abrasion of the superficial epithelium. Abraded corneal epithelium readily accepts stain. However, although corneal staining is an indirect measure of inflammation and immunoreactivity, it is a commonly used diagnostic test for chronic

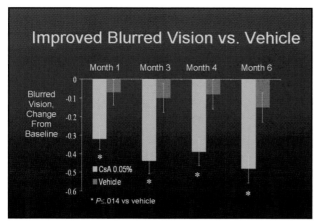

Figure 13-13. Graph showing the change from baseline in blurred vision. (Adapted from Sall K, Stevenson OD, Mundorf TK, Reis BL. Two multicenter, randomized studies of the efficacy and safety of cyclosporine ophthalmic emulsion in moderate to severe dry eye disease. CsA Phase 3 Study Group. *Ophthalmology.* 2000;107:631–639.)

dry eye syndrome and is considered clinically important. Significant differences relative to the vehicle were seen for corneal staining for both the 0.05% and 0.1% cyclosporine at month 4.

Significant differences relative to the vehicle were seen for 0.05% cyclosporine at month 6, with a trend toward significance for the 0.1% emulsion. With the 0.05% emulsion, both patients showed statistically and clinically significant mean reductions of ≥30% versus baseline in corneal staining at all time points.

Changes also occurred from baseline blurred vision. Blurring of vision occurs in chronic dry eye syndrome because of desiccation of corneal epithelial cells, causing them to shrink, crease, and opacify. This makes a reduction in blurred vision an important efficacy measure. The 0.05% cyclosporine-treated patients exhibited statistically and clinically significant reductions versus baseline and vehicle in complaints of blurred vision at all time points. At 6 months, 44% of the 0.05% cyclosporine-treated patients experienced a mean improvement in blurred vision of 24%, indicating a significant difference in normalizing ocular surface improvement compared to the vehicle at months 1, 3, 4, and 6 (Figure 13-13).

Reliance on the administration of artificial tears was also tested, whereby a reduction in the volume of artificial tears used can be a gauge of symptomatic relief. Patients in all study groups were allowed to instill artificial tears between study medication doses throughout the trial. A trend toward decreased artificial tear use in all groups was observed. After 6 months, a reduction in artificial tear use was seen in all cyclosporine groups versus baseline. The decrease was statistically significant for the 0.05% cyclosporine group at month 6. A total of 33% of patients reduced concomitant tear use by at least 5 times daily. A total of 51% reduced tear use by at least 3 times daily. The overall use of artificial tears fell by one-third at month 6. These data indicate that the condition of the patients' eyes was improving (Figure 13-14).

Clinical presentation of dry eye syndrome can have significant variation. Patients range from mildly to extremely symptomatic, and staining can be very mild or pronounced. One patient may have severe corneal staining and a very low Schirmer's score, whereas another with severe corneal staining may have a normal Schirmer's score. Therefore, the need for laboratory assessments is vital because there is current-

Figure 13-14. Graph showing the change from baseline in the use of artificial tears. (Adapted from Sall K, Stevenson OD, Mundorf TK, Reis BL. Two multicenter, randomized studies of the efficacy and safety of cyclosporine ophthalmic emulsion in moderate to severe dry eye disease. CsA Phase 3 Study Group. *Ophthalmology.* 2000;107:631–639.)

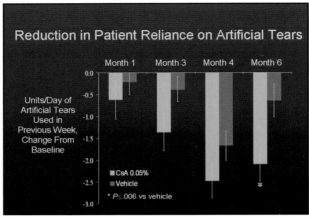

ly no good, single test in order to assess function or even that which correlates well with common complaints.

Severe dry eye may have no effect on vision in one patient, whereas another might complain of blurring despite only minor corneal staining. The condition may have just reached clinical level, or it may be severe end stage disease with complete lacrimal gland shutdown and severe corneal and conjunctival signs. Signs and symptoms may be the result of the primary disease, or they may be secondary to autoimmune disorder, trauma, or other factors. All these factors warrant the performance of laboratory assessments, which include the following: CD3 levels (staining for immune T lymphocyte cell marker CD3 in chronic dry eye syndrome patients both in non-Sjögren's and Sjögren's syndrome). Comparing baseline (Figure 13-15) to 6-month values in a Sjögren's patient, a significant decrease is again seen in the number of CD3-positive T cells in the conjunctiva with 0.05% cyclosporine. Similar results occurred in non-Sjögren's patients (see Figure 13-15).

Consistent with a similar path physiology for both conditions, there was a reduction in the inflammatory markers HLA-DR and CD11a determined by conjunctival biopsy. Baseline values were found to be significantly elevated in both Sjögren's and non-Sjögren's patients in the pivotal clinical trials, as well as a separate biopsy study performed by Allergan in collaboration with the NEI. After 6 months of 0.05% cyclosporine treatment, statistically significant decreases in the levels of HLA-DR and CD11a were seen, compared with increases in the vehicle group.

The final laboratory efficacy measure, goblet cell density, may be the most sensitive measure of overall ocular surface health. The number of mucin-producing goblet cells is decreased in patients with moderate-to-severe chronic dry eye syndrome. As goblet cells die, their density decreases, resulting in decreased mucin production, which further destabilizes tear film. Increases in goblet cell density indicate a normalization of the ocular surface. Cyclosporine treatment resulted in a significant increase in goblet cells. The increase over the 6-month treatment period was 191% in the cyclosporine-treated patients, compared with only 13% in the vehicle-treated group (p = 0.013). The vehicle provided only symptomatic relief and had no effect on goblet cell density (Figure 13-16).

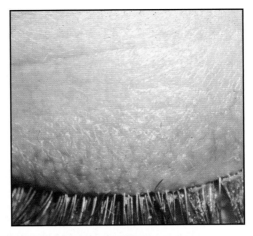

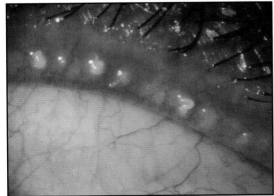

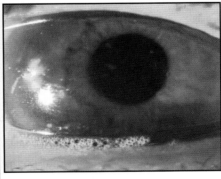

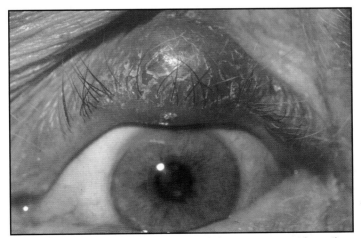

Figure 13-22. Clinical photos of eyelids in patients with meibomian gland dysfunction.

Figure 13-23. Bar graph demonstrating cyclosporine-reduced meibomian gland inclusions.

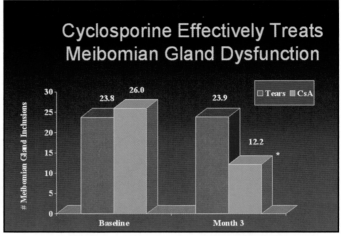

The reason that TCSA may ameliorate posterior blepharitis is because underlying the pathophysiology of posterior blepharitis is meibomian gland dysfunction. The signs and symptoms of this disease are exacerbated by abnormalities in the lipid layer of the tear film, which is produced by the meibomian glands. Obstruction of the meibomian ducts causes accumulation of meibomian secretions known as meibum (Figure 13-24). Accumulation of meibum within the meibomian gland can lead to inflammation of the gland and bacterial colonization.[1,3,68,75–79] The colonizing bacteria have lipases that break the nonpolar wax and sterol esters into triglycerides and free fatty acids (polar lipids), thus altering the normal composition of the meibum.[33,80] The polar lipids diffuse more easily through the aqueous layer and contaminate the mucin layer, making it hydrophobic.[81] This causes the tear film to become unstable, and the surface of the eye becomes unwettable. The abnormal meibum has a melting point above the ocular surface temperature, in contrast to normal meibum, which has a melting point equal to or lower than the ocular surface temperature.[75,79,82] The abnormal meibum, therefore, solidifies and obstructs the ducts, leading to further inflammation and perpetuating the vicious cycle. TCSA, as a highly specific immunomodulator that affects primarily T lymphocytes, may decrease the inflammation of the meibomian glands and thus reduce their plugging and dysfunction.

RESTASIS AND OCULAR ROSACEA

Rosacea is a common oculodermal disorder primarily affecting the sebaceous glands of the face and the meibomian glands of the eyelids. Recent studies estimate the prevalence of potentially blinding ocular pathology to be between 6% and 18% of patients with acne rosacea (Figures 13-25 and 13-26).[83] Ocular signs and symptoms are common and include foreign body sensation, photophobia, lid margin telangiectasia, meibomian gland inflammation and inspissation, decreased tear BUT, conjunctival hyperemia, and marginal corneal ulcers and vascularization. In addition, this autoimmune disease routinely produces tear film abnormalities, which result in complaints of blurred vision, tearing, and burning. Tear film instability, characterized by rapid tear BUT, leads to decreased tear production and function.[84] As a result, the

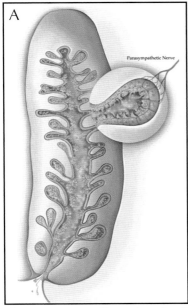
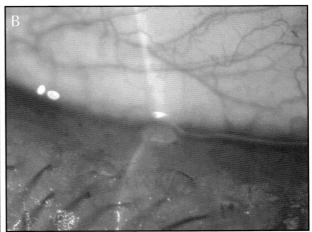

Figure 13-24. (A) Illustration of meibomian gland demonstrating secretion of lipid layer of tear film. (Reprinted with permission from Pflugfelder SC, Beuerman RW, Stern ME. *Dry Eye and Ocular Surface Disorders*. New York: Marcel Dekker; 2004:248.) (B) Clinical photograph of inspissated meibomian gland.

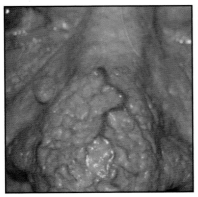

Figure 13-25. Clinical photograph of severe dermatological effect of rosacea.

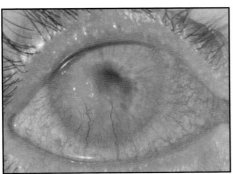

Figure 13-26. Clinical photograph of severe effects of ocular rosacea.

corneal and conjunctival epithelium of these patients often exhibits significant pathology compared with normal subjects.[85] Artificial tears have been used for chronic management of dry eye symptoms; however, these drops provide insufficient long-term symptomatic relief in most patients and fail to address the underlying pathology. Traditional treatment for ocular rosacea has included lid hygiene with warm soaks, use of the oral tetracycline family of antibiotics, application of topical antibiotics to lid margins, or short courses of corticosteroids.

Two recent studies were performed examining the role of TCSA in the management of ocular rosacea. One investigation was a retrospective chart review that surveyed patients with chronic ocular rosacea, refractory to traditional treatments, who were subsequently administered cyclosporine 0.05% ophthalmic emulsion.[86] The second recent study investigated the efficacy of TCSA compared to an artificial tear solution (Refresh Plus) used as a control for the treatment of rosacea-associated eyelid and corneal pathology.[87]

In the first study, a retrospective chart review of patients diagnosed with ocular rosacea, all patients had active inflammation of lids and ocular surface (many for several months prior to the study). All patients from a large group practice treated with cyclosporine ophthalmic emulsion over a 17-month period were included, and they all failed to respond to other currently available treatments (including oral tetracycline, warm soaks with lid hygiene, topical antibiotics, or short courses of topical steroids).

The treatment regimen for the initial 1 to 2 weeks consisted of loteprednol etabonate 0.5% (Lotemax, Bausch & Lomb, Rochester, NY) or fluorometholone 0.1% ophthalmic suspension (FML, Allergan, Inc, Irvine, Calif) twice daily, oral tetracycline (250 mg) or doxycycline (100 mg) once daily, and gatifloxacin 0.3% ophthalmic solution (Zymar, Allergan, Inc, Irvine, Calif) 4 times daily if conjunctivitis was present. The treatment regimen thereafter consisted of TCSA twice daily. After starting cyclosporine, oral tetracycline/doxycycline was continued, while loteprednol or fluorometholone tapered off over 2 weeks.

Evaluation of treatment efficacy consisted of a patient symptom assessment, clinical examination, including supravital staining with lissamine green and/or fluorescein, and follow-up for at least 6 months.

The results of the study showed that 18% (10/55) of patients with ocular rosacea refractory to other treatments showed complete resolution when treated with cyclosporine 0.05% ophthalmic emulsion, 31% (17/55) showed significant improvement, 31% (17/55) experienced mild (4) to moderate (13) relief of symptoms and improved clinical signs, 4% (2/55) had recurrence of symptoms while on treatment despite initial improvement, and 20% (11/55) of patients showed poor response to the treatment and withdrew before 6 months (Figure 13-27). At last follow-up visit, 5% of the patients who responded to cyclosporine (2/44) were able to discontinue all medications without recurrence of rosacea. TCSA was sufficient to control ocular rosacea in 68% of responsive patients (30/44). They required no additional medications 27% (12/44) and continued low-dose tetracycline along with topical cyclosporine (Figure 13-28).

This study demonstrated that TCSA effectively treated signs and symptoms of ocular rosacea in patients who failed to respond to other treatments. The majority of patients were able to discontinue oral tetracyclines, but most required continued treatment with cyclosporine 0.05% to manage the condition.

In the second investigation, a double-masked clinical trial of 37 patients with rosacea-associated eyelid and corneal changes were enrolled in a study comparing the

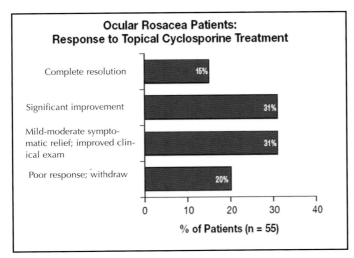

Figure 13-27. Response to topical cyclosporine after at least 6 months of treatment.

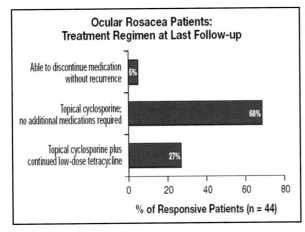

Figure 13-28. Ocular rosacea patients: treatment regimen at last follow-up.

efficacy of TCSA with artificial tear solution in treating rosacea-associated eyelid and corneal pathology. Patients were enrolled after any active infections were treated with lid scrubs and antibiotics. Once the infection was clinically controlled, patients were randomized to cyclosporine or artificial tears for 3 months. All patients were withdrawn from oral doxycycline for at least 2 weeks prior to the study, and patients with eyelid defects or lagophthalmos were excluded.

At each visit, patients were assessed by the OSDI questionnaire, Schirmer's testing with anesthesia, measurement of corneal staining, and tear BUT. The number of meibomian glands expressed (due to inspissation) and the quality of the excreta were also evaluated at each study visit. Changes from baseline were described at follow-up visits, and final patient success was evaluated at the month 3 visit. Patients who were still symptomatic after their initial regimen (at the month 3 evaluation) were offered a switch to the alternate regimen and returned for a follow-up assessment after 1 month.

Table 13-5 EXPECTATIONS FOR THE FIRST MONTHS OF THERAPY WITH TOPICAL CYCLOSPORIN A		
One Month	*Three Months*	*Six Months*
Significant improvement in signs and symptoms • Dryness • Itching • Blurred vision • Photophobia • Corneal staining	Key signs and symptoms continue to improve	Improvement maintained with continued therapy

The results of the study demonstrated that TCSA provided statistically significantly greater improvements in Schirmer's scores, TBUT, corneal staining, and OSDI scores compared with artificial tears after 3 months of treatment. TCSA produced a statistically significant increase in Schirmer's (with anesthesia) scores of 2.7 ± 2.2 mm after 3 months of treatment ($P < .001$). Conversely, Schirmer's scores worsened in the artificial tears group, with a mean decrease of 1.4 ± 4.6 mm ($P = .271$). Similarly, the mean TBUT score also significantly improved in the cyclosporine-treated patients (a mean increase of 3.56 ± 1.5 seconds, $P < .001$) but worsened in the control group (a mean decrease of 0.04 ± 1.6 seconds, $P = .929$). Cyclosporine-treated patients exhibited a significantly greater mean reduction in corneal staining (-1.3 ± 0.53) compared with artificial tears (-0.2 ± 0.83) after 3 months of treatment ($P < .001$). Moreover, TCSA provided significantly greater improvement in OSDI scores than did artificial tears (mean reduction of 11.5 ± 8.8 with cyclosporine versus a mean decrease of 2.9 ± 11.6 with artificial tears, $P = .022$). The study demonstrated that TCSA is superior to artificial tears for the treatment of rosacea-associated lid and corneal changes.

RECOMMENDED TOPICAL CYCLOSPORIN A REGIMEN

The recommended dosing for TCSA is 1 drop in each eye every 12 hours. It is important to inform patients to not use "as needed" like traditional drops. Patients may concomitantly use aqueous tears. Nonpreserved tears were used in clinical trials. Patients should allow a 15-minute interval between instillations and realize that additional application of a topical emulsion agent may be poorly tolerated. For patients who wear contact lenses, they should be instructed to remove their contact lenses before administering TCSA and to wait 15 minutes before replacing the lenses.

While it is common to advise patients that it may take 3 months to see an improvement in symptoms after starting TCSA (Table 13-5), a recent study has demonstrated that a positive effect may be seen after only a few weeks of therapy[72] to 30 days of therapy.[88] However, to ensure patient compliance, it is important to caution patients that it could take as much as 90 days of continual use of TCSA to experience improvement.

Patients should be informed that the most common adverse event reported following TCSA use was ocular burning (17%). Other ocular adverse events reported by 1% to 5% of cyclosporine patients included conjunctival hyperemia, discharge, epiphora, eye pain, foreign body sensation, stinging, and visual disturbance. To increase patient comfort, ketorolac 0.4% (Acular LS, Allergan, Inc, Irvine, Calif) could be applied 10 minutes preceding instillation of TCSA and has been demonstrated to increase patient comfort and improve patient compliance in the induction phase of using TCSA (first 6 weeks).[89] Long-term treatment with TCSA over a period of up to 3 years has been demonstrated to be well tolerated and not associated with systemic side effects.[90]

SUMMARY

Topical cyclosporin A ophthalmic emulsion (Restasis) is the first treatment that targets an underlying pathological mechanism for chronic dry eye: immune-mediated inflammation. Furthermore, it is the only purpose-designed topical drug therapy for chronic dry eye syndrome. Restasis has been demonstrated to be safe and effective in animal and human clinical trials. TCSA reduces signs and symptoms of dry eye syndrome, has a favorable pharmacokinetic profile, and is well tolerated, with few and minor ocular adverse effects.

TCSA has no effect on IOP and does not inhibit the phagocytic system as greatly as do corticosteroids, allowing the antimicrobial arm of the immune system to fight infection. Furthermore, TCSA does not inhibit wound healing or produce lens changes. These characteristics create a wide safety profile for this drug.[26] There were no systemic side effects from the topical Restasis, and no detectable serum levels in the phase III trial.

No microbial overgrowth or ocular infections occurred during clinical studies. Restasis is well accepted by patients, and they can expect results in 3 to 6 months of treatment. Most importantly, this agent provides rational pharmacological therapy where none currently exists.

CONCLUSION

In conclusion, the difficulty of diagnosing and treating dry eye syndrome remains problematic. However, a breakthrough in our understanding of the pathogenesis of dry eye syndrome has led to the first drug therapy aimed at treating the cause of dry eye, rather than merely signs or symptoms. Restasis is also useful for a variety of disorders related to dry eye disease, including posterior blepharitis and ocular rosacea. In addition, Restasis has been demonstrated to be effective or has shown promise in the treatment of management of a wide variety of additional ophthalmic disorders. Restasis offers the advantage of immunomodulation without the risk of corticosteroid side effects.

Key Points

1. One major advance in dry eye over the past decade is the understanding that the ocular surface and lacrimal glands function as an integrated unit.
2. Restasis is a 0.05% emulsion of the active ingredient cyclosporin A formulated in a castor oil-based topical emulsion vehicle containing glycerin, polysorbate 80, carbomer 1342, purified water, and sodium hydroxide.
3. The reason that Restasis may ameliorate posterior blepharitis is because underlying the pathophysiology of posterior blepharitis is meibomian gland dysfunction.
4. Restasis effectively treats signs and symptoms of ocular rosacea in patients who failed to respond to other treatments.
5. The recommended dosing for Restasis is 1 drop in each eye every 12 hours.

REFERENCES

1. Schaumberg DA, Sullivan DA, Buring JE, Dana MR. Prevalence of dry eye syndrome among US women. *Am J Ophthalmol.* 2003;136:318–326.
2. Fox RI, Howell FV, Bone RC, Michelson P. Primary Sjögren's syndrome: clinical and immunopathologic features. *Sem Arthritis Rheumatol.* 1984;14:77–105.
3. Lin PY, Tsai SY, Cheng CY, Liu JH, Chou P, Hsu WM. Prevalence of dry eye among an elderly Chinese population in Taiwan: the Shihpai Eye Study. *Ophthalmology.* 2003;110:1096–1101.
4. Schein OD, Tielsch JM, Munoz B, et al. Relationship between signs and symptoms of dry eye in the elderly: a population-based perspective. *Ophthalmology.* 1997;104:1395–1401.
5. Afonso AA, Monroy D, Tseng SCG, Stern M, Pflugflelder SC. Diagnostic sensitivity and specificity of Schirmer's test and fluorescein clearance test for ocular irritation. *Ophthalmology.* 1999;106:803–810.
6. Macri A, Pflugfelder S. Correlation of the Schirmer's 1 and fluorescein clearance tests with the severity of corneal epithelial and eyelid disease. *Arch Ophthalmol.* 2000;118:1632.
7. Chodosh J, Dix R, Howell RC, Stoop WG, Tseng SCG. Staining characteristics and antiviral activities of sulfonhodamine B and lissamine green. *Invest Ophthalmol Vis Sci.* 1994;35:1046–1058.
8. Feenstra RBG, Tseng SCG. Comparison of fluorescein and rose bengal staining. *Ophthalmology.* 1992;110:984–993.
9. Kim J, Foulks G. Evaluation of the effect of lissamine green and rose bengal on human corneal epithelial cells. *Cornea.* 1999;183:328–332.
10. Manning FJ, Wehely SR, Foulks GN. Patient tolerance and ocular surface staining characteristics of lissamine green versus rose bengal. *Ophthalmology.* 1995;102:1953–1957.
11. Lemp MA. Report of the National Eye Institute/Industry workshop on clinical trials on dry eyes. *CLAO J.* 1995;21:221–232.
12. Huang B, Mirza MA, Qazi MA, Pepose JS. The effect of punctual occlusion on wavefront aberrations in dry eye patients after laser in situ keratomileusis. *Am J Ophthalmol.* 2004;137:52–61.
13. Sade De Paiva C, Pflugfelder SC. Corneal epitheliopathy of dry eye induces hyperesthesia to mechanical air jet stimulation. *Am J Ophthalmol.* 2004;137:109–115.
14. Pflugfelder SC, Jones D, Ji Z, Afonso A, Monroy D. Altered cytokine balance in the tear fluid and conjunctiva of patients with Sjogren's syndrome keratoconjunctivitis sicca. *Curr Eye Res.* 1999;19:201–211.

15. McDonnell PJ, Doyle J, Stern L, Behrens A, and Dysfunctional Tear Syndrome Group. A modified Delphi technique to obtain consensus on the treatment of dysfunctional tear syndrome. *Invest Ophthalmol Vis Sci.* 2004; E-Abstract 3909, available at www.arvo.org.

16. Behrens A, Pirouzmanesh A, Almeda TI, et al. Dysfunctional tear syndrome therapy: an evidence–based review. *Invest Ophthalmol Vis Sci.* 2004; E-Abstract 3459, available at www.arvo.org.

17. Song XJ, Li DQ, Farley W, Luo LH, et al. Neurturin-deficient mice develop dry eye and keratoconjunctivitis sicca. *Invest Ophthalmol Vis Sci.* 2003;44:4223–4229.

18. Prabhasawat P, Tseng SC. Frequent association of delayed tear clearance in ocular irritation. *Br J Ophthalmol.* 1998;82:666–675.

19. Stern ME, Gao J, Siemasko KF, Beuerman RW, Pflugfelder SC. The role of the lacrimal functional unit in the pathophysiology of dry eye. *Exp Eye Res.* 2004;78:409–416.

20. Pflugfelder SC. Antiinflammatory therapy for dry eye. *Am J Ophthalmol.* 2004;137:337–342.

21. Marsh P, Pflugfelder SC. Topical non-preserved methylprednisolone therapy of keratoconjunctivitis sicca. *Ophthalmology.* 1999;106:939–943.

22. Solomon R, Perry HD, Donnenfeld ED, Greenman HE. Slit-lamp biomicroscopy of the tear film of patients using topical Restasis and Refresh Endura. *J Cataract Refract Surg.* 2005;31:661–663.

23. Calne RY, White PJG. The use of cyclosporine A in clinical organ grafting. *Ann Surg.* 1982; 9:330–335.

24. Kirby B, Harrison PV. Combination low-dose cyclosporine (Neoral) hydroxyurea for severe recalcitrant psoriasis. *Br J Dermatol.* 1999;140:186–187.

25. Popovic M, Stefanovic D, Pejnovic N, et al. Comparative study of the clinical efficacy of four DMARDs (leflunomide, methotrexate, cyclosporine, and levamisole) in patients with rheumatoid arthritis. *Transplant Proc.* 1998;30:4135–4136.

26. Perry HD, Donnenfeld ED, Kanellopoulos AJ, Grossman GA. Topical cyclosporine A in the management of post-keratoplasty glaucoma. *Cornea.* 1997;16:284–288.

27. Bar-Ilan A, Neumann R. Basic considerations of ocular drug-delivery systems. In: Zimmerman TJ, Kooner KS, Sharir M, Fechtner RD, eds. *Textbook of Ocular Pharmacology.* Philadelphia: Lippincott-Raven; 1997:139–150.

28. *Stedman's Medical Dictionary.* 25th ed. Baltimore, Md: Williams and Wilkins; 1990:505.

29. Sall K, Stevenson OD, Mundorf TK, Reis BL. Two multicenter, randomized studies of the efficacy and safety of cyclosporine ophthalmic emulsion in moderate to severe dry eye disease. CsA Phase 3 Study Group. *Ophthalmology.* 2000;107:631–639.

30. Stevenson D, Tauber J, Reis BL. Efficacy and safety of cyclosporin A ophthalmic emulsion in the treatment of moderate-to-severe dry eye disease: a dose-ranging, randomized trial. The cyclosporin A phase 2 study group. *Ophthalmology.* 2000;107:967–974.

31. Nelson JD, Helms H, Fiscella R, et al. A new look at dry eye disease and its treatment. *Adv Ther.* 2000;17:84–93.

32. Rao SN. Comparison of the efficacy of topical cyclosporine 0.05% compared with tobradex for the treatment of posterior blepharitis. *Invest Ophthalmol Vis Sci.* 2005; E-Abstract 2662, available at www.arvo.org.

33. Perry HD, Doshi-Carnevale S, Donnenfeld ED, et al. Efficacy of topical cyclosporin A 0.05% in the treatment of meibomian gland dysfunction. *Cornea.* 2006;25:171–175.

34. Perry HD, Wittpenn JR, D'Aversa G, Donnenfeld ED. Topical cyclosporine 0.05% for the treatment of chronic, active ocular rosacea. *Invest Ophthalmol Vis Sci.* 2005; E-Abstract 2660, available at www.arvo.org.

35. Wittpenn JR, Schechter B. Efficacy of cyclosporin A for the treatment of ocular rosacea. *Invest Ophthalmol Vis Sci.* 2005; E-Abstract 2846, available at www.arvo.org.

36. Mendicute J, Aranzasti C, Eder F, Ostolaza JI, Salaberria M. Topical cyclosporin A 2% in the treatment of vernal keratoconjunctivitis. *Eye.* 1997;11:75–78.

37. Manvikar S, Figueiredo FC. Thygeson's superficial punctate keratitis: topical cyclosporin A drops use in patients resistant to topical steroids. *Invest Ophthalmol Vis Sci.* 2003; E-Abstract 3745, available at www.arvo.org.

38. Reinhard T, Sundmacher R. Topical cyclosporin A in Thygeson's superficial punctuate keratitis. *Graefes Arch Clin Exp Ophthalmol.* 1999;237:109–112.

39. Perry HD, Doshi S, Donnenfeld ED, et al. Topical cyclosporin A 0.5% as a possible new treatment for superior limbic keratoconjunctivitis. *Ophthalmology.* 2003;110:1578–1581.

40. Saib G, McDonald M. Use of cyclosporine 0.05% drops versus unpreserved artificial tears in dry-eye patients having LASIK. Presented at the American Society of Cataract and Refractive Surgery Symposium on Cataract, IOL, and Refractive Surgery; San Diego, Calif; 2003.

41. Perry HD, Donnenfeld ED, Acheampong A, et al. Topical cyclosporin A in the management of postkeratoplasty glaucoma and corticosteroid-induced ocular hypertension (CIOH) and the penetration of topical 0.5% cyclosporine A into the cornea and anterior chamber. *CLAO J.* 1998;24:159–165.

42. Heiligenhaus A, Steuhl KP. Treatment of HSV-1 stromal keratitis with topical cyclosporin A: a pilot study. *Graefes Arch Clin Exp Ophthalmol.* 1999;237:435–438.

43. Akpek EK, Dart JK, Watson S, et al. A randomized trial of topical cyclosporin 0.05% in topical steroid-resistant atopic keratoconjunctivitis. *Ophthalmology.* 2004;111:476–482.

44. Gunduz K, Ozdemir O. Topical cyclosporin treatment of keratoconjunctivitis sicca in secondary Sjogren's syndrome. *Acta Ophthalmol (Copenh).* 1994;72:438–442.

45. Sharma A, Gupta A, Ram J, Nirankari VS. Topical cyclosporin A: an adjunct in severe keratomycosis. Presented as a poster at the American Academy of Ophthalmology Annual Meeting; Anaheim, Calif; 2003.

46. Bell NP, Karp CL, Alfonso EC, et al. Effects of methylprednisolone and cyclosporine A on fungal growth in vitro. *Cornea.* 1999;18:306–313.

47. Roberts CW, Carniglia PE, Brazzo BG. Comparison of cyclosporine to punctal plugs in relieving the signs and symptoms of dry eyes. *Invest Ophthalmol Vis Sci.* 2005; E-Abstract 2027, available at www.arvo.org.

48. Behar-Cohen FF, Bourges J-L, Agla E, et al. Prevention of corneal graft rejection by eye drop instillation of UNIL088, a hydrosoluble prodrug of cyclosporin A. *Invest Ophthalmol Vis Sci.* 2004; E-Abstract 598, available at www.arvo.org.

49. Xi XH, Qin B, Jiang DY. Cyclosporin A combined with dexamethasone in preventing and treating immune rejection after penetrating keratoplasty. *Hunan Yi Ke Da Xue Xue Bao.* 2003;28:627–630.

50. Holland EJ, Olsen TW, Ketcham JM, et al. Topical cyclosporine A in the treatment of anterior segment inflammatory disease. *Cornea.* 1993;12:413–419.

51. Bouzas E, Karadimas P, Kotsiras I, Mastorakos G. Topical cyclosporin 0.05% ophthalmic emulsion in patients with dysthyroid ophthalmopathy. *Invest Ophthalmol Vis Sci.* 2005; E-Abstract 2659, available at www.arvo.org.

52. Velasco P, Baca O, Velasco R. Topic cyclosporin "A" in the management of allergic conjunctivitis. *Invest Ophthalmol Vis Sci.* 2003; E-Abstract 3798, available at www.arvo.org.

53. Akpek EK, Tatlipinar S. Topical cyclosporin in the treatment of ocular surface disorders: an evidence-based update. *Invest Ophthalmol Vis Sci.* 2005; E-Abstract 2642, available at www.arvo.org.

54. Doan S, Elbim C, Gabison E. Efficacy of topical cyclosporin A in phlyctenular keratoconjunctivitis associated with severe corneal inflammation. *Invest Ophthalmol Vis Sci.* 2003; E-Abstract 681, available at www.arvo.org.

55. Lelli GJ, Mian S. Ophthalmic cyclosporine use in ocular graft versus host disease. *Invest Ophthalmol Vis Sci.* 2004; E-Abstract 1472, available at www.arvo.org. Accessed May 30, 2005.

56. McCarthy JM, Dubord PJ, Chalmers A, et al. Cyclosporin A for the treatment of necrotizing scleritis and corneal melting in patients with rheumatoid arthritis. *J Rheumatol.* 1992;19:1358–1361.

57. Wu H, Chen G. Cyclosporin A and thiotepa in prevention of postoperative recurrence of pterygium. *Yan Ke Xue Bao.* 1999;91–92.

58. Dios E, Herreras JM, Mayo A, Blanco G. Efficacy of systemic cyclosporin A and amniotic membrane on rabbit conjunctival limbal allograft rejection. *Cornea.* 2005;24:182–188.

59. Perry HD, Doshi SJ, Donnenfeld ED, Bai GS. Topical cyclosporin A in the management of therapeutic keratoplasty for mycotic keratitis. *Cornea.* 2002;21:161–163.

60. Hom MM, Comparison of cyclosporin A versus a contact lens rewetter for contact lens intolerance: a pilot study. Presented as a poster at the American Academy of Optometry; Tampa, Fla; December 11, 2004.

61. Gottsch JD, Akpeka EK. Topical cyclosporine stimulates neovascularization in resolving sterile rheumatoid central corneal ulcers. *Tr Am Ophth Soc.* 2000;98:81–90.

62. Belin MW, Bouchard CS, Phillips TM. Update on topical cyclosporin A. Background, immunology, and pharmacology. *Cornea.* 1990;184–195.

63. Kaswan RL, Salisbury MA, Ward DA. Spontaneous canine keratoconjunctivitis sicca. A useful model for human keratoconjunctivitis sicca: treatment with cyclosporine eye drops. *Arch Ophthalmol.* 1989;107:1210–1216.

64. Gao J, Schwalb TA, Addeo JV. The role of apoptosis in the pathogenesis of canine keratoconjunctivitis sicca: the effect of topical cyclosporin A therapy. *Cornea.* 1998;17:654–663.

65. Tsubota K, Saito I, Ishimaru N, Hayashi Y. Use of topical cyclosporin A in a primary Sjögren's syndrome mouse model. *Invest Ophthalmol Vis Sci.* 1998;39:1551–1559.

66. Power WJ, Mullaney P, Farrell M, Collum LM. Effect of topical cyclosporin A on conjunctival T-cells in patients with secondary Sjögren's syndrome. *Cornea.* 1993;12:507–511.

67. Laibovitz RA, Solch S, Andriano K, et al. Pilot trial of cyclosporine 1 percent ophthalmic ointment in the treatment of keratoconjunctivitis sicca. *Cornea.* 1993;124:311–323.

68. Kunert KS, Tisdale AS, Gipson IK. Goblet cell numbers and epithelial proliferation in the conjunctiva of patients with dry eye syndrome treated with cyclosporine. *Arch Ophthalmol.* 2002;120:330–337.

69. Turner K, Pflugfelder SC, Ji Z, Feuer WJ, Stern M. Interleukin-6 levels in the conjunctival epithelium of patients with dry eye disease treated with cyclosporine ophthalmic emulsion. *Cornea.* 2000;19:492–496.

70. Kunert KS, Tisdale AS, Stern ME, Smith JA, Gipson IK. Analysis of topical cyclosporine treatment of patients with dry eye syndrome: effect on conjunctival lymphocytes. *Arch Ophthalmol.* 2000;118:1489–1496.

71. Perry HD, Donnenfeld ED, Perry AR, et al. Evaluation of topical cyclosporin A 0.05% for the treatment of dry eye disease. Presented at the American Academy of Ophthalmology Annual Meeting; New Orleans, La; 2004.

72. Stonecipher K, Perry HK, Gross RG, Kerney DL. The impact of topical cyclosporin A emulsion 0.05% (TCSA) on the outcomes of patients with keratoconjunctivitis sicca (KCS). *Curr Med Res Opin.* 2005;21:1057–1063.

73. Tauber J. A dose-ranging clinical trial to assess the safety and efficacy of cyclosporine ophthalmic emulsion in patients with keratoconjunctivitis sicca. The cyclosporine study group. *Adv Exp Med Biol.* 1998;438:969–972.

74. Perry HD, Doshi S, Donnenfeld ED, et al. Double masked randomized controlled study evaluating topical 0.05% cyclosporin A in the treatment of meibomian gland dysfunction (posterior blepharitis). *Invest Ophthalmol Vis Sci.* 2003; E-Abstract 1395, Available at www. arvo.org.

75. Hori Y, Spurr-Michaud S, Russo CL, et al. Differentiation regulation of membrane-associated mucins in the human ocular surface epithelium. *Invest Ophthalmol Vis Sci.* 2004;45:112–117.

76. Smith RE, Flowers CW. Chronic blepharitis: a review. *CLAO J.* 1995;21:200–207.

77. Driver PJ, Lemp MA. Meibomian gland dysfunction. *Surv Ophthalmol.* 1996;40:343–367.

78. Zengin N, Tol H, Gunduz K, Okundan S, Balevi S, Endogru H. Meibomian gland dysfunction and tear film abnormalities in rosacea. *Cornea.* 1995;14:144–146.

79. McCulley JP, Shine WE. Meibomian secretions in chronic blepharitis. *Adv Exp Med Biol.* 1998; 438:319–326.

80. Shine WE, Silvany R, McCulley JP. Relation of cholesterol-stimulated *Staphylococcus aureus* growth to chronic blepharitis. *Invest Ophthalmol Vis Sci.* 1993;34:2291–2296.

81. Shine WE, McCulley JP. Keratoconjunctivitis sicca associated with meibomian secretion polar lipid abnormality. *Arch Ophthalmol.* 1998;116:849–852.

82. Shine WE, McCulley JP. Meibomian gland triglyceride fatty acid differences in chronic blepharitis patients. *Cornea.* 1996;15:340–346.

83. Stone DU, Chodosh J. Ocular rosacea: an update on pathogenesis and therapy. *Curr Opin Ophthalmol.* 2004;15:499–502.

84. Bowman RW, McCulley JP, Jester JV. Meibomian gland dysfunction and rosacea. In: Pepose J, Holland G, Wilhelmus K, eds. *Ocular Infection and Immunity.* St. Louis, Mo: Mosby-Year Book; 1996:334–343.

85. Kocak-Altintas AG, Kocak-Midillioglu I, Gul U, Bilezikci B, Isiksacan O, Duman S. Impression cytology and ocular characteristics in ocular rosacea. *Eur J Ophthalmol.* 2003;13:351–359.

86. Perry HD, Wittpenn JR, D'Aversa G, Donnenfeld ED. Topical cyclosporine 0.05% for the treatment of chronic, active ocular rosacea. *Invest Ophthalmol Vis Sci.* 2005; E-Abstract 2660, available at www.arvo.org.

87. Wittpenn JR, Schechter B. Efficacy of cyclosporin A for the treatment of ocular rosacea. *Invest Ophthalmol Vis Sci.* 2005; E-Abstract 2846, available at www.arvo.org.

88. Herrygers L, Noecker R. Efficacy of cyclosporin A (Restasis) for the treatment of dry eye symptoms in the first 30 days of therapy. *Invest Ophthalmol Vis Sci.* 2005; E-Abstract 2026, available at www.arvo.org.

89. Schechter B, Wittpenn J. Evaluation of ketorolac 0.4% (Acular LS) during the induction phase of cyclosporin A (Restasis) therapy to improve patient comfort. *Invest Ophthalmol Vis Sci.* 2005; E-Abstract 2033, available at www.arvo.org.

90. Barber LG, Foulks GN, Pflugfelder SC, Tauber J. Phase 3 safety evaluation of cyclosporine 0.1% ophthalmic emulsion instilled twice daily for up to 3 Years. *Ophthalmology.* 2005;112: 1790–1794.

Disclaimer of financial interest: Drs. Perry, Wittpenn, and Donnenfeld are paid consultants for Allergan, Inc, Irvine, Calif.

14

Management: Miscellaneous Modalities

Soosan Jacob, MS, FRCS, Dip NB;
C. Sujatha, DO; Juan Murube, MD; and
Amar Agarwal, MS, FRCS, FRCOphth

INTRODUCTION

Over 10 million Americans suffer from dry eyes. Many different factors contribute to dry eye syndrome. It is usually caused by a problem with the quality of the tear film that lubricates the eyes. The tear film is composed of 3 layers (Figure 14-1). The innermost mucus layer forms a foundation for the tear film to adhere to the eye. The middle aqueous layer provides moisture and supplies oxygen and other important nutrients to the cornea. This layer is made of 98% water along with small amounts of salt, proteins, and other compounds. The outer lipid layer is an oily film that seals the tear film on the eye and helps to prevent evaporation as well as spillage of tears onto the lids.

The normal aging of tear glands, as well as extended use of contact lenses, environmental pollutants, prescription drugs, refractive surgery, autoimmune diseases, nutrient deficiencies, and other disorders can cause abnormalities in tear production and retention process. The typical symptoms of dry eye syndrome include dryness; grittiness; itching; burning; irritation; redness; blurred vision that improves with blinking; excessive tearing or watering; increased discomfort after periods of reading, watching TV, or working on a computer; and difficulty in reading for long periods of time. In severe cases, there may be photosensitivity, pain, and defective vision. Successful treatment is thus essential to avoid permanent damage.

Three characteristics are included in the triple classification of dry eye and this is in the classification of Madrid:

1. Etiopathogenesis.
2. Clinical severity.
3. The histologically affected subsystem (ALMEN classification).

Figure 14-1. The tear film is composed of 3 layers: innermost mucin layer, middle aqueous layer, and outermost lipid layer.

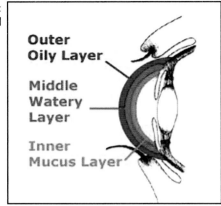

Lifestyle Changes

Many factors, such as high altitudes; hot, dry, or windy climates; air-conditioning; and cigarette smoke cause dry eyes. Drinking plenty of water each day keeps the body hydrated and flushes impurities. Rubbing the eyes should be avoided because it may worsen the irritation. Many people suffer from computer vision syndrome (CVS) or the visual display unit syndrome in which their eyes become irritated during reading or working on a computer. Ergonomic seating and stopping periodically to rest and blink keeps the eyes more comfortable. Making a conscious effort to blink frequently is also especially important when reading or watching television.

Treatment of Precipitating Factors

Certain medications, thyroid conditions, vitamin A deficiency, and diseases such as Parkinson's and Sjögren's can also cause dryness. These underlying conditions should be treated to help in decreasing the severity of the dry eyes.

Contact Lens Care

This patient population may suffer from dryness because the contact lenses absorb the tears and cause protein deposition on the lens surface. For patients with dry eyes, contact lens wear can be very uncomfortable. The eye normally needs tears for lubrication and with contact lens wear, this lubrication is even more essential.

Cleaning and maintenance of the contact lenses is extremely important. Proteins and other airborne particles can build up deposits on the contact lens when not properly washed and this can cause irritation, redness, and allergic reactions, more pronounced in the dry eye patient. A dry lens with deposits can rub and cause damage to the ocular surface. Proper care of the contact lens along with storing the lens in the solution overnight replenishes the moisture and durability of the lens. Patients with borderline dryness may need to discontinue contact lens wear or change over to other types of contact lens materials. They can also use daily disposable lenses to decrease deposit build up, which in turn leads to a decrease in the symptoms.

HORMONAL THERAPY

Dryness commonly occurs secondary to the normal aging process. With aging, especially in females, the body produces less oil. This also affects the lipid layer of the tear film. In the presence of a defective lipid layer, the tear film evaporates much faster, leaving dry spots on the cornea and a decreased tear BUT. Women frequently experience dry eyes as they enter menopause because of hormonal changes. HRT, especially the use of estrogen alone, leads to increased risk of dry eye syndrome.[1] The odds of having dry eyes were 70% more if postmenopausal women used HRT. Each 3-year increase in the duration of HRT use was associated with a 15% increase in the risk of having dry eyes. It is thought to promote both meibomian gland dysfunction and evaporative dry eye. Estrogens have been shown to induce a significant decrease in the size, activity, and lipid production by sebaceous glands whereas androgens appear to modulate meibomian gland function, improve the quality and/or quantity of lipids produced by this tissue, and promote the formation of the tear film's lipid layer.[2–5] The meibomian gland, like other sebaceous glands, is an androgen target organ. Estrogens enhance the polyclonal B cell activation, autoantibody formation, and tissue abnormalities encountered in Sjögren's syndrome.[6] They have also been used clinically to reduce sebaceous gland function and secretion in humans.[2]

Androgen deficiency is also thought to contribute to aqueous-deficient dry eye in Sjögren's syndrome, menopause, and aging. Systemic androgen administration alleviates dry eye signs and symptoms and stimulates tear flow in Sjögren's syndrome patients.[7] The hormone actions seem to be mediated through androgen receptors within epithelial cell nuclei and involves the regulation of numerous genes (including those related to lipid, sex steroid, and other cellular metabolic pathways).[8]

Certain studies have found no significant influence of estrogens on the lacrimal gland or the tear film.[9] Some studies have even proposed that estrogens may promote lacrimal gland function, suppress lacrimal tissue inflammation in Sjögren's syndrome, and serve as a treatment for dry eye signs and symptoms.[9,10]

OTHER DRUGS/FORMULATIONS

Vitamin A

Hypovitaminosis A should be suspected in severe cases of dry eye.[11,12] Topical retinoids significantly reduced the symptoms and increased the goblet cell density.[12] In relatively high concentrations, it may be used topically for severe dry eye conditions. It may be used as drops or as ointment.

Oral Tetracyclines

In severe dry eyes, chronic inflammation of the lacrimal glands, ocular surface, and lids may be seen due to release of cytokines from the ocular surface. Oral tetracyclines may be useful as an anti-inflammatory in these cases.[12]

Botulinum Toxin Injection

Injection into the medial part of the lids may act by interfering with the lacrimal pump mechanism, and thus inhibit tear drainage.[13] This is not very popular as of now due to unpleasant associated side effects of botulinum toxin. Further studies are required to assess the clinical value of this treatment.

Oral Antioxidants

These have been used for the treatment of dry eyes. They are required for the normal production and secretion of tears and tear constituents. Oral antioxidants improved both tear stability and conjunctival health.[14,15] Vitamins A, C, E, B$_6$, zinc, selenium, molybdenum, and carotenoids amongst others are especially important.

Essential Fatty Acids

The body does not produce essential fatty acids (EFAs), so they must be supplied through diet. The 2 basic categories of EFAs are omega-3 and omega-6. An ideal diet includes a ratio of 4 parts omega-6 to 1 part omega-3. The omega-6 EFAs are found in raw nuts (almonds, walnuts, and their oils), seeds (sesame, sunflower, and their oils), borage oil, grape seed oil, primrose oil, soybean oil, whole grains, and legumes. Omega-3 EFAs are found in cold water fish such as salmon, mackerel, sardines, and herring. They are also in certain vegetables, flaxseeds, walnuts, and canola oil. It is essential to consume EFAs properly for the body to receive their full benefit. EFAs are destroyed with heat, causing free radicals to form, which may cause damage to healthy cells.

Therapy with essential fatty acids such as systemic linoleic (LA) and gamma-linolenic acid (GLA) and tear substitutes reduces ocular surface inflammation and improves dry eye symptoms. Long-term studies are needed to confirm the role of this new therapy for KCS.[16]

Diquafosol Tetrasodium

This is a new treatment agent that has recently been approved by the FDA. It is a second-generation uridine nucleotide analog, P2Y2 purinergic receptor agonist, acting on P2Y2 receptors on the ocular surface to stimulate the fluid pump mechanism of the accessory lacrimal glands on the conjunctival surface.[17-19] Goblet cell secretion of ocular mucins is stimulated and there may be some increase in ocular lipid (the outer most layer of the tear film) production. It is claimed to provide rapid, receptor-mediated rehydration of the ocular surface through the coordinated production of salt, water, mucin, and possibly lipid, thus restoring major tear film components (Figure 14-2). It is an unpreserved, sterile, aqueous eye drop administered QID for dry eye and can be used for treatment of dry eye patients who have failed to respond to lubricants or as a supplementary treatment for patients with severe dry eye who may be using other treatments such as topical cyclosporine.

Miscellaneous Oral Formulations

Preparations containing ingredients such as mucopolysaccharides, turmeric extract and lactoferrin, black currant seed oil, and cod liver oil are available in the market as various proprietary formulations for dry eyes.

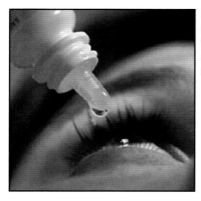

Figure 14-2. Diquafasol tetrasodium provides rapid, receptor-mediated rehydration of the ocular surface through the coordinated production of salt, water, mucin, and possibly lipid, thus restoring major tear film components.

Herbal Extracts

These have recently received propaganda as being useful for relieving symptoms. They are claimed to be able to boost intracellular metabolism, membrane permeability, and blood microcirculation to the eye. Ingredients include beta carotene, bilberry, chrysanthemum, copper, fructus lycii, semen cassiae, etc.

IODIDE IONTOPHORESIS

Oxidative damage may have a role in the pathogenesis of dry eye disorder. Antioxidants, such as iodide, have shown a strong effect in preventing this damage to the ocular surface.[20] Iodide iontophoresis has been demonstrated to be a safe and well tolerated method of improving subjective and objective dry eye factors in patients with ocular surface disease.[20]

BANDAGE LENSES

Bandage contact lenses worn on an extended wear basis are useful in severe dry eye, leading to painful ocular surface disorder and recurrent corneal erosion. They have a protective action when the blink mechanism may damage the corneal epithelium or in cases of weak adhesion of the corneal epithelium to the basement membrane. The lipid layer is extremely thin over a soft lens. This leads to the aqueous layer evaporating rapidly from the bandage contact lens surface.[21] High water content bandage lenses dehydrate on use and draw fluid from the tears into the bandage lens. This leads to a continuous flow of fluid from tears into the bandage contact lens and out into the surrounding air. In dry eye patients, this leads to an exacerbation of symptoms.

OINTMENTS AND LUBRICANTS

Ointments and lubricants act by preventing frictional damage to the ocular surface secondary to lid movement or extraocular movements. They also act by retaining fluid and maintaining hydration of the ocular surface.[21] It can be used for patients with lagophthalmos, especially if they sleep with the eyes partially open. Ointments and gels are also useful in superficial ocular surface damage.

LID THERAPY

Lid therapy is of use in dry eye of environmental origin. Gentle pinching of the lower or upper lid margin squeezes meibomian oils out onto the ocular surface. This extra lipid is spread over the precorneal tear film with blinking action, thus thickening the lipid layer,[22] which in turn reduces evaporation of tears from the ocular surface.

Lid scrubs are especially useful in cases of mild blepharitis or meibomitis. They are useful for cleaning the lid margin; unblocking meibomian gland openings; and for removing environmental debris (pollution), make up, dry skin, denatured skin, and mucosal secretions.[21] Lid massaging expresses fresh meibomian secretions through the duct openings. If meibomian secretions are too viscid, hot compresses can be used to soften the secretions, which eases the passage of meibomian oils to the ocular surface.

LIPOSOMAL SPRAYS

Liposomal sprays are claimed, by the manufacturers, to enhance skin and mucous membranes. The spray is made of microvesicles[21] consisting of an inner aqueous phase and an outer phospholipid bilayer floating in an aqueous outer phase. Proper clinical trials are required for validating these claims.

MOISTURE RETENTION

The use of goggles are helpful in maintaining high levels of humidity around the eyes. Flexible side shields can be fitted to the patient's spectacles to enhance retention of moisture.[21] Semirigid goggles that fit over one eye are available in the rare cases of monocular dry eye. Swimmer's goggles are a cheap and very good alternative. The disadvantage is condensation of moisture behind the lenses, reducing vision.

SYSTANE

Alcon Laboratories has introduced Systane, a new artificial tear that provides long-lasting relief from distressing dry eye symptoms.[23,24] Systane is derived from "system" to sustain moisture on the eye. It has a polymerizing protective property that helps to form a gel-like coat over the surface, which creates an environment for healing of the epithelial cells. It is the first lubricant to relieve signs and symptoms of dry eye. It gives temporary relief of burning and irritation due to dryness of eyes.

Systane is a multidose aqueous tear containing hydroxypropyl guar (HP-guar) derived from guar, a form of gum; preservative is polyguad relatively nontoxic preservative. The contents are polyethylene glycol 400–0.4% (lubricants), propylene glycol–0.3% (lubricants), boric acid, hydroxypropyl GUAR, calcium chloride, magnesium chloride, potassium chloride, sodium chloride, zinc chloride, polyquaternium-1 (preservative), and purified water.

Systane is a colloidal solution containing HP guar, which is a gelling agent that binds with boric acid to form a cross link. This complex binds to the hydrophobic surface of the cornea, forming a network that is a gel-like consistency. This layer can bind to any kind of desiccation, especially to damaged epithelial cells, creating an ocular shield that allows epithelial repair in a healthy environment. It has been noted that Systane produces 51%

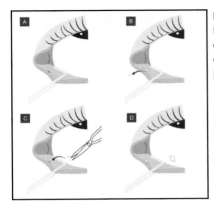

Figure 14-3. Punctal patching with autologous conjunctiva. (A) The punctum is exposed. (B) A square of tissue is excised around the punctum. (C) A corresponding square of bulbar conjunctiva is harvested. (D) The autologous patch is sutured onto the punctum.

decrease in corneal staining from baseline. Statistically significant decrease in morning dryness, end of the day dryness, and foreign body sensation is noted. Because of the increase in viscosity caused by guar, the tear BUT is increased to 20 to 30 seconds. Systane is claimed to be superior to Refresh Tears with respect to preservatives, demulcents, viscosity, and active ingredients. The preservative used in Systane is polyquad, whereas in Refresh Tears, it is purite. The main advantage of Systane is HP-guar, which is pH sensitive. When exposed to ocular pH, viscosity is increased significantly.

It comes in single use and multidose packs and needs to be applied 2 to 3 times per day. Because of its polymerizing protective action that changes according to each individual tear properties and preservative free, Systane is suitable for all eyes without adverse effects.

Punctal Patching With Autologous Conjunctiva

A 2 mm x 2 mm patch of conjunctiva including epithelium and subconjunctival tissue is removed from around the punctum and a similar size graft taken from the same patient's bulbar conjunctiva is sutured in place (Figure 14-3). This causes permanent closure of the punctum. It can be reversed if required by piercing or excising the conjunctival patch over the punctum.[24]

Salivary Supplementation to Tears

The biochemical and physical properties of saliva is such that it is well tolerated by the ocular surface. Hence, surgeries that supplement tears with saliva have been utilized, though only in severe cases of dry eyes.

Stenson's Duct Transposition

The mouth of the Stenson's duct is identified opposite the upper second molar and is dissected including a 1 cm radius of buccal mucosa. The duct is then dissected for 33.5 cm and is then passed via a subcutaneous tunnel through a linear incision in the inferolateral conjunctival fornix where it is then sutured. Interocular decantation can be done by transposition of the nasolacrimal duct of one eye to the conjunctival fornix

Figure 14-4. Stenson's duct transposition with interocular decantation.

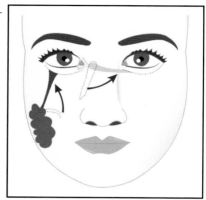

Figure 14-5. Salivary gland transplantation with vascular anastomosis.

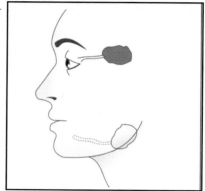

of the other eye (Figure 14-4). A side effect is the crocodile tear syndrome which occurs while eating or thinking of food. This can be taken care of by denervation of the auriculotemporal nerve.

Salivary Gland Transplantation With Vascular Anastomosis

The submandibular gland is dissected and is placed in the temporal fossa where vascular anastomosis is done to the superficial temporal artery and vein (Figure 14-5). This cannot be done in immunological causes of dry eyes such as Sjögren's syndrome where salivary damage is great. It can be done in cases of mild salivary disease.

Salivary Gland Transplantation Without Vascular Anastomosis

One or several pieces of a major or minor salivary gland are transplanted under the preseptal conjunctiva. Spontaneous vascularization of these transplanted tissues has to take place and so a larger area of contact is required (Figure 14-6).

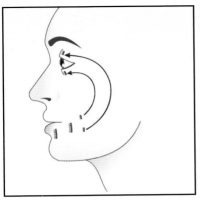

Figure 14-6. Salivary gland transplantation without vascular anastomosis.

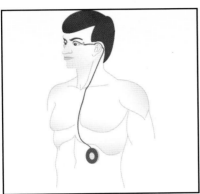

Figure 14-7. Subcutaneous abdominal dacryoreservoir.

DACRYORESERVOIRS

These are done in severe cases of dry eyes and can also be done prior to keratoplasty in severe dry eyes. Here continuous delivery of artificial tears is done into the conjunctival sac from either an external or a subcutaneous abdominal reservoir (Figure 14-7). A pump delivers artificial tears continuously at around 1.5 mL/day. It is refilled via a percutaneous abdominal injection every 45 days.

SUMMARY

There is no perfect cure for dry eye syndrome, but appropriate care along with other treatments can give relief from the frustrating symptoms.

Key Points

1. Ergonomic seating and stopping periodically to rest and blink helps in avoiding CVS. Making a conscious effort to blink frequently is also especially important when reading or watching television.
2. Certain medications, thyroid conditions, vitamin A deficiency, and diseases such as Parkinson's and Sjögren's can cause dryness.
3. Patients with borderline dryness may need to discontinue contact lens wear or change over to other types of contact lens materials or use daily disposable lenses.
4. Bandage contact lenses worn on an extended wear basis are useful in severe dry eye leading to painful ocular surface disorder and recurrent corneal erosion.
5. HRT, especially the use of estrogen alone, leads to increased risk of dry eye syndrome.
6. Diquafosol tetrasodium is claimed to provide rapid, receptor-mediated rehydration of the ocular surface through the coordinated production of salt, water, mucin, and possibly lipid, thus restoring major tear film components.
7. Alcon Laboratories has introduced Systane, a new artificial tear that provides long lasting relief from distressing dry eye symptoms.

REFERENCES

1. Schaumberg DA, Buring JE, Sullivan DA, Dana MR. Hormone replacement therapy and the prevalence of dry eye syndrome. *JAMA.* 2001;286:2114–2119.
2. Sullivan DA, Yamagami H, Liu M, et al. Sex steroids, the meibomian gland and evaporative dry eye. *Adv Exp Med Biol.* 2002;506(Pt A):389–399.
3. Krenzer KL, Dana MR, Ullman MD, Cermak JM. Effect of androgen deficiency on the human meibomian gland and ocular surface. *J Clin Endocr Metab.* 2000;85:4874–4882.
4. Sullivan BD, Evans JE, Krenzer KL, Dana MR, Sullivan DA. Impact of anti-androgen treatment on the fatty acid profile of neutral lipids in human meibomian gland secretions. *J Clin Endocr Metab.* 2000;85:4866–4873.
5. Sullivan BD, Evans JE, Dana MR, Sullivan DA. Impact of androgen deficiency on the lipid profiles in human meibomian gland secretions. *Adv Exp Med Biol.* 2002;506(Pt A):449–458.
6. Sullivan DA. Sex hormones and Sjögren's syndrome. *J Rheumatol.* 1997;24(Suppl 50):17–32.
7. Sullivan DA, Wickham LA, Krenzer KL, et al. *Aqueous Tear Deficiency in Sjögren's Syndrome: Possible Causes and Potential Treatment.* The Netherlands: Aeolus Press; 1997:95–152.
8. Schirra F, Liu M, Sullivan DA. Androgen regulation of gene expression in the mouse meibomian gland. *Invest Ophthalmol Vis Sci.* 2005;46(10):3666–3675.
9. Sullivan DA, Wickham LA, Rocha EM, et al. Influence of gender, sex steroid hormones and the hypothalamic-pituitary axis on the structure and function of the lacrimal gland. *Adv Exp Med Biol.* 1998;438:11–42.
10. Sator MO, Joura EA, Golaszewski T, Gruber D. Treatment of menopausal KCS with topical oestradiol. *Br J Obstet Gynaecol.* 1998;105:100–102.
11. Qureshi SH, Selva-Nayagam DN, Crompton JL. Hypovitaminosis A in metropolitan Adelaide. *Clin Experiment Ophthalmol.* 2000;28(1):62–64.

12. Heiligenhaus A, Koch JM, Kemper D, Kruse FE, Waubke TN. Therapy of dry eye disorders. *Klin Monatsbl Augenheilkd.* 1994;204(3):162–168.

13. Sahlin S, Chen E, Kaugesaar T, Almqvist H, Kjellberg K, Lennerstrand G. Effect of eyelid botulinum toxin injection on lacrimal drainage. *Am J Ophthalmol.* 2000;129(4):481–486.

14. Blades KJ, Patel S, Aidoo KE. Oral antioxidant therapy for marginal dry eye. *Eur J Clin Nutr.* 2001; 55(7):589–597.

15. Brown NA, Bron AJ, Harding JJ, Dewar HM. Nutrition supplements and the eye. *Eye.* 1998;12 (Pt 1):127–133.

16. Barabino S, Rolando M, Camicione P, et al. Systemic linoleic and gamma-linolenic acid therapy in dry eye syndrome with an inflammatory component. *Cornea.* 2003;22(2):97–101.

17. Tauber J, Davitt WF, Bokosky JE, et al. Double-masked, placebo-controlled safety and efficacy trial of diquafosol tetrasodium (INS365) ophthalmic solution for the treatment of dry eye. *Cornea.* 2004;23(8):784–792.

18. Nichols KK, Yerxa B, Kellerman DJ. Diquafosol tetrasodium: a novel dry eye therapy. *Expert Opin Investig Drugs.* 2004;13(1):47–54.

19. Fischbarg J. Diquafosol tetrasodium. Inspire/Allergan/Santen. *Curr Opin Invest Drugs.* 2003;4(11):1377–1383.

20. Horwath-Winter J, Schmut O, Haller-Schober EM, Gruber A, Rieger G. Iodide iontophoresis as a treatment for dry eye syndrome. *Br J Ophthalmol.* 2005;89(1):40–44.

21. Patel S, Blades KJ. *The Dry Eye: A Practical Approach.* Boston: Butterworth-Heinemann Publications; 2003.

22. Craig J, Blades KJ, Patel S. Tear lipid layer structure and stability following expression of the meibomian glands. *Ophthalmol Physiol Opt.* 1995;15:569–574.

23. Ubels JL, Clousing DP, Van Haitsma TA. Preclinical investigation of the efficiency of an artifical tear solution containing hydroxypropyl-guar as a gelling agent. *Curr Eye Res.* 2004;28(6):437–444.

24. Murube J. Surgical treatment of dry eye. *Orbit.* 2003;22(3):203–232.

15

Punctal Occlusion: Plugs, Cautery, and Suturing

Sanjay V. Patel, MD and H. Kaz Soong, MD

INTRODUCTION

Therapeutic occlusion of the lacrimal canalicular system was first performed in 1877 to seal off the lacrimal sac from the ocular surface in patients with infectious dacryocystitis.[1] It was not until the 1890s that therapeutic punctal occlusion was used to prevent the drainage of tears in patients with xerophthalmus.[2–4] This simple procedure is the most common surgical treatment of dry eye today and is indispensable in the management of tear insufficiency associated with KCS, GVHD, Sjögren's syndrome, neurotrophic and exposure keratitides, cicatricial conjunctivitis, post-LASIK dry eyes, and SLK.[5] The lacrimal puncta can be occluded by thermal methods, by implantation of plugs, or with more complex surgical methods requiring incisions and sutures.

Punctal and canalicular closure increases mainly the aqueous component of natural tears, but also has secondary beneficial effects on goblet cell density, tear film stability, and tear osmolality.[6–8] The procedure also increases the retention of artificial tears. Objective and subjective signs and symptoms of xerophthalmus are both improved. This, in turn, results in improved visual acuity, reduced punctate staining of the ocular surface, diminished mucous discharge, relief from foreign body sensation, improved tolerance of contact lenses, and reduction in the frequency of artificial tears.

The procedure is associated with very few complications. These include epiphora, spontaneous reopening of the punctum, canaliculitis, dacryocystitis,[9] and toxic medicamentosus (from increased retention of topical medications).[10] Additionally, complications unique to punctal and canalicular plugs include abrasion of the ocular surface by the exposed ends of the implants,[8,11] pruritus,[10,12] dacryocystitis (from the migration of plugs into the common canaliculus),[13] pyogenic granuloma,[13] and extrusion.

Although upper and lower canaliculi have very similar drainage capabilities, the inferior canaliculi may have slightly more activity.[14] Closure of one canaliculus may not necessarily translate to a 50% improvement in objective and subjective measures because the unoccluded side may increase its drainage activity in response.

THERMAL OCCLUSION AND LASER PHOTOCOAGULATION

Thermal punctal and canalicular occlusion may be performed with a hot cautery, diathermy, or argon laser to cause destruction, shrinkage, and scarring of the punctal opening and the wall of the proximal lumen. Thermal cautery is the oldest technique, dating back to the late 1800s,[1] and is simpler, quicker, and less costly than diathermy or laser photocoagulation. It is currently the most common method of thermal punctal occlusion.

The hot cautery method utilizes the direct transmission of heat from a hot probe to produce a controlled burn injury to the punctal opening. It is most frequently performed with a battery-operated unit with an electrically-heated nichrome wire tip (galvanocautery) (Figure 15-1), although wall-current units are also available. In some parts of the world, punctal cauterization is still performed with a hot needle heated with an alcohol lamp. Although low temperature cauterization may provide better control of tissue destruction, some surgeons prefer higher temperatures to produce deeper scarring and shrinkage for longer-lasting results. The procedure is performed in the outpatient clinic under local infiltrative anesthesia with a lidocaine injection into the tissues surrounding the punctum. Cauterization may be performed at the slit lamp, under an operating microscope, or with magnifying loupes. It is important to treat not only the surface of the punctum, but to also insert the tip of the cautery gently into the proximal lumen to achieve a more effective and permanent closure. In many successful occlusions, a clear membrane eventually covers the surface of the punctal opening. In cases of late punctal occlusion failure, the wall of the canalicular lumen becomes re-epithelialized through the normal reparative process of cell migration. Temporary tissue edema postoperatively may sometimes functionally obstruct the punctum and canaliculus, but with resolution of the edema, the channel may reopen.

Diathermy utilizes radiofrequency (455 kHz to 100 mHz) energy to heat the tissues in the area of the punctal opening and proximal lumen. Some diathermy units employ a second electrode on the patient's torso or limb to complete the electrical circuit. In others, the electrodes are placed in close proximity to each other (eg, bipolar pencil or forceps-style cautery tips), thus negating the need for a remote, second electrode pad. The diathermy procedure is performed under local infiltrative anesthesia. A fine-needle electrode is introduced into the canaliculus through the punctum and the electromagnetic current is activated until the surrounding tissues blanch and contract. Available commercial diathermy units include the Hyfrecator (ConMed Corp, Utica, NY), Mentor Diathermy (Mentor Ophthalmics, Santa Barbara, Calif), and Surgitron (Ellman International, Oceanside, NY).

Argon laser photocoagulation for punctal occlusion[15,16] may be done under either topical or local anesthesia. After the punctal opening is first encircled with laser spots, additional spots are then delivered into the punctum itself (Figure 15-2). Laser treatment on average has a shorter duration of effect compared to thermal cautery.[16,17]

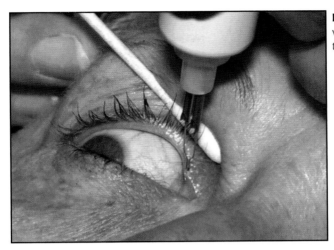

Figure 15-1. Punctal occlusion with hand-held, battery-operated thermal cautery.

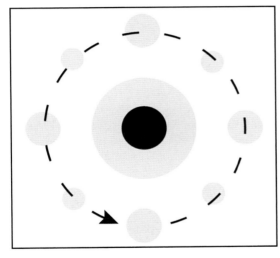

Figure 15-2. Laser punctal occlusion. Argon laser spot (gray circle) pattern at and around central punctal opening (black circle).

If the patient experiences significant epiphora after any of the aforementioned thermal punctal occlusion methods, the obstruction may be reversed in some cases by using a punctal dilator to probe and dilate the punctal opening and the proximal canaliculus.[9] If this fails, more invasive methods, such as passage of a pigtail probe, incision of the eyelid margin medial to the punctum with marsupialization of the canaliculus, or (in extremely rare instances) a full dacryocystorhinostomy, may become necessary.

PUNCTAL OBSTRUCTION

The lacrimal punctum and canaliculus may be occluded temporarily or permanently with tissue glue or implanted foreign bodies. Temporary occlusive procedures are useful in assessing the beneficial effects of lacrimal obstruction prior to resorting to permanent occlusion.

Figure 15-3. Insertion of absorbable collagen canalicular implant with jeweler's forceps. (Courtesy of Medennium, Inc, Irvine, Calif.)

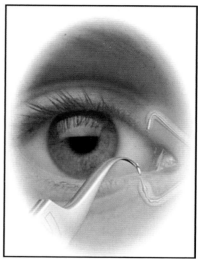

PUNCTAL OBSTRUCTION WITH GLUE

Cyanoacrylate tissue adhesive may be applied to the punctal opening or into the proximal canaliculus, using a 25- to 27-gauge cannula or needle.[7,18] A new fibrin surgical glue (Tisseel VH, Baxter Healthcare, Deerfield, Ill) is now available and may possibly be used as an alternative to cyanoacrylate adhesive. Typically, occlusion with glue lasts only several days to week because the epithelial cells lining the punctal opening and the walls of the proximal lumen slough during the natural cell-turnover cycle.

PUNCTAL OBSTRUCTION WITH ABSORBABLE IMPLANTS

Although most absorbable implants are made of collagen, other absorbable materials are also available. Collagen implants are inserted into the canaliculus and typically degrade over 3 to 7 days,[19] although total degradation may take as long as 14 days.[20] These implants may be inserted to temporarily enhance the retention of the ocular surface tear film, thus permitting the clinician to assess whether or not permanent occlusion might improve subjective comfort and objective clinical findings. If epiphora results, permanent occlusion with nonabsorbable canalicular implants, thermal methods, or suture techniques would be contraindicated.

Implantation of absorbable plugs may be performed with or without topical anesthesia. Small punctal openings may require dilation before insertion of plugs, but care should be taken to not excessively dilate and damage the fibrous ring surrounding the punctal opening. Plugs are inserted with toothless pincers, such as the jeweler's forceps (Figure 15-3). The insertion may be facilitated by gentle lateral traction on the eyelid. Absorbable collagen punctal plugs and canalicular implants are available from Alcon Laboratories (Fort Worth, Tex), Ciba Vision (Atlanta, Ga), FCI Ophthalmics (Marshfield Hills, Mass), Lacrimedics (Eastsound, Wash), and Oasis Products (Glendora, Calif).

Catgut (2–0) or chromic catgut (4–0) sutures are absorbable materials (collagen matrix) that can be used instead of collagen plugs. Any desired length of suture may be

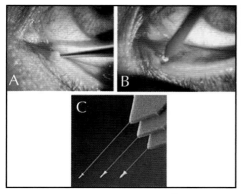

Figure 15-4. Nonabsorbable punctal plugs with flange to prevent distal migration. Punctal dilation (A), plug insertion (B), and different size plugs (C).

cut and inserted into the canaliculus. This inexpensive material is used by some surgeons to temporarily enhance the tear film in the immediate postoperative phase after corneal surgery.

PUNCTAL OBSTRUCTION WITH NONABSORBABLE IMPLANTS AND PLUGS

Nonabsorbable implant materials include polyethylene, silicone, and acrylic. Silicone and polyethylene implants are made in a variety of shapes and sizes to facilitate insertion, prevent extrusion, and inhibit distal migration. The implant shape may determine whether the punctum is partially or completely occluded. Silicone and polyethylene implants are generally safe and effective. Although they are considered "permanent," they are usually removable with varying degrees of difficulty.[21]

Insertion of silicone and polyethylene plugs is performed with or without topical anesthesia and magnification (Figure 15-4). Punctal dilation is typically required before insertion. The implants are typically preloaded on an inserter for direct placement into the punctal orifice. Gentle horizontal eyelid traction helps evert the punctum to facilitate insertion. When the shaft of the implant is located in the vertical portion of the canaliculus and the head (flange) of the implant protrudes above the punctum, the implant is released from the inserter. Some inserters have a built-in button to release the implants, while others require forceps to hold the implant in position while the inserter is withdrawn. This type of punctal plug implant is visible under slit lamp biomicroscopy and can readily be removed with jeweler's forceps.

A newer, nonabsorbable implant made from hydrophobic acrylic (SmartPlug, Medennium Inc, Irvine, Calif) is now available. This material is heat responsive and its physical dimensions undergo transition from 9.0 x 0.4 mm to 2.0 x 1.0 mm at temperatures above 32°C. No sizing of the punctal opening is required because one plug size fits all puncta before heat activation. Insertion may be done with or without topical anesthesia and magnification. The implant is inserted approximately two-thirds of its length into the canaliculus with special SmartPlug forceps. The implant retracts itself into the canaliculus as the heat-activated conformational change pulls it distally. As the implant molds to the dimensions of the vertical canaliculus, the exposed portion retracts completely into the punctum. The SmartPlug is not visible once it attains its final position.

Removing the SmartPlug requires grasping the implant at the punctal orifice with jeweler's forceps if it is visible or flushing the implant distally into the lacrimal sac with saline solution. Other companies in the United States (Form Fit, Oasis Products, Glendora, Calif) and Japan have now developed similar heat-sensitive plugs. Recurrent extrusion of flanged surface punctal plugs may be an indication for switching to these heat-sensitive implants or to thermal occlusion.

PUNCTAL AND CANALICULAR IMPLANT INFECTIONS AND INFLAMMATION

Serious but rare complications of both punctal plugs and canalicular implants include canaliculitis (infectious or noninfectious) and implant migration.[22] Initial treatment of the former requires systemic antibiotics, irrigation of the canaliculus, and drainage of suppurative material; however, recurrences after the initial episode are very common. Surgical removal of the implant via an incision through the palpebral conjunctiva into the canaliculus or a full dacryocystorhinostomy may be necessary in recalcitrant cases. Distal implant migration may occur spontaneously or following forceful insertion. Diagnosis may be aided by checking for canalicular patency with punctal irrigation and by ultrasound biomicroscopy.[23] Initial management of implant intrusion involves observation, but if the implant causes complications, canalicular surgery or dacryocystorhinostomy would be warranted to remove the problematic implant.[22] Punctal surface implants with inserter holes may collect debris that may become colonized with microorganisms. Rarely, tear stasis from the punctal obstruction may predispose the patient to ocular infection.[24]

PUNCTAL OCCLUSION TECHNIQUES REQUIRING SUTURES AND INCISIONS

If punctal occlusion fails multiple times, it may become necessary to resort to more extensive surgical procedures that involve suturing and incision. These procedures are more time consuming and may commensurately be associated with greater surgical morbidity and complications.

The punctum may be occluded first with a hot cautery and then sutured shut with a single nylon stitch. Alternatively, the vertical canaliculus may be sutured shut with a single 8–0 polyglactin full-thickness eyelid mattress suture tied on the skin side. If desired, these techniques can also be combined with nonthermal punctal epithelial debridement. A more extensive procedure employs surgical laceration of the horizontal canaliculus medial to the punctum on the eyelid margin, thermal cauterization of the exposed canalicular and punctal surfaces, and suture closure of both the canaliculus and punctum (Figure 15-5).[25] Complete canalicular excision is a rarely performed procedure in which the canaliculus is identified with a probe and extirpated through either a lid margin or palpebral conjunctival incision.[26] The operation is associated with a risk of eyelid distortion and is best performed by a surgeon experienced in canalicular and cosmetic eyelid procedures.

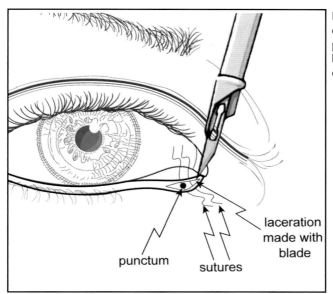

Figure 15-5. Incisional punctal occlusion. Thermally cauterized punctum is incorporated into blade incision, which is then closed with sutures.

punctum   sutures   laceration made with blade

A medial tarsorrhaphy procedure can be modified to incorporate simultaneous occlusion of the upper and lower puncta.[27] In this technique, a rectangle of epithelial tissue is removed from around both the upper and lower puncta. The denuded surfaces of the medial eyelid margins are approximated with 8–0 polyglactin sutures, resulting in occlusion of both puncta. A standard medial temporary tarsorrhaphy is then performed with a mattress suture over protective bolsters. This procedure is ideal for patients with severe tear deficiency and in cases of severe neurotrophic or exposure keratitis.

There are several less complicated surgical techniques that are also more readily reversible.[27] A bulbar conjunctival autograft taken from one of the fornices can be sutured as a patch over the punctal orifice after a similar sheet of epithelial tissue surrounding the punctum is excised. The patch graft is secured with 4 polyglactin (8–0) or nylon (10–0) sutures (the latter are removed after 1 week). The procedure may be reversed by simply removing the tissue patch. Another technique is the translocation of the punctal orifice away from the tear lake. The vertical canaliculus is identified with a probe and moved anteriorly through the anterior lamellae of the eyelid, in effect moving the punctal orifice to the eyelash line. Reversal involves translocation of the punctum back to its original position.

CONCLUSION

Punctal occlusion is a very effective invasive method of treating dry eye and other ocular surface disorders. Methods of occlusion include tamponade by implants, as well as thermal and surgical occlusion. In general, the latter methods should be reserved for severe cases of tear deficiency.

Key Points

1. Punctal and canalicular closure increases mainly the aqueous component of natural tears but also has secondary beneficial effects on goblet cell density, tear-film stability, and tear osmolality. The procedure also increases the retention of artificial tears.
2. The procedure is associated with very few complications. These include epiphora, spontaneous reopening of the punctum, canaliculitis, dacryocystitis, and toxic medicamentosus (from increased retention of topical medications).
3. Thermal punctal and canalicular occlusion may be performed with a hot cautery, diathermy, or argon laser to cause destruction, shrinkage, and scarring of the punctal opening and the wall of the proximal lumen.
4. The lacrimal punctum and canaliculus may be occluded temporarily or permanently with tissue glue or implanted foreign bodies.
5. Serious but rare complications of both punctal plugs and canalicular implants include canaliculitis (infectious or noninfectious) and implant migration.
6. If punctal occlusion fails multiple times, it may become necessary to resort to more extensive surgical procedures that involve suturing and incision.

REFERENCES

1. Panas F, Chamoin É. *Leçons sur les affections de l'appareil lachrymal comprenant la glande lacrymale et les voies d'excrétion des larmes.* Paris: Delahaye et Cie; 1877:168–169.
2. Römer P. Experimentelle untersuchungen über Infektionen vom Konjunktivalsack. *Zeitschr Hygiene.* 1899;32:295–326.
3. Záboj-Bruckner A. Lacrymal passages in the guinea-pig and rabbit. *Br J Ophthalmol.* 1924; 8:158–165.
4. Beetham WP. Filamentary keratitis. *Tr Am Ophthalmol Soc.* 1935;33:413–435.
5. Yang HY, Fujishima H, Toda I, et al. Lacrimal punctal occlusion for the treatment of superior limbic keratoconjunctivitis. *Am J Ophthalmol.* 1997;124:80–87.
6. Fayet B, Bernard JA, Ammar J, et al. Traitement des sécheresses lacrymales par occlusion réversible des méats lacrymaux. Résultats comparés à un groupe témoin. *J Fr Ophtalmol.* 1990;13:123–133.
7. Turss R, Adolf HJ. Vorübergehender verschlub der tränenkanälchen mit gewebekleber. *Forsch Oftalmol.* 1982;79:266–269.
8. Willis RM, Folberg R, Krachmer JH, Holland EJ. The treatment of aqueous-deficient dry eye with removable punctal plugs. A clinical and impression-cytologic study. *Ophthalmology.* 1987; 94:514–518.
9. Glatt HJ. Acute dacryocystitis after punctal occlusion for keratoconjunctivitis sicca. *Am J Ophthalmol.* 1991;111:769–770.
10. Huang TC, Lee DA. Punctal occlusion and topical medications for glaucoma. *Am J Ophthalmol.* 1989;107:151–155.
11. Nelson CC. Complications of Freeman plugs. *Arch Ophthalmol.* 1991;109:923–924.
12. Fayet B, Bernard JA. Tolérance et complications des bouchons lacrymaux. *Bull Soc Belg Ophtalmol.* 1990;238:53–56.

13. Fayet B, Bernard JA, Ammar J, et al. Complications des bouchons lacrymaux employés dans le traitement symptomatique des sécheresses oculaires. *J Fr Ophtalmol.* 1990;13:135–142.

14. Ogut MS, Bavbek T, Kazokoglu H. Assessment of tear drainage by fluorescein dye disappearance test after experimental canalicular obstruction. *Acta Ophtalmologica.* 1993;71:69–72.

15. Benson DR, Hemmady PB, Snyder RW. Efficacy of laser punctal occlusion. *Ophthalmology.* 1992;99:618–621.

16. Vrabec MP, Elsing SH, Aitken PA. A prospective, randomized comparison of thermal cautery and argon laser for permanent punctal occlusion. *Am J Ophthalmol.* 1993;116:469–471.

17. Beisel JG. Treatment of dry eye with punctal plugs. *Optom Clin.* 1991;1:103–117.

18. Köhler U. Komplikationen nach vorübergegendem trännennasenwegverschlub mit Gewebekleber (Histoacryl). *Klin Monatsbl Augenheilkd.* 1986;189:486–490.

19. Herrick RS. A subjective approach to the treatment of dry eye syndrome. In: Sullivan DA, ed. *Lacrimal Gland, Tear Film, and Dry Eye Syndromes.* New York: Plenum Press; 1994.

20. Lamberts D. Punctal occlusion. *Int Ophthalmol Clin.* 1987;27:44–46.

21. Tai MC, Cosar CB, Cohen EJ, et al. The clinical efficacy of silicone punctal plug therapy. *Cornea.* 2002;21:135–139.

22. Sopakar CNS, Patrinely JR, Junts J, et al. The perils of permanent punctal plugs. *Am J Ophthalmol.* 1997;123:120–121.

23. Hurwitz JJ, Pavlin CJ, Rhemtulla el K. Identification of retained intracanalicular plugs with ultrasound biomicroscopy. *Can J Ophthalmol.* 2004;39:533–537.

24. Yokoi N, Okada K, Sugita J, Kinoshita S. Acute conjunctivitis associated with biofilm formation on a punctal plug. *Jap J Ophthalmol.* 2000;44:559–560.

25. Frueh BR. Exposure keratitis. In: Waltman SR, Keates RH, Hoyt CS, eds. *Surgery of the Eye.* New York: Churchill Livingstone; 1988.

26. Putterman AM. Caniculectomy in the treatment of keratitis sicca. *Ophthalmic Surg.* 1991;22:478–480.

27. Murube J, Murube E. Treatment of dry eye by blocking the lacrimal canaliculi. *Surv Ophthalmol.* 1996;40:463–480.

16

Amniotic Membrane Transplantation

Oscar Gris, MD and José Luis Güell, MD

HISTOLOGY OF THE AMNIOTIC MEMBRANE

The amnion, the innermost layer of the amniotic cavity, is formed by a single layer of epithelial cells overlying a basement membrane. The basement membrane is attached to a thin layer of underlying connective tissue.[1] Although the amnion is adjacent to the chorion, it is not completely fused to it, so they can be easily separated by means of blunt dissection. Observation with an optical microscope shows a single layer of cuboidal cells, similar to those of the epidermis, overlying the basement membrane. This epithelium sits on a layer of mesenchyma containing large amounts of collagen and few cells—mostly fibroblasts. The height of the amniotic epithelial cells varies widely between the different regions. Thus, columnar cells are found in the placental amnion, whereas the extra-placental amnion contains cuboid and flattened cells. Epithelial cells of the mature amnion have numerous microvilli on the surface and lateral walls.[2] In the lower part of the lateral membranes, these microvilli form labyrinth-like intercellular caniculim that contribute to intercellular adhesion, together with desmosomes, which are also found in the lateral cell membranes.[3] The underside of the amniotic epithelial cells is attached to the basement membrane by hemidesmosomes.[4]

Underneath the amniotic epithelial basement membrane is the connective tissue stroma, which is divided into a compact layer and a fibroblast layer. Macrophages are found among the collagen, particularly in the first trimester of pregnancy.[5]

IMMUNOLOGY OF THE AMNIOTIC MEMBRANE

Immunofluorescence techniques have shown that human amniotic epithelial cells do not express HLA-A, B, C, or DR antigens on their surface.[6] This may explain why different studies have shown that the amniotic membrane implant produces no significant local immune response at the site of the implant and why HLA antibodies have not been detected in the serum of recipients.[7]

When the human amnion is implanted subcutaneously as an autograft in the newborn, it is incorporated into the tissues as a permanent graft[8] without vascularizing and is probably fed by simple diffusion. When the amnion is implanted subcutaneously as an allograft, it behaves in the same way for the first 14 to 17 days. The graft is subsequently reabsorbed slowly with a very mild inflammatory reaction.[8] Other authors[9] using the amnion as a subcutaneous allograft have not observed local signs of rejection in the implant and have shown that the amniotic epithelial cells survive and can even proliferate 30 days after the graft has been performed. This last result indicates that the immune response to the graft, if present, is mild and ineffective.

However, when the chorion is used as an allograft, it triggers a considerable inflammatory reaction with neovascularization, finally leading to a typical phenomenon of rejection of the graft by the recipient.[10] It has recently been shown that this tissue possesses considerable antigenicity, which leads to an intense cellular response and a lesser response involving antibodies.

OBTAINING AND PRESERVING THE AMNIOTIC MEMBRANE

Selection of Placenta Donors

Placenta donors must be healthy women with no significant pathological history who have been monitored throughout pregnancy without presenting complications. Shortly before delivery, a serological study of the donor must be performed to exclude infection caused by the hepatitis B virus (HBV), hepatitis C virus (HCV), human immunodeficiency virus (HIV), and syphilis. Because the donor is alive, the serological study must be repeated 3 months after birth in order to cover the window period of these infections. Where studies are performed using polymerase chain reaction (PCR), this interval can be reduced to 2 to 3 weeks.

Before delivery, the donor must have signed an informed consent form authorizing extraction of blood samples for the serological study and extraction of the placenta for transplantation purposes.

Obtaining, Processing, and Preserving the Amniotic Membrane

The placenta may be obtained in delivery via cesarean section or via the vagina. However, it has been shown that bacterial contamination is higher in number and pathogenicity in placentas obtained via the vagina.[11] For this reason, all placentas intended for transplantation should be obtained by means of elective cesarean section. The placenta is obtained in the operating room during the cesarean section under strictly sterile conditions and is subsequently processed in the tissue bank. We prepare and preserve the amniotic membrane using the method described by Tseng et al.[12] The placenta is cleaned of any remaining blood and clots under a laminar-flow hood, using a sterile BSS containing 50 mL/mL penicillin, 50 mL/mL streptomycin, 100 mL/mL neomycin, and 2.5 mL/mL amphotericin B. The amnion is then separated from the chorion by means of blunt dissection via the virtual spaces between the 2 tissues and is flattened onto nitrocellulose paper with the epithelial/basement membrane surface face up. The discs of nitrocellulose paper with the fragment of amniotic membrane are then stored at -80°C in sterile vials containing Dulbecco's Modified Eagle's Medium (Life Technologies Ltd, Paisley, Scotland) and glycerol in a proportion of 1/1 (vol/vol). Dimethyl sulfoxide can also be used as a cryoprotective agent instead of glycerol.

A small fragment of amniotic membrane should be sent for microbiological testing, including bacterial and fungal cultures. Only placentas with negative microbiological cultures and negative serological results in the donor should be used for transplantation. The membrane can be removed from the freezer between 10 and 15 minutes prior to surgery because thawing takes little time at room temperature.

HISTORY OF AMNIOTIC MEMBRANE TRANSPLANTATION IN OPHTHALMOLOGY

The first author in the literature to use fetal membranes in ophthalmology was De Rotth in 1940.[13] De Rotth implanted fresh fetal membranes (including both the amnion and the chorion) for reconstruction of the conjunctival surface. Of the 6 cases of symblepharon and conjunctival defects he treated, only one was successful, probably because the chorion was included in the graft. In 1941, Brown[14] proposed using rabbit peritoneum as a temporary covering for the ocular surface following acute lime burns in an attempt to accelerate epithelialization and slow down or prevent tissue necrosis. Using this idea, in 1946 and 1947, Sorsby et al[15,16] used preserved amniotic membrane (which they called amnioplastin) as a temporary covering in the treatment of acute caustic soda burns of the eye. They achieved positive results with this technique, although they observed that frequent applications of the amnioplastin were required. They also showed that the sooner the amniotic membrane was applied, the shorter the healing time. However, for reasons that are not clear, the use of amniotic membrane disappeared from the ophthalmology literature for a long period of time. Some authors believe that this could have been due to problems with preserving the tissue.

In 1995, Kim and Tseng[17] reintroduced the use of amniotic membrane in ophthalmology. In an animal model using rabbits, they showed that 40% of corneas with limbal deficiency could be reconstructed by replacing the conjunctivalized surfaces with preserved human amniotic membrane. Since the work of these authors was published, interest has revived in the use of amniotic membrane in ophthalmology and numerous studies have appeared regarding its efficacy in different pathologies of the ocular surface.

MECHANISMS OF ACTION OF AMNIOTIC MEMBRANE

Preserved amniotic membrane can be used for a large number of indications, whether as a graft, a patch, or a combination of both. When implanted as a graft (Figures 16-1 and 16-2), it covers a tissue defect, replacing the missing stromal matrix and providing a basement membrane on which epithelialization can take place. When used as a covering (Figures 16-3 and 16-4), it protects the ocular surface from possible external insults and provides biological substances that reduce inflammation and promote epithelial regeneration beneath the implant.

Figure 16-1. Implantation of amniotic membrane as a graft in a case of corneal ulceration. The amniotic membrane is grafted on the stromal defect (in one or more layers) and sutured without exceeding the borders of the ulcer (amniotic membrane is shown in black and corneal-conjunctival epithelium in grey).

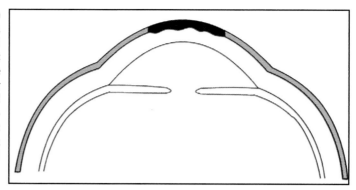

Figure 16-2. Implantation of amniotic membrane as a graft in a case of corneal ulceration. The epithelialization, in these cases, occurs over the amniotic membrane, which remains trapped within the stroma until reabsorption is completed (amniotic membrane is shown in black).

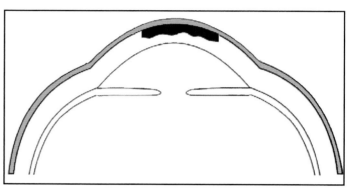

Figure 16-3. Implantation of amniotic membrane as a patch in a case of persistent epithelial defect. Bowman's membrane is conserved in these cases, and the amniotic membrane is used to cover the entire corneal surface, exceeding the limits of the epithelial defect (amniotic membrane is shown in black and corneal-conjunctival epithelium in gray).

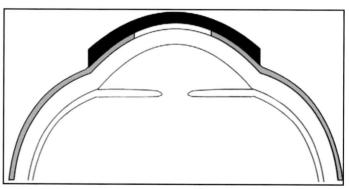

Figure 16-4. Implantation of amniotic membrane as a patch in a case of persistent epithelial defect. Once epithelialization has been achieved, the amniotic membrane can be completely removed, such that corneal transparency is not affected (amniotic membrane is shown in black).

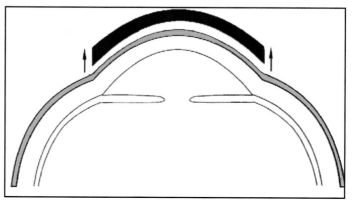

Amniotic Epithelium

The role of the epithelium of preserved amniotic membrane is still not fully understood. Some laboratory results suggest that it contains a large amount of growth factors, since preserved amniotic membrane with the epithelium intact has been shown to have a greater amount of growth factors than the amniotic membrane denuded of the epithelium.[18] Furthermore, the epithelium of the amniotic membrane can provide cytokines, which play an important role in maintaining the microenvironment of the stem cells of the corneal epithelium.[19] In cultures of epithelial stem cells of the limbus, amniotic membrane with intact epithelium has been shown to be a better substrate than amniotic membrane with no epithelium because only the former manages to maintain an epithelial phenotype with little differentiation, comparable to that found in the basement epithelium of the human limbus.[20]

Basement Membrane

The basement membrane of the amniotic membrane contains type-IV collagen, laminin-1, laminin-5, fibronectin, and type-VII collagen. Its composition is very similar to that of the conjunctiva,[21] and the laminins are particularly effective at improving the adhesion of corneal epithelial cells.[22] In general, the basement membrane of the amniotic membrane facilitates migration of the epithelial cells, reinforces adhesion of the basement epithelial cells, promotes epithelial differentiation, and prevents apoptosis. The basement membrane of the amniotic membrane also constitutes an ideal substrate for growing epithelial stem cells, prolonging their lifespan, and maintaining their clonal behavior. These actions explain why transplantation of amniotic membrane can be used to stimulate residual stem cells in the limbus and transitory amplifier cells in the peripheral cornea in the treatment of partial deficiencies of the limbus[12] and to facilitate epithelialization in persistent defects of the corneal epithelium with stromal ulceration.[23–25] In tissue cultures, amniotic membrane has also been shown to be a good substrate for growing cultured epithelial cells,[26,27] while maintaining normal epithelial differentiation and morphology.[28] Subsequently, amniotic membrane, together with the epithelial cells that have grown on it, has been successfully reimplanted to reconstruct injured corneal surfaces, both in humans[26,29,30] and animals.[31] Amniotic membrane can also be used to encourage differentiation of the caliciform cells of the conjunctival epithelium.[28] These results explain why, *in vivo*, following transplantation of the amniotic membrane to the conjunctival surface, the epithelium—which has regenerated over the graft—presents a higher density of caliciform cells.[32]

Stromal Matrix

The stromal portion of amniotic membrane contains a component of the matrix that suppresses signaling via TGF-β, and the proliferation and differentiation of normal human corneal myofibroblasts and limbal fibroblast.[33] This component also suppresses the proliferation and differentiation of normal conjunctival fibroblasts and pterygial body fibroblasts.[34] These actions explain why amniotic-membrane transplantations reduce the formation of scar tissue when used in the reconstruction of the conjunctival surface,[35,36] prevent recurrent scarring following pterygium resection,[37–40] and reduce stromal opacity following phototherapeutic and photorefractive keratectomy.[41–43] Although these effects are more marked when the fibroblasts are in direct contact with the stromal matrix, a lesser effect has also been shown when the fibroblasts are separated from the membrane by a moderate distance,[33] suggesting that one of the factors present in the stromal matrix may have the ability to diffuse and act at a distance.

The stromal matrix of the amniotic membrane can also trap inflammatory cells,[44] thus excluding them from the other tissues and inducing them to undergo rapid apoptosis.[43] It also contains anti-inflammatory and antiangiogenic proteins[45] and substances that inhibit several protease.[46] These properties explain why stromal inflammation[23,35] and corneal neovascularization[17] are reduced following AMT. Both actions are very important in preparing the stroma before receiving a transplant of limbal stem cells,[12,38,47] and they also explain why apoptosis of keratocytes and hence residual stromal opacity are reduced following transplantation in corneal ablation using an excimer laser.[41–43]

Finally, different growth factors have been identified in the amniotic membrane[18] that also contribute to facilitating tissue epithelialization.

CLINICAL EFFECTS FOLLOWING AMNIOTIC MEMBRANE TRANSPLANTATION

All these biological properties shown by the amniotic membrane can be summarized as a series of clinical effects, which can be expected following transplantation of the amniotic membrane onto the ocular surface:

- It facilitates epithelization of the tissues (cornea and/or conjunctiva) using the healthy surrounding epithelium, maintaining the epithelial phenotype present in the area.
- It reduces inflammation of the tissues under the implant and in the surrounding area.
- It reduces neovascularization in the corneal stroma.
- It reduces residual scarring following tissue regeneration, both in the conjunctiva and in the cornea.

INDICATIONS FOR AMNIOTIC MEMBRANE TRANSPLANTATION IN PATHOLOGIES OF THE OCULAR SURFACE

Amniotic Membrane as a Graft in Conjunctival Reconstruction

Amniotic membrane facilitates epithelialization while maintaining a normal epithelial phenotype (with caliciform cells when performed on the conjunctiva) and reduces inflammation, neovascularization, and the formation of scar tissue. For these reasons, amniotic membrane can be used in the reconstruction of the conjunctival surface. When implanted as a graft in areas with conjunctival tissue defects, amniotic membrane helps restore a normal stroma and provides a suitable basement membrane for new epithelial proliferation and differentiation (Figures 16-5 and 16-6). Papers published in recent years show that AMT can be used in the reconstruction of the conjunctival surface as an alternative to conjunctival transplantation following resection of extensive conjunctival lesions. It has been successfully used to treat pterygium,[37–40]

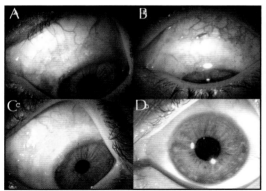

Figure 16-5. (A) Patient with conjunctival nevus affecting 180 degrees of the corneal limbus. (B) Appearance of the superior area 24 hours after complete resection of the lesion and AMT. (C) Nasal area 3 weeks after the surgery. (D) Final appearance 3 months after AMT: observe the minimal scarring.

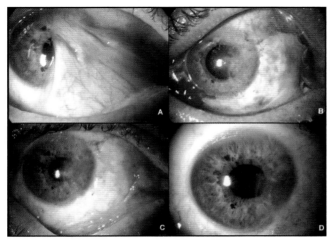

Figure 16-6. (A) Three time recurrent pterygium, with extensive conjunctival lesion, not suitable for conjunctival graft. (B) Next day postoperative image after pterygium surgery and amniotic membrane graft. (C) Three weeks and (D) 3 months postoperative, healthy conjunctival regeneration without recurrence of the lesion.

conjunctival tumors,[35,48,49] conjunctival scarring and symblepharon,[35,36] and conjunctivochalasis.[50] Some articles have shown the efficacy of amniotic membrane in conjunctival reconstruction even over ischemic sclera, provided the surrounding conjunctiva is viable and vascularized.[51]

As a substitute for a conjunctival autograft, an amniotic membrane graft can be used to close perforated blebs after glaucoma filtering surgery[52] and, combined with a scleral graft, it can help repair scleral perforations.[53] Amniotic membrane can also be used as an acceptable alternative to conjunctival or mucous membrane autografts in palpebral surgery[54] and orbital surgery.[55]

Amniotic Membrane as a Graft in Corneal Surface Reconstruction

In recent years, advances have been made in the diagnosis and treatment of sclerocorneal limbus deficiencies in which limbal and AMTs are prominent. In cases of limbal hypofunction or partial limbal deficiency, amniotic membrane re-establishes the stem cell environment in the stroma of the sclerocorneal limbus, reduces inflammation, and stimulates proliferation of these cells. In situations in which there is a total lack of stem cells, limbal transplant is essential to re-establish the population of limbal stem cells. Some studies have shown the efficacy of this combined treatment in varying degrees of limbal deficiency.[12]

Figure 16-7. (A) Neurotrophic cor-neal ulcer not responsive to medical treatment. (B) After surgical clean up of the ulcer bed and border, an amniotic membrane coverage was done, protecting the corneal surface. (C) One month and (D) 4 months after surgery.

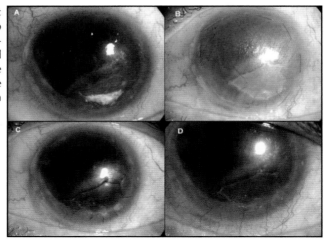

A major advance achieved with amniotic membrane is that partial limbal deficiencies can currently be treated using this technique without requiring a limbal transplant.[12,56]

Another advance is the considerable reduction achieved in the percentage of limbal allografts that are rejected when AMT is performed as a prior procedure to restore the microenvironment of the sclerocorneal limbal stroma.[12] This effect is attributed to reduced inflammation of the stroma in the area. Furthermore, when amniotic membrane is implanted in association with a limbal transplant, it increases the proliferation and activity of stem cells, thus substantially improving results in this type of pathology.

Amniotic membrane applied as a graft is also useful in treating pathologies of the corneal surface because it encourages healing of persistent corneal ulcers of different etiologies.[23–25,49,57,58] In these cases, the technique using an amniotic membrane graft provides a stroma and basement membrane on which epithelialization is encouraged, thus closing the ulcer (Figure 16-7). Its other advantage over alternative surgical techniques such as tarsorrhaphy and conjunctival autografts is that the appearance of the patient's eye is much more aesthetically acceptable. We recently described the behavior of the amniotic membrane in the corneal stroma from the histological point of view following its implantation as a graft in cases of neurotrophic ulcers.[59] We saw that the amniotic membrane was an excellent substrate for epithelialization in these ulcers because normal corneal epithelium was able to grow on the basement membrane. In the absence of corneal neovascularization, the fragment of amniotic membrane remained on the stroma for months without producing any inflammatory reaction or rejection. This is why reabsorption of the graft is so slow in these cases and is probably due to the process of phagocytosis and collagenolysis by the activated surrounding keratocytes. Conversely, in corneas with stromal neovascularization, abundant inflammatory infiltrate was observed (consisting mainly of histiocytes and T lymphocytes), which easily reached the area from the neovessels and led to rapid reabsorption of the graft. In both situations, following reabsorption of the amniotic membrane, the space it had initially occupied was later replaced by a neoformed corneal stroma with fibrotic characteristics. Although this helped recover part of the corneal

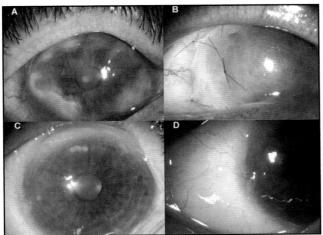

Figure 16-8. (A) Preoperative nod-ular degeneration. (B) Post-operative image after superficial keratectomy and amniotic membrane graft coverage. (C and D) Normal epithelialization and absence of inflammation on the corneal surface 3 weeks postoperatively, after amniotic membrane re-moval.

thickness lost through ulceration, it did not have the transparency of normal corneal stroma.

Some authors recommend AMT in eyes with painful bullous keratopathy and poor visual outcome in which penetrating keratoplasty is not indicated. According to these authors,[60,61] AMT is an effective technique for reducing symptoms in these cases. In comparative studies,[62] it has been shown to be a superior option to isolated de-epithelialization. Other studies,[63] however, state that it is an ineffective procedure.

Amniotic Membrane as a Patch

Amniotic membrane can be used as a patch for both the conjunctiva and the cornea. When used as a patch over the cornea, amniotic membrane is effective in the treatment of persistent corneal epithelial defects that have not responded to medical treatment and in promoting postoperative epithelialization (Figure 16-8) in cases with neurotrophic problems.[64] It also reduces the corneal opacities that may appear following stromal ablation using an excimer laser.[41–43] When implanted on the corneal and conjunctival surfaces, it reduces inflammation and facilitates epithelialization[65] and has, therefore, been used in acute chemical burns to prevent the formation of scar tissue.[66]

Amniotic Membrane as a Substrate for Culturing Epithelial Stem Cells of the Sclerocorneal Limbus

In recent years, amniotic membrane has been the most commonly used element as a substrate for growing epithelial stem cells of the sclerocorneal limbus *in vitro*. This is a major advance in the treatment of patients with severe unilateral limbal deficiency. Using this technique, a small sample of limbus from the healthy eye can, in culture, provide a large number of epithelial cells on the amniotic membrane, which is then transplanted as an autograft to the affected eye in order to restore the corneal surface. This technique, which prevents the risk of rejection and the need for systemic immunosuppression, has been used in both animals[31] and humans.[26,29,30]

On the other hand, it might also be useful to expand donor cadaver limbal cells in order to get a higher density at the time of their transplantation.

Key Points

1. Immunofluorescence techniques have shown that human amniotic epithelial cells do not express HLA-A, B, C or DR antigens on their surface. This may explain why different studies have shown that the amniotic membrane implant produces no significant local immune response at the site of the implant and why HLA antibodies have not been detected in the serum of recipients.
2. The placenta may be obtained in delivery via cesarean section or via the vagina. However, it has been shown that bacterial contamination is higher in number and pathogenicity in placentas obtained via the vagina. For this reason, all placentas intended for transplantation should be obtained by means of elective cesarean section.
3. Amniotic membrane facilitates epithelialization while maintaining a normal epithelial phenotype (with caliciform cells when performed on the conjunctiva) and reduces inflammation, neovascularization, and the formation of scar tissue. For these reasons, amniotic membrane can be used in the reconstruction of the conjunctival surface.
4. As a substitute for a conjunctival autograft, an amniotic membrane graft can be used to close perforated blebs after glaucoma filtering surgery and, combined with a scleral graft, it can help repair scleral perforations. Amniotic membrane can also be used as an acceptable alternative to conjunctival or mucous-membrane autografts in palpebral surgery and orbital surgery.
5. In cases of limbal hypofunction or partial limbal deficiency, amniotic membrane re-establishes the stem cell environment in the stroma of the sclerocorneal limbus, reduces inflammation, and stimulates proliferation of these cells.

REFERENCES

1. Danforth DM, Hull RW. The microscopic anatomy of the fetal membranes with particular reference to the detailed structure of the amnion. *Am J Obstet Gynecol*. 1958;75:536–550.
2. Mukaida T, Yoshida K, Kikyokawa T, Soma H. Surface structure of the placental membranes. *J Clin Electron Microsc*. 1977;10:447–448.
3. Bartels H, Wang T. Intercellular junctions in the human fetal membranes. *Anat Embryol*. 1983;166:103–120.
4. Robinson HL, Anhalt GJ, Patel HP, et al. Pemphigus and pemphigoid antigens are expressed in human amnion epithelium. *J Invest Dermatol*. 1984;83:234–237.
5. Schwarzacher HG. Beitrag zur histogenese des menschilichen amnion. *Acta Anat*. 1960;43:303–311.
6. Adinolfi M, Akle CA, McColl I, et al. Expression of HLA antigens, beta 2-microglobulin and enzymes by human amniotic epithelial cells. *Nature*. 1982;295:325–327.

17

Limbal Stem Cell Disease and Management

W. Barry Lee, MD and
Ivan R. Schwab, MD

INTRODUCTION

Normal health and function of the corneal epithelial stem cells is vital for maintenance and stabilization of a healthy ocular surface. Any process or disease that compromises the integrity of these stem cells can create subsequent breakdown and instability of the ocular surface, leading to asperity of the cornea with scarring, vascularization, and subsequent decreased vision. A myriad of disorders have the potential to create such damage to the stem cells with severe adverse ocular sequelae.

HISTORICAL CONCEPTS

Stem cells are defined as undifferentiated cells that are found in all self-renewing tissues.[1] They possess the ability to proliferate, produce differentiated daughter cells, self-maintain, and regenerate after injury. Our knowledge of corneal epithelial stem cell origin, location, and function has remained a relatively new discovery in evolution since Friedenwald's observation that the corneal epithelium regenerated fully after total de-epithelialization in 1951.[2] The connection between the limbal papillary structures and their importance in corneal epithelial regeneration was proposed in 1971.[3] Additional research with 64 K corneal keratin, 3H-labeled thymidine, and additional corneal keratins provided evidence for the location of stem cells in the limbal basal epithelium.[4–7] Additional studies postulated the migratory pattern of epithelial cells following repair after injury.[8,9] Thoft and Friend proposed the X, Y, Z hypothesis of corneal epithelial maintenance in which basal epithelial cells (X) and cells from the periphery (Y) divide and replace the desquamated surface cells (Z)[8] (see Figure 19-1).

Cells known as transient amplifying cells, daughter cells of the limbal stem cells, migrate centripetally from the limbus and vertically from the basal epithelial layers forward.[8–10] This process of epithelial cell migration is critical in maintenance of the corneal epithelial mass and its ability to regenerate after injury.

CAUSES/CLASSIFICATION

A variety of ocular surface diseases can contribute to stem dell damage with division into primary and secondary causes (Table 17-1). Primary stem cell disease includes congenital disorders, many of which have a hereditary component. Secondary stem cell disorders develop from external factors that damage stem cells with insult over time.

While stem cell disorders are commonly thought of as an acquired disease, several types of congenital causes exist. These conditions lead to improper development of the anterior segment with resultant decreased number of viable stem cells and/or dysfunctional stem cells that are unable to maintain a stable ocular surface with aging. The ocular surface is typically normal early in life and stem cell deficiency develops with increasing age. Examples of these disorders include aniridia, autosomal dominant keratitis, and sclerocornea. Aniridia represents the most common cause of congenital stem cell deficiency. Both aniridia and autosomal dominant keratitis are inherited disorders related to a PAX6 gene mutation, a gene that is essential for appropriate ocular embryogenesis, while the development of sclerocornea is not completely understood. Other congenital stem cell diseases include multiple endocrine neoplasia, chronic mucocutaneous candidiasis, and ectodermal dysplasia syndromes, of which over 150 separate forms exist. Ectodermal dysplasia syndromes include a heterogeneous group of disorders that involve the epidermis and at least one of its appendages such as hair, nails, teeth, or sweat glands. Ichthyosis-related diseases are included in this category with disorders such as Conradi-Hünermann syndrome, keratitis-ichthyosis-deafness (KID) syndrome (Figure 17-1), and Sjögren-Larsson syndrome.

Secondary, or acquired, stem cell diseases include a multitude of external factors that destroy limbal stem cells. The disorders can be divided into conditions that lead to conjunctival tissue loss, direct stem cell loss, chronic nonautoimmune inflammation, autoimmune disease, and iatrogenic stem cell deficiency. Disorders that cause conjunctival tissue loss include Stevens-Johnson syndrome, toxic epidermal necrolysis, and mucous membrane pemphigoid (ocular pemphigoid). Collagen vascular diseases can also cause stem cell deficiency. Direct stem cell loss is caused by chemical injury, thermal injury, radiation damage, and long-term use of certain topical medications. Chronic nonautoimmune inflammatory conditions include damage from contact lens wear as well as ocular surface diseases such as rosacea, staph marginal disease, herpetic keratitis, pterygia, and limbal neoplasias. Iatrogenic stem cell damage is created from multiple surgeries, cryotherapy to the limbus, large limbal lesion excisions from pterygium surgery or limbal neoplasias, and medication toxicity (Table 17-2).

A staging system of limbal stem cell deficiency was proposed by Schwartz and Holland that accounts for the status of limbal stem cells and the conjunctival surface.[11,12] The authors suggest this system can be useful for establishing medical and surgical treatments for ocular surface diseases. The system involves 2 stages with the first stage categorizing the degree of limbal stem cell lost with stage 1 representing less than 50% loss and stage II representing more than 50% stem cell loss. The second

Table 17-1
CAUSES OF STEM CELL DEFICIENCY

Primary

- Aniridia.
- Autosomal dominant keratitis.
- Sclerocornea.
- Multiple endocrine neoplasia.
- Chronic mucocutaneous candidiasis.
- Ectodermal dysplasia syndromes

Secondary

- Autoimmune disease:
  * Stevens-Johnson syndrome.
  * Toxic epidermal necrolysis.
  * Mucous membrane pemphigoid.
  * Collagen vascular disease.
- Direct stem cell loss:
  * Alkali or acid injury.
  * Thermal injury.
  * Radiation injury.
- Chronic nonautoimmune inflammatory disorders:
  * Contact lenses.
  * Neurotrophic keratitis.
  * KCS.
  * Ocular rosacea
  * Staph marginal disease.
  * Bacterial and fungal keratitis.
  * Viral keratitis (Epstein Barr, herpes simplex, herpes zoster).
  * Pterygia/pseudopterygia.
  * Limbal neoplasm
- Iatrogenic stem cell deficiency:
  * Multiple ocular surgeries.
  * Excision of pterygia.
  * Excision of limbal neoplasm.
  * Cryotherapy of limbus.
  * Medication toxicity.

Figure 17-1. A slit lamp photograph of extensive corneal neovascularization from primary stem cell damage in KID syndrome.

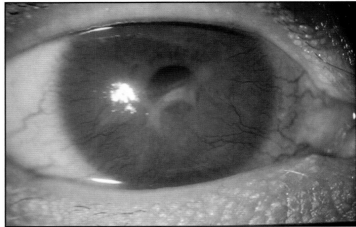

Table 17-2
COMMON MEDICATIONS CAUSING STEM CELL DEFICIENCY

- Pilocarpine.
- Silver nitrate.
- Beta blockers.
- Mitomycin.
- 5-fluorouracil.
- Topical anesthetics.
- Oral medications causing Stevens-Johnson syndrome/TEN.
- Preservatives (thimerosal, benzalkonium chloride)

stage categorizes the level of conjunctival involvement. Normal conjunctiva falls under stage "A," quiet conjunctiva with signs of previous inflammation or injury is stage "B," and stage "C" involves active conjunctival inflammation (Table 17-3).[12]

DIAGNOSIS

Stem cell deficiency can present with a variety of symptoms, many of which are shared with KCS. Symptoms at presentation may include foreign body sensation, pain, dryness, increased tearing, redness, photophobia, decreased vision, and blepharospasm. A review of ocular history may elicit a history of painful corneal erosions resulting from epithelial breakdown or chronic inflammatory episodes with redness, dryness, and surface irritation. Biomicroscopy findings at the slit lamp can reveal important findings indicative of stem cell disease within the eyelids, bulbar and palpebral conjunctiva, and the corneal surface. Eyelid margins can develop trichiasis, distichiasis, entropion, ectropion, chronic injection, keratinization, symblepharon, and ankyloblepharon. Conjunctival findings may include similar findings of inflammation including subepithelial fibrosis and scarring, shortened fornices, hyperemia, and symblepharon. Persistent

Table 17-3
CLASSIFICATION OF OCULAR SURFACE DISEASE

	Normal Conjunctiva (Stage A)	*Previously Inflamed Conjunctiva (Stage B)*	*Inflamed Conjunctiva (Stage C)*
Partial stem cell deficiency (stage 1)	Iatrogenic, conjunctival intraepithelial neoplasia (CIN), contact lens	Chemical or thermal injury	Mild Stevens-Johnson syndrome, pemphigoid, recent chemical injury
Total/subtotal stem cell deficiency (stage 2)	Aniridia, severe contact lens, iatrogenic	Severe chemical or thermal injury	Severe Stevens-Johnson syndrome, pemphigoid, chemical or thermal injury

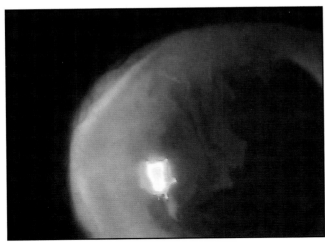

Figure 17-2. A slit lamp photograph demonstrating late fluorescein staining of the cornea from superior stem cell deficiency.

conjunctival inflammation leads to goblet cell and accessory lacrimal gland damage, resulting in mucin tear deficiency and aqueous tear deficiency. Early slit lamp findings of the cornea include loss of palisades of Vogt, late staining of the corneal epithelium with fluorescein, corneal neovascularization, and localized or diffuse pannus formation (Figure 17-2). As stem cell disease progresses, the corneal epithelial mass cannot maintain its regenerative functions and the epithelium becomes irregular and hazy. Punctate keratitis and epithelial defects can develop with subsequent corneal scarring and calcification. Presence of chronic epithelial defects can predispose to corneal ulceration, melting, perforation, and/or infection. As conjunctivalization of the cornea develops, histological diagnosis of stem cell disease can be made by demonstrating the presence of conjunctival goblet cells in the corneal epithelium with excisional corneal biopsy or impression cytology. Alcian blue and periodic acid-Schiff stains identify glycosaminoglycans within the goblet cells of the tissue specimens.

Treatment

Management of ocular surface disease patients can present a frustrating and challenging dilemma in regards to treatment regimens and successful outcomes. A variety of medical treatments can alleviate symptoms of stem cell disease and delay complications; however, specific treatment of stem cell disease requires surgical intervention. Preservative-free artificial tear supplements (liquid and ointment) and punctal occlusion can temporarily increase tear film volume. Selective use of topical prescription medications such as cyclosporine, corticosteroids, autologous serum drops, vitamin A, and hyaluronic acid compounds can prove efficacious in regards to ocular surface improvement. Cyclosporine 0.05% received FDA approval in the United States for treatment of KCS in December 2002 based on studies that showed an increase in Schirmer values over 10 mm in 15% of dry eye patients and decreased punctate keratitis at 6 months after treatment.[13] Additional therapies can include oral omega-3 fatty acid supplements and topical or oral mucin secretagogues. Oral secretagogues, such as pilocarpine and cevimeline, may provide benefit of symptoms in patients with ocular surface disease in association with dry mouth, while topical secretagogues continue to remain under investigational trials for approval. Unfortunately, oral secretagogues have considerable and often intolerable side effects. Minor surgical treatments may include tarsorrhaphy, punctal cautery, and bandage contact lenses for temporary treatment of ocular surface disease. As mentioned before, surgical treatment remains the only definitive method for treating the underlying abnormalities of stem cell disease.

Stem Cell Surgery Evolution

Restoration of the ocular surface in stem cell diseases has remained a difficult and challenging task for ocular surface surgeons. A variety of surgical treatments have been proposed over the last several decades with varying or limited success. As our knowledge of the corneal epithelial stem cell and its importance to the ocular surface has evolved, our understanding of how to repair and adequately restore a damaged surface has expanded. Barraquer is credited with performing the first stem cell autograft 40 years previously by treating unilateral chemically-damaged ocular surfaces with 3 clock hours of conjunctival, limbal, and peripheral corneal epithelium from unaffected fellow eyes.[14] Thoft was instrumental in the development of our understanding of severe ocular surface disease and treatment with his published works on conjunctival transplantation and later keratoepithelioplasty to treat severe ocular surface disease.[15,16] In 1977, he described treating severe ocular surface disease with conjunctival transplantation resulting in improved ocular surfaces in 19 of 22 eyes with severe stem cell disease following transplantation of bulbar conjunctival grafts from the opposite normal eye to the diseased eye.[15] In 1984, Thoft discussed a technique referred to as keratoepithelioplasty in which he improved ocular surfaces in 3 of 4 eyes following transplantation of cadaveric corneal tissue with lenticules of peripheral cornea (Figure 17-3). The technique required harvesting 4 lenticules from the midperipheral cornea of a donor globe including epithelium and a thin layer of stroma. These 4 tissue segments were secured around the corneoscleral limbus of the damaged ocular surface.[16] The keratoepithelioplasty procedure was the first attempt to transplant corneal epithelial stem cells in patients with severe bilateral ocular surface disease although the knowledge of limbal stem cell importance was not completely understood at that time.

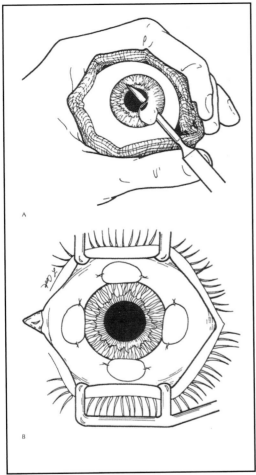

Figure 17-3. Keratoepithelioplasty as described by Thoft. (A) Four lenticules are harvested from a donor globe. (B) The lenticules are secured to the diseased corneoscleral limbus in equidistant positions. (Reproduced with permission from Thoft RA. Keratoepithelioplasty. *Am J Ophthalmol.* 1984;97:1–6.)

As our knowledge of the location and function of stem cells broadened, improved treatments were developed. Once the location of the stem cells was confirmed at the limbus, techniques of limbal transplantation emerged as a treatment for ocular surface restoration. Kenyon and Tseng used theories derived from Thoft's earlier conjunctival transplantation to include limbal stem cells in their grafts.[17] They described success with a limbal autograft technique using donor conjunctiva extending 0.5 mm onto the peripheral cornea from the normal fellow eye with transplantation to the diseased eye. They reported stable ocular surfaces in 20 of 21 eyes with improvement in vision in 17 eyes.[17] Tsai and Tseng, followed by Tsubota and colleagues, further modified the technique by using a cadaveric keratolimbal graft harvested from a whole globe to create a donor keratolimbal ring.[18,19] The ring of tissue was transplanted to the diseased corneoscleral limbus after appropriate preparation. This technique avoided the potential complications of autologous grafts and creation of iatrogenic stem cell deficiency in the fellow donor eye. Tsubota and colleagues further modified this technique, referred to as "limbal allograft transplantation," by using stored corneoscleral rims for

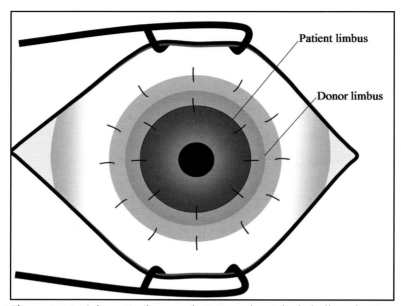

Figure 17-4. Schematic diagram depicting a keratolimbal allograft using an entire ring of donor keratolimbal tissue from the donor cadaveric globe. The donor graft contains a portion of the peripheral donor cornea, the donor limbus, and the anterior portion of donor conjunctiva and episclera. (Illustration by Annette Joglar.)

transplantation to the limbus of the diseased eye (Figure 17-4).[19] Holland developed a similar technique in which he used 2 cadaveric corneoscleral rims for transplantation.[20] His technique called for division of the 2 rims, making 4 total segments. The stem cells were harvested from all 4 quadrants and 3 of the 4 segments of stem cells were transplanted to the diseased limbus. This method completely surrounded the host limbus, avoiding gaps of exposed conjunctiva, and it provided 1.5 times more stem cells to the host limbus than a single donor corneoscleral rim.[20]

SURGICAL TECHNIQUES

As stem cell surgical procedures have evolved, a variety of surgical techniques have developed with designated procedure classifications. Current nomenclature for stem cell transplant procedures includes conjunctival limbal autograft (CLAU), living-related conjunctival limbal allograft (LR-CLAL), cadaveric keratolimbal allograft (KLAL), and combined conjunctival-keratolimbal allograft (C-KLAL).[21]

Conjunctival Limbal Autografting

CLAU is the procedure of choice for unilateral limbal stem cell disease in which the fellow eye has completely normal stem cells. The procedure involves preparation of 2 trapezoidal grafts from the superior and inferior limbus of the unaffected fellow eye, each of which includes limbal stem cells within a conjunctival carrier. Each graft should include approximately 4 clock hours of limbal tissue with extension of approximately 6 mm of conjunctiva posteriorly and approximately 0.5 mm of corneal extension anteriorly. The grafts are then transferred to the same anatomical location of the affected contralateral eye after appropriate recipient beds are constructed. A marking pen is used to place an irreversible letter on the surface of the graft to maintain alignment during transfer. The recipient bed is created by a superior and inferior conjunctival peritomy with undermining of the conjunctiva to allow tissue recession. This often avoids the need to resect conjunctiva. The fibrovascular pannus and diseased epithelium can then be removed, and grafts can be secured to the recipient bed with 10–0 nylon sutures. Sutures should not be placed at the limbal margin in order to prevent any additional stem cell damage (Figure 17-5). This procedure does not require systemic immunosuppression but can potentially create stem cell deficiency in the donor eye.

Living-Related Conjunctival Limbal Allografting

LR-CLAL is indicated for treatment of bilateral stem cell disease or unilateral stem cell damage in which the fellow eye does not have completely normal stem cell function. Consideration must be given to fewer stem cells transplanted in this technique versus KLAL, thus patients with limited stem cell function as opposed to severe stem cell deficiency have better potential for success. The advantage of this procedure includes transplantation of conjunctiva with the stem cells, which may provide more advantage than KLAL in diseases with conjunctival tissue loss. This procedure requires 2 separate surgeries with harvesting of 2 trapezoidal grafts from the living-related donor eye in identical fashion to CLAU. Careful maintenance of tissue orientation is imperative during transfer to the patient with stem cell deficiency. An irreversible letter is placed on the surface of the grafts prior to complete removal and transfer to maintain proper alignment. The tissue can be placed on glove paper and immersed in colloidal storage solution during transfer. The donor bed of the diseased eye is prepared in a similar fashion to the diseased eye in CLAU. The grafts are secured to the host tissue in the same anatomical fashion using 10–0 nylon suture (see Figure 17-5). This procedure does require systemic and topical immunosuppression unlike CLAU and has the potential to create stem cell deficiency in the living-related donor eye.

Cadaveric Keratolimbal Allografting

KLAL is indicated for treatment of unilateral stem cell deficiency in which damage to the contralateral or living-related stem cells is feared and for bilateral severe stem cell deficiency. This procedure affords a high number of stem cells for transplantation to the diseased eye. The current technique described by Holland and colleagues delivers 1.5 times more stem cells than previous stem cell transplant techniques (Figure 17-6). KLAL is more effective for stem cell disorders that have little or mild conjunctival loss or inflammation, and it can be effective for complete stem cell deficiency or sectoral stem cell deficiency to localized regions of disease. Several considerations are critical before attempting KLAL. Success of KLAL is improved with absence or mild active conjunctival inflammation, a stable tear film, normal lid apposition, normal corneal sensation, and lack of ocular surface keratinization. For eyes with conjunctival inflammation, success of surgery is improved if the inflammation is maximally controlled prior to surgery. Tear film

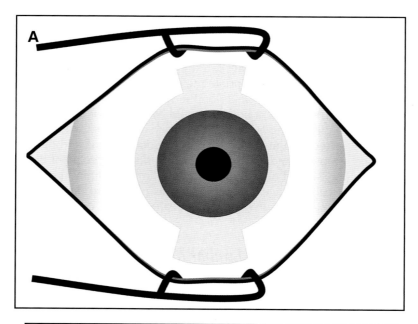

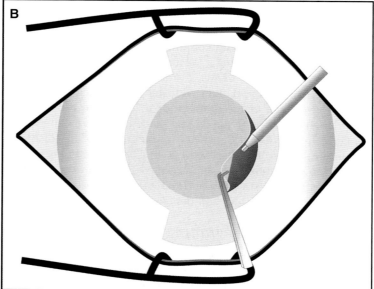

Figure 17-5. Schematic diagram depicting a CLAU. (A) The recipient eye is prepared with a 360-degree conjunctival peritomy and conjunctival resection is performed as shown. (B) The abnormal epithelium and pannus are removed as shown. (Illustrations by Annette Joglar.)

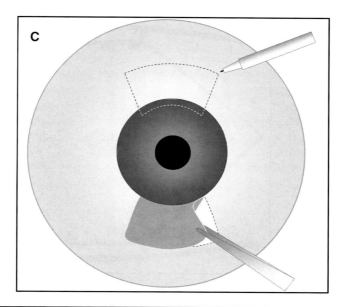

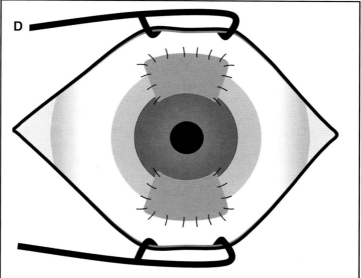

Figure 17-5. (C) Two conjunctival grafts are harvested from the uninvolved eye (in CLAU) or a living-related donor eye (in LR-CLAL), including 6 mm of conjunctiva and approximately 0.5 mm of peripheral cornea as shown. The grafts are marked for identification. (D) The donor conjunctival graft is secured to the recipient bed with 10–0 nylon suture as shown. (Illustrations by Annette Joglar.)

Figure 17-6. A schematic diagram depicting a KLAL. After a 360-degree conjunctival peritomy and conjunctival resection, 3 of 4 segments are positioned around the limbus and secured with 10–0 nylon sutures, one segment at a time with avoidance of gaps between tissue segments. (Illustration by Annette Joglar.)

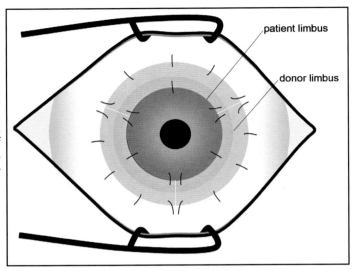

and lid abnormalities must be corrected before attempting KLAL because persistent surface defects following surgery hamper surgical results. Neurotrophic corneas, ocular surface keratinization, and severe aqueous tear deficiency are relative contraindications to KLAL because corneal sensation and a normal tear layer are crucial for survival of the cadaveric donor stem cells. Systemic and topical immunosuppression is critical for survival of KLAL.

In our current technique, the recipient bed is first prepared by a 360-degree limbal conjunctival peritomy with undermining of the conjunctiva. If significant conjunctival loss or symblepharon is present, minimal to no conjunctival resection may be needed to expose the recipient bed because this conjunctiva can be used for self-reconstruction of the damaged conjunctiva once the graft is in place. If the conjunctiva is relatively preserved, a resection of 4 mm can be made to allow for recipient bed exposure. Ocular surface bleeding is not modest during these cases, thus topical thrombin and sympathomimetics along with wet field cautery are often needed to achieve hemostasis. A superficial keratectomy is performed with removal of all fibrovascular pannus and abnormal epithelium. A diamond-dusted corneal burr can be used to smooth the ocular surface after removal, but care must be given to avoid penetration into deep layers of the corneal stroma. Our current technique for stem cell harvesting requires 2 corneoscleral donor tissues preserved in Optisol GS storage medium (Bausch & Lomb, Rochester, NY) at 4°C with large scleral rims measuring 14 mm in diameter. Routine keratoplasty techniques using any trephination system can be employed to remove a 7.5- to 8.0-mm central button within each donor for adult cases and smaller sizes for pediatric cases. We harvest our stem cells as described by Mannis and colleagues using a 22-mm silicone orbital sizing sphere in adults and 3 25-gauge needles for fixation of the rims (Figure 17-7).[22] The posterior two-thirds of each circular rim are dissected from the anterior one-third of the rim using lamellar dissection with a rounded crescent blade. The posterior tissue is discarded and the residual anterior one-third of both circular rims is bisected with scissors, making 4 stem cell segments. The healthiest 3 pieces are then fashioned in the recipient bed in the same anatomical alignment encir-

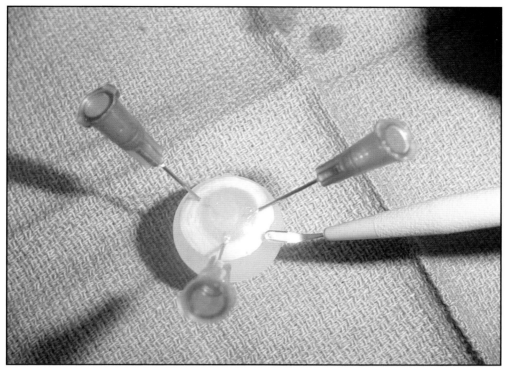

Figure 17-7. Harvesting of limbal stem cells from a cadaveric corneoscleral rim using stabilization with a 22-mm silicone orbital sizing sphere and 3 25-gauge needles placed at the apices of an imaginary isosceles triangle in clear cornea. A crescent blade is used to remove the posterior two-thirds of the donor tissue. The posterior tissue is discarded and the residual anterior one-third of both circular rims is bisected with scissors, making 4 stem cell segments.

cling the limbus. The stem cell segments are secured one at a time at the 4 corners using 10–0 nylon to the host corneal border, followed by securing the conjunctival borders. Segments may be trimmed for appropriate sizing around the limbus, but meticulous attention to avoid gaps in the 3 segments is essential to avoid conjunctival extension toward the cornea postoperatively. Additional sutures may be placed to ensure appropriate fixation of each of the segments (Figure 17-8). A bandage contact lens and pressure patch are applied after topical and subconjunctival medications have been administered.

Combined Conjunctival-Keratolimbal Allografting

C-KLAL is indicated for unilateral or bilateral stem cell disease with cicatricial conjunctival disease in which tissue loss and conjunctival inflammation are pronounced. This procedure is extensive and also requires 2 surgeries, yet it affords transplantation of significant amounts of conjunctiva in addition to stem cells. Systemic and topical immunosuppression is essential in this procedure. The recipient bed is prepared in a similar manner to KLAL; however, conjunctival tissue is undermined rather than resected after the conjunctival peritomy to prevent further

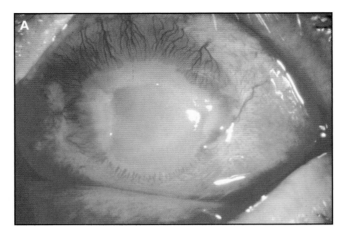

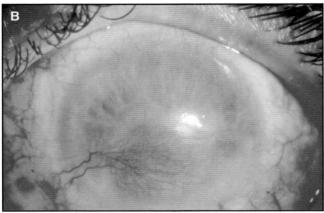

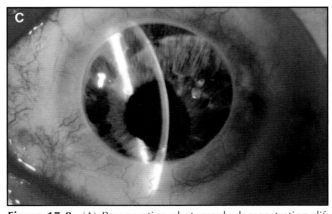

Figure 17-8. (A) Preoperative photograph demonstrating diffuse limbal stem cell deficiency with 360 degrees of peripheral corneal neovascularization, diffuse corneal haze, and central ulceration. (B) A slit lamp photograph demonstrating a keratolimbal allograft in the same eye 3 months postoperatively. (C) A slit lamp photograph demonstrating a restored ocular surface 2 years after keratolimbal allografting and a subsequent penetrating keratoplasty.

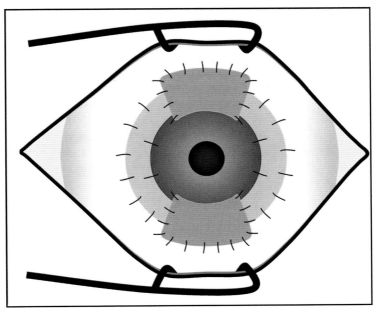

Figure 17-9. A schematic diagram depicting a conjunctival-keratolimbal allograft procedure. The conjunctival grafts are constructed first as seen in Figure 17-5. After dissection and subsequent bisection of a corneoscleral donor rim, the anterior one-third of the 2 keratolimbal grafts are secured along the nasal and temporal limbus with 10–0 nylon suture. (Illustration by Annette Joglar.)

conjunctival tissue loss. Stem cells are harvested from a living-related donor eye as with LR-CLAL and placed in storage medium. Once again, meticulous attention to preservation of appropriate anatomical alignment is essential. Stem cells are then harvested from one corneoscleral rim as described with KLAL. The circular rim of dissected stem cells are bisected and placed in storage medium. The LR-CLAL segments are secured to the superior and inferior limbus as with KLAL using 10–0 nylon suture. The bisected cadaveric tissue is placed along the bare nasal and temporal limbus adjacent to the conjunctival grafts with care to avoid gaps. It is essential to avoid gaps because conjunctiva will otherwise stream through these breaks. The segments can be trimmed for appropriate sizing and secured to the recipient as with KLAL (Figure 17-9). A bandage lens and pressure patch are placed over the eye after topical and subconjunctival medications are administered. Postoperative follow-up is typically performed at 1 day, 1 week, 2 weeks, and every 2 to 3 weeks until the 6-month visit at which time follow-up can be extended to every 4 weeks for the next year. More numerous visits may be needed if postoperative problems arise. Patients with poor epithelialization may be followed with several visits during the first postoperative week.

IMMUNOSUPPRESSION

Immunosuppression is a crucial component of successful management in limbal transplantation. Transplanted limbal tissue differs from corneal grafts in that it has increased vascularity and lack of immune privilege. These factors contribute to the increased accessibility of immune cells and subsequent higher risk of limbal transplant rejection in comparison to penetrating keratoplasty. Because of the heightened risk of immunologic rejection, anti-inflammatory and immunosuppressive agents can significantly enhance graft survival. Several studies have shown improved ocular surfaces following limbal transplantation with institution of topical and systemic immunosuppression. Sixty-three of 73 eyes (86.3%) receiving systemic immunosuppression following limbal transplantation had stable ocular surfaces with mean follow-up of 4.7 years, while only 6 of 21 eyes (28.6%) not receiving systemic immunosuppression obtained a stable ocular surface.[23] Other studies have confirmed similar improvement in limbal transplantation survival in patients taking systemic immunosuppression.[24,25] Recent work by Daya et al suggests that long-term continuation of immunosuppression may not be necessary. These investigators documented that few if any of the donor cells remained at 1 year, although the fate of the donor cells is unknown.[26]

Current immunosuppressive therapies available today include medications with a variety of underlying mechanisms of action. This group of medications includes corticosteroids, immunophilin binders, antimetabolites, and polyclonal and monoclonal antibodies.

Corticosteroids have both anti-inflammatory and immunosuppressive properties and remain an integral part of all organ transplant protocols. Corticosteroids have a variety of direct and indirect modes of action, including inhibition of phospholipase A, a key initial component of the inflammatory cascade, and inhibition of T cell lymphokines, which leads to decreased activity of macrophage and T lymphocytes. Indirect effects include lymphopenia, monocyte migration inhibition, and blockage of vasodilating factors. Corticosteroids are used topically and systemically in limbal transplantation. Topical dosing is usually 3 to 4 times daily with tapered dosing and indefinite use. Oral dosing is 1 mg/kg/day with attempted tapering over 3 to 6 months if no signs of tissue rejection occur.

Immunophilin binders include cyclosporine, tacrolimus, sirolimus, and everolimus (SDZ-RAD). They are typically used in combination with corticosteroids and an antimetabolite in limbal transplantation. Cyclosporine is derivative of a Norwegian soil fungus, *Beauveria nivea*, first discovered in 1970.[27] It was the first medication used in this drug class for organ transplantation. The mode of action includes binding to cyclophilin within cellular cytoplasm and this complex creates inhibition of calcineurin. Calcineurin inhibition prevents lymphokine production and directly blocks T lymphocyte activity. Topical cyclosporine is administered with dosing of 3 to 4 times a day for an indefinite amount of time and orally at 3 mg/kg/day in 2 divided doses with a typical adult dose of 100 to 150 mg 2 times a day. The systemic dose is adjusted by monitoring serum trough levels with a therapeutic range between 100 to 150 ng/mL. Tacrolimus was first described in 1987 and is derived from the soil fungus, *Streptomyces tsukubaensis*.[27] It has a similar mode of action to cyclosporine by binding to an immunophilin known as FK-506. This complex inhibits calcineurin and blocks lymphokine production and T lymphocyte activation. Tacrolimus is 10 to 100 times more potent than cyclosporine on a per gram basis. Oral dosing is 0.5 to 0.1

mg/kg/day every 12 hours with a common starting dose of 1 mg 2 times daily. The dose may be adjusted by monitoring serum trough levels with a therapeutic range between 5 to 10 mg/mL. Sirolimus is a derivative of a macrolide antibiotic obtained from a soil actinomycete. Sirolimus is similar to tacrolimus in structure and binds to the same immunophilin; however, it does not block calcineurin and thus works a step beyond calcineurin by blocking production of proteins essential for lymphokine production, particularly interleukin 2. Sirolimus involves both T and B lymphocyte inhibition because of its different mechanism of action. Oral dosing ranges from 1 to 5 mg/m^2/day beginning with a loading dose of 15 mg on the first day followed by 5 mg daily for subsequent doses. Therapeutic drug monitoring is performed with desired levels at 8 to 10 ng/mL. Everolimus (SDZ-RAD) is a sirolimus derivative that is currently under investigational trial for prevention of organ transplant rejection. Its mode of action is identical to that of sirolimus.

Antimetabolites are typically used in combination with corticosteroids and an immunophilin-binding agent. Azathioprine is a derivative of 6-mercaptopurine and was first introduced clinically in 1962. This purine analog is metabolized in the liver to activate 6-mercaptopurine, the active compound. The active drug interferes with DNA synthesis, causing suppression of both T and B lymphocytes. Oral dosing is 1 to 2 mg/kg/day, and a typical adult dose is 100 mg/day. Mycophenolate mofetil is a relatively new semisynthetic derivative of mycophenolate acid, isolated from the mold *Penicillium glaucum*. It was developed in 1982 and directly inhibits an enzyme important for DNA synthesis, inosine monophosphate dehydrogenase.[27] This inhibition causes selective and reversible suppression of both T and B lymphocytes, an advantage over the diffuse inhibition of all lymphocytes, neutrophils, and platelets as seen with azathioprine. Oral dosing is 1 to 3 grams per day in 2 divided doses with typical adult doses of 500 to 1000 mg 2 times daily. Some patients may require dosing as high as 3 g per day to achieve appropriate immunosuppression. Other antimetabolites under investigation include mizoribine, brequinar, leflunomide, and deoxyspergualin.

Production of polyclonal and monoclonal antibodies in limbal transplantation may prove a useful adjunct to current immunosuppression regimens in the future. Polyclonal antibodies are produced by immunizing animals with human lymphoid tissue and isolating the resultant immune serum created after an immune response. This serum is purified and used to recognize specific human lymphocytes for immunosuppression. Monoclonal antibodies are produced by hybridization of a myeloma cell line and murine antibody-secreting B lymphocytes to produce specific antibodies directed at different components of the immune system. These therapeutic modalities remain under investigation and their use in prevention of immunologic rejection in tissue transplantation remains to be seen.

Although systemic immunosuppression is a necessary component of limbal transplantation, devastating potential systemic side effects can occur. Side effects are numerous and can include drug-drug interactions, hyperglycemia, hyperlipidemia, hypertension, nephrotoxicity, hepatotoxicity, myelosuppression, anemia, electrolyte and urine abnormalities, gastrointestinal effects, and bone density changes depending on the particular drug in use. Proper understanding of these side effects and understanding of appropriate laboratory monitoring is essential when using immunosuppression medications. Collaboration and consultation with a trained specialist knowledgeable of medication side effects and appropriate laboratory monitoring may be advisable in postoperative management.

Our typical immunosuppressive regimen after allogeneic stem cell replacement includes indefinite topical therapy with a corticosteroid and cyclosporine starting at dosing of 4 times a day with a slow tapering dose. Oral therapy typically includes oral prednisone at 1 mg/kg/day with attempted taper at 6 months along with oral tacrolimus 1 mg 2 times a day and oral mycophenolate 1000 mg 2 times a day begun 2 weeks before surgery. A slow taper off oral prednisone can be attempted at 4 to 6 months. Tapering of mycophenolate can be attempted at 18 months followed by attempted taper of tacrolimus at 2 years. These medications may be needed indefinitely if signs of rejection occur with attempted tapering doses.

Ex Vivo Stem Cell Expansion

Current conjunctival stem cell transplantation techniques create loss of almost half of the corneal epithelial stem cell population in the living-related or contralateral healthy donor eye, thus a major limitation of these procedures includes potential risk of iatrogenic stem cell deficiency in a normal eye. Ex vivo composite grafting procedures avoid the limitations of conjunctival limbal autografts and allografts by preservation of the majority of stem cells in the donor eye. Harvested limbal conjunctiva can be obtained from a small biopsy from the patient or a living-related donor eye. Disadvantages of this technique include time, preparation, need for extensive laboratory facilities, and expense; therefore, it should only be considered in cases where alternative stem cell transplantation techniques carry a poor prognosis.

Ex vivo stem cell expansion, as outlined by Torfi and colleagues, requires a 2-mm^2 conjunctival biopsy of the donor superotemporal conjunctiva that must include limbal conjunctiva for harvesting of stem cells.[28] The cells are transferred to a laboratory in cellular transport medium and cultivated on modified amniotic membrane. This complex is placed within enriched medium and the stem cells are allowed to attach to the amniotic membrane over the next 10 to 14 days (Figure 17-10). The medium is changed every 2 days during the attachment phase, and the graft is ready for transplantation after the allotted time.[28,29]

Surgical technique includes a 360-degree conjunctival peritomy and a 2- to 4-mm conjunctival resection followed by removal of the diseased corneal pannus and epithelium. The edges of the amniotic membrane carrier are then sutured to the conjunctival edges with 10–0 nylon suture, and a bandage lens is placed to allow for adhesion of the stem cells to the underlying tissue (see Figure 17-10). The lens is left in place for 2 to 3 months with careful observation. All allogeneic ex vivo expansions require systemic and topical immunosuppression as with other allogeneic limbal grafting procedures.

While the idea of cultured corneal epithelial stem cells was considered in 1982,[30] the first clinical reports of cultured autologous limbal stem cell transplantation occurred in 1996.[28] Torfi and colleagues reported improvement in 3 of 4 patients with severe ocular surface disease, and a follow-up study using the same technique showed ocular surface improvement in 10 of 16 patients with mean follow-up of 13

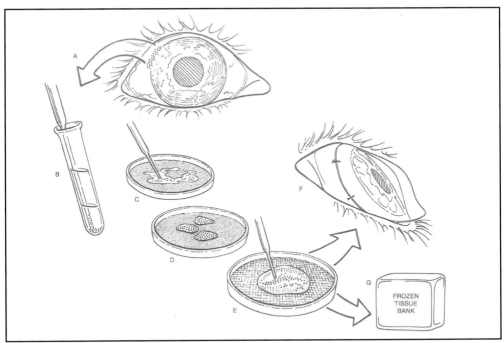

Figure 17-10. Schematic of ex vivo stem cell transplantation. (A) Stem cells are harvested from a 2-mm² limbal biopsy. (B) Harvested stem cells are transported to the laboratory in storage medium. (C) Stem cells and epithelial cells are grown in culture medium. (D) Stem cells are selected from the formed colonies. (E) The pure stem cell/epithelial cell culture is transported to amniotic membrane and allowed to grow and attach. (F) The amniotic membrane and attached stem cells are transplanted to a diseased recipient eye with stem cell deficiency with placement of the membrane across the entire cornea or in a "doughnut" fashion encircling the limbus. (G) The remaining cells can be frozen. (Reprinted with permission from Schwab IR, Isseroff, RR. Ex vivo stem cell expansion. In: Holland EJ, Mannis MJ, eds. *Ocular Surface Disease: Medical and Surgical Management.* New York: Springer-Verlag; 2002:238.)

months.[28,31] Several studies have shown similar results with improved ocular surfaces following ex vivo expansion of limbal stem cells using different harvesting techniques.[26,32,33] Daya et al found improved ocular surfaces in 7 of 10 eyes with a mean follow-up at 28 months.[26] They cultivated stem cells harvested from a corneoscleral rim and transplanted the cultured cell sheet to the diseased recipient eye, followed by coverage with amniotic membrane.[26] Additional successful bioengineered tissue replacements have included a fibrin gel carrier, a carrier-free cultivated corneal epithelial sheet, and cultivated oral mucosal epithelial stem cells.[34–37]

FUTURE TECHNOLOGY

As our knowledge of stem cells evolves, we can expect improved clinical success following autologous and allogeneic stem cell replacement surgery in the future. Additional advancements in stem cell surgical technique and new immunosuppressive agents will contribute to future success. A variety of laboratories across the world continue to contribute new laboratory and surgical techniques for procedures such as bioengineered tissue replacement. Perhaps additional carriers or improved laboratory cultivation techniques for ex vivo expansion stem cell replacement will improve clinical outcomes in ocular surface diseases. Discovery of a bone marrow-derived pluripotent stem cell for use in ocular surface transplantation may provide utility for future improvements in stem cell deficient eyes in addition to the evolution of ex vivo expansion stem cell replacement techniques.

Key Points

1. Stem cells are defined as undifferentiated cells that are found in all self-renewing tissues. They possess the ability to proliferate, produce differentiated daughter cells, self-maintain, and regenerate after injury.
2. Current nomenclature for stem cell transplant procedures includes CLAU, LR-CLAL, KLAL, and C-KLAL.
3. CLAU is the procedure of choice for unilateral limbal stem cell disease in which the fellow eye has completely normal stem cells.
4. LR-CLAL is indicated for treatment of bilateral stem cell disease or unilateral stem cell damage in which the fellow eye does not have completely normal stem cell function.
5. KLAL is indicated for both treatment of unilateral stem cell deficiency in which damage to the contralateral or living-related stem cells is feared and for bilateral severe stem cell deficiency.
6. C-KLAL is indicated for unilateral or bilateral stem cell disease with cicatricial conjunctival disease in which tissue loss and conjunctival inflammation are pronounced.
7. Immunosuppression is a crucial component of successful management in limbal transplantation.

References

1. Potten CS, Loeffler M. Stem cells: attributes, cycles, spirals, pitfalls and uncertainties. Lessons for and from the crypt. *Development*. 1990;110:1001–1020.

2. Friedenwald JS. Growth pressure and metaplasia of conjunctival and corneal epithelium. *Doc Ophthalmol*. 1951;5:184–192.

3. Davanger M, Evensen A. A role of pericorneal papillary structure in renewal of corneal epithelium. *Nature*. 1971;229:560–561.

4. Schermer A, Galvin S, Sun TT. Differentiation-related expression of major 64K corneal keratin in vivo and in culture suggests limbal location of corneal epithelial stem cells. *J Cell Biol*. 1986;103:49–62.

5. Cotsarelis G, Cheng SZ, Dong G, et al. Existence of slow-cycling limbal epithelial basal cells that can be preferentially stimulated to proliferate: implications on epithelial stem cells. *Cell*. 1989;57:201–209.

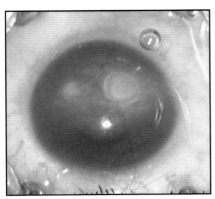

Figure 18-3. Patient to undergo limbal stem cell transplantation. Note the corneal vascularization and corneal opacity.

LIMBAL STEM CELL TRANSPLANTATION

A variety of techniques of limbal transplantation have been reported.[30–41] All these procedures remove the host's altered corneal epithelium and pannus and provide a new source of epithelium for a diseased ocular surface. From the donor tissue, transient amplifying cells are generated that migrate onto the denuded corneal surface of the host. A successful transplantation leads to the host's cornea (or grafted cornea) being permanently covered by epithelium from the donor. The donor tissue can be obtained from the other eye (limbal autograft) in cases of unilateral disease. In case of bilateral disease, the cadaveric whole globe or corneoscleral rim of a living relative (limbal allograft) can be used. Limbal transplantation procedures may also be classified depending on the carrier tissue used for the transfer of the limbal stem cells. Either conjunctiva (conjunctival limbal graft) or corneal/limbal stroma (keratolimbal graft) has been used as carrier tissue for limbal stem cells.[36]

PREOPERATIVE PREPARATION

Any pre-existing problem such as dry eye, corneal anesthesia, conjunctival scarring, corneal epithelial keratinization, mucous depletion, meibomitis, entropion, ectropion, trichiasis, etc should be taken care of. Procedures like punctal occlusion, autologous serum eye drops, lid margin eversion, scleral contact lens, and topical retinoid acid ointment may be used preoperatively to augment ocular surface defense. The patient (Figure 18-3) can be put on preoperative steroids and immunosuppressives to decrease coexisting inflammation. In the case of allograft, HLA typing and matching can be done.

SURGICAL TECHNIQUE FOR LIMBAL ALLOGRAFT

From a Cadaver Eye

Because success depends on transplantation of healthy limbal stem cells, fresh donor eyes are preferred. In the case of the cadaver eye, the whole globe is preferred because it provides better stability while dissecting the donor tissue. Several variations of limbal

Figure 18-4. Dissection done in the live, related donor eye to get a limbal graft.

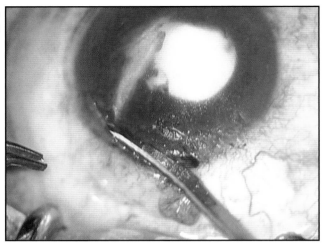

autografts[30–37]and allografts[32–41] have been reported. Dua et al have described a modified procedure for limbal allograft.[42] The eye is first made tense by injecting air into the vitreous cavity through the optic nerve using a 26-gauge needle and the nerve is clamped. The eye is held in a Tudor Thomas stand. A trephine 3 mm smaller than the corneal diameter is used to make a well centered, superficial, partial thickness cut in the donor tissue (approximately 150 mm depth). The cornea peripheral to the cut is then dissected using a bevel up dissector. The dissection is carried all the way through the limbus into a small peripheral rim of sclera, approximately 1 mm. Any conjunctiva, if present, is retained. This corneoscleral rim is then cut free from the cadaver globe.

The recipient bed is prepared by doing a 360-degree peritomy and removing the conjuctivalized epithelium and underlying scar tissue off the cornea by blunt dissection. The donor graft is then placed at the host limbus and sutured in place using 10–0 nylon. Any gap is filled with a "spacer" made from donor corneal stroma or a piece of donor limbal tissue from the other eye of the same donor. The host conjunctiva is reapproximated to the limbus using interrupted sutures. If required, a tarsorrhaphy can be done.

The advantages of cadaver eye are that a 360-degree limbal graft can be taken, thus providing more limbal stem cells. The larger graft also acts as a barrier for migration of conjunctivally derived epithelium over the cornea. The disadvantage is that there is a greater chance of rejection of the graft, and the patient may even be required to take immunosuppressives for his or her lifetime.

From a Live Related Donor

The procedure followed is the same as limbal autograft (explained next) except that the donor tissue is taken from a live, related donor (Figures 18-4 and 18-5), preferably after HLA typing and matching. This is done in case of bilateral limbal stem cell deficiency. Even though this theoretically decreases the chances of rejection as compared to cadaver graft, postoperative systemic immunosuppressive therapy may be required for the patient's lifetime.

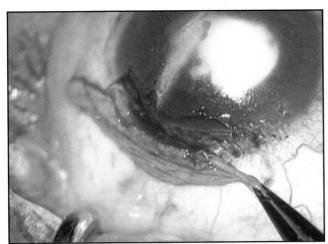

Figure 18-5. Limbal graft dissection complete.

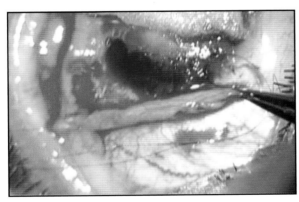

Figure 18-6. Dissection done in the recipient eye and graft kept over the area for suturing to start.

RECIPIENT EYE

The recipient bed is then prepared by doing a peritomy in the involved area and removing the conjuctivalized epithelium and underlying scar tissue off the cornea by blunt dissection. A bed is prepared for the graft by excising a rim of corneolimbal tissue corresponding in size to the donor. A thin rim of conjunctiva is also excised. The donor graft is then kept in place (Figure 18-6) and sutured in place using 10–0 nylon (Figure 18-7). The host conjunctiva is approximated to the donor conjunctiva using interrupted sutures. If required, a tarsorrhaphy can be done. An AMT can also be done at the end if necessary (Figure 18-8).

AMNIOGRAFT

Amniotic membrane can be acquired from a maternity ward. This way one can use fresh amniotic membrane. One can also use Amniograft (Bio-Tissue Inc, Miami, Fla). This has been recovered aseptically from a donated placental tissue through elective caesarean section delivery and processed under class 100 condition. The donor is screened for HIV, HBsAg, etc. Amniograft is preserved in a validated and patented stor-

Figure 18-7. Suturing done of the limbal graft.

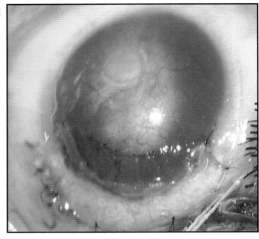

Figure 18-8. Amniotic membrane transplantation.

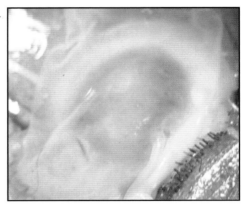

age medium made of Dulbecco's Modified Eagle Medium and glycerol (1:1) with antibiotics. No preservatives or additives are added. The tissue is stored at -80°C prior to distribution.

Amniograft is attached to a white nitrocellulose paper with the (sticky) stromal side adherent to the filter paper and the basement membrane side away from the paper. If orientation is questionable after detaching the membrane from the paper, one can use a dry Weckcel or cotton tip to check. Weckcel will only adhere to the (sticky) stromal side.

Bio-Tissue has also introduced Prokera, a clinically proven amniograft that is mounted on a corneal-shaped ring so that you can use a sutureless graft for ocular surface reconstruction. This way there is quicker healing, no scars, and less time.

SURGICAL TECHNIQUE FOR LIMBAL AUTOGRAFT

The donor tissue is taken from the same or the opposite eye.[43,44] Hence, it can be performed only in conditions with limited or unilateral limbal stem cell deficiency.[22] The advantage is that the risk of graft rejection is very low.

Dua et al have described a modified procedure for limbal allograft.[22] The donor tissue is taken from the contralateral eye and transplanted onto the diseased eye. It may also be taken from a different site on the same eye in case of localized disease. Approximately 2 clock hours of the donor tissue consisting of 2 mm of superficial (about 150 mm) peripheral cornea, limbus, and 3 mm of conjunctiva is dissected from the donor eye.

The number of grafts taken depends on the severity and extent of involvement of the diseased eye. A maximum of up to 180 degrees of limbal tissue may be excised from the donor eye without inducing iatrogenic limbal stem cell deficiency.

LIMBAL STEM CELL TRANSPLANTATION WITH KERATOPLASTY

In case of both allografts and autografts, if a penetrating keratoplasty is also planned for the same sitting, it is done after the limbal grafts are sutured in place. The corneal graft generally has to be kept to within 7 mm in size to avoid encroaching onto the limbal graft.

LIMBAL STEM CELL TRANSPLANTATION WITH AMNIOTIC MEMBRANE GRAFT

Limbal stem cell transplantation can be combined with an amniotic membrane graft in severe cases (see Figure 18-8). Amniotic membrane graft may be sufficient by itself in cases with partial limbal stem cell deficiency but in cases with total stem cell deficiency, it is combined with limbal stem cell transplantation.

Amniotic membrane serves as a "transplanted basement membrane." It facilitates migration of epithelial cells and reinforces epithelial cell adhesion. It provides a potential substrate and is a source of various growth factors that promote epithelialization and enhance wound healing.[13,23,24]

POSTOPERATIVE COURSE

Patients should be on frequent follow-up until epithelialization is complete. Generally, the epithelium starts growing from the graft within 2 to 3 days and becomes complete within 2 weeks.[42] If, at any stage, conjunctival epithelium is seen to grow over the limbus or cornea again, it is scraped off to allow the epithelialization to occur from the graft. Signs indicative of graft rejection include graft edema, graft neovascularization, vascularization over the graft onto the cornea, focal conjunctival injection, or focal corneal epithelial defect in the sector of rejection.

POSTOPERATIVE DRUG THERAPY

Postoperatively, the patient is maintained on topical antibiotic steroid drops and preservative-free artificial tears. Autologous serum eye drops have also been found to be useful. In case of allografts, steroids may be continued for a longer period at a low dosage (1 drop per day). Immunosuppressive therapy is also given postoperatively for allografts.

SUCCESS RATES

Tsubota and coauthors[45] published a large case series in the *New England Journal of Medicine* in which they used a cadaver source for the donor limbal stem cell and all patients underwent concomitant amniotic membrane grafting. Success rates as denoted by successful epithelialization with phenotypic corneal epithelium, presence of a clear cornea, and visual acuity were 71%, 50%, and 0.04 % (count fingers), respectively, in burn patients and were lower (50%, 28%, and 0.02) [hand motion], respectively), in OCP/Stevens-Johnson syndrome group. Their conclusion was that limbal stem cell transplantation with amniotic membrane grafting was successful in certain patients. These results, though not as satisfactory from the point of final visual acuity, are acceptable because the only other alternative for these patients would be a keratoprosthesis.

RECENT ADVANCES

Transplantation of Ex Vivo Expanded Limbal Epithelial Stem Cells

USING COLLAGEN SHIELD AS TRANSFER SUBSTRATE

He and McCulley[46] documented that limbal epithelial stem cells can be grown in vitro and stratified on collagen gel substrate. They transferred these collagen shields with epithelial cells to denuded ex vivo human corneal stroma in organic cultures. The 3T3 coculture system allows clonal growth of corneal epithelial cells and maintains them in the relatively undifferentiated state.[47]

USING AMNIOTIC MEMBRANE AS TRANSFER SUBSTRATE

Pellegrini et al[25] transplanted a sheet of in vitro cultured autologous limbal corneal epithelial cell layer to stem cell deficient cornea and reported successful long-term restoration of the corneal epithelial surface in 2 cases. A small piece of limbal tissue obtained from a biopsy from the contralateral eye was digested enzymatically and the epithelium was then expanded in special medium. Three weeks later, the confluent epithelial sheet was grafted to the diseased cornea. They found difficulties in handling this fragile sheet of epithelium and hence the search for a suitable carrier was begun, the role being fulfilled by amniotic membrane. When the expanded cell population reached 40% to 50% confluence, they were passed onto human amniotic membrane and allowed to attach to the amniotic membrane for 10 to 14 days. This was then used for limbal stem cell transplantation. The biopsy can be taken from the same patient in case of unilateral or limited disease and from a living, related donor or a cadaver eye[28,48] in case of bilateral total involvement. Culturing the cells takes 3 to 4 weeks. It may then be cryopreserved for any length of time in liquid nitrogen. In case of allografts, the patient may need to be placed on immunosuppressive therapy postoperatively.

USING FIBRIN AS TRANSFER SUBSTRATE

Limbal stem cells can be cultured using fibrin as a medium and can be transferred to the eye.[49]

19

Large Diameter Lamellar Keratoplasty and Stem Cell Transplantation

Javier Mendicute, MD, PhD;
Itziar Martínez-Soroa, MD;
Aritz Bidaguren, MD; Ane Gibelalde, MD;
and Ana Blanco, MD

Introduction

The ocular surface, according to the concept introduced by Thoft and Friend[1] in 1977, comprises the inner surface of the eyelid, the conjunctival fornix, the bulbar conjunctiva, and the cornea.[2] In recent years, the relationship between the corneal and conjunctival epithelium has been and continues to be the subject of increasing interest. While both epitheliums have similar functions, protecting against infection and maintaining sensory alertness in the face of trauma, they are different histologically and biochemically. The corneal epithelium is a multilayer nonkeratinized epithelium. On the contrary, the conjunctival epithelium has fewer layers, the cells are less attached, and they contain fewer desmosomes and hemidesmosomes. One of the most peculiar characteristics is the presence of mucin-producing goblet cells, which are absent in the healthy corneal epithelium.[1]

The corneal epithelium not only serves as a layer of protection for the underlying cornea, it also plays an important role in maintaining the basal membrane and the optical transparency of the stroma.

The processes of epithelium repair are also peculiar in the cornea in that the epithelium is an avascular tissue. It has been proven that in corneal epithelial defects, regardless of their etiology, initial healing takes place through the migration of adjacent cells.[3] Also characteristic in such processes is the centripetal movement of corneal epithelial cell from the corneoscleral limbus toward the center of the cornea. Given that corneal epithelium is a self-renewing tissue, a number of clinical trials and studies support the existence of a source of stem cells as its proliferative reserve. These cells are thought to be located in the basal layers of the corneoscleral limbus[4,5] and to be ultimately responsible for cell replacement and tissue regeneration.[6]

We know that the sclerocorneal junction or limbus is a narrow annular transition zone of epithelium and connective tissue between the cornea and the bulbar conjunctiva that represents the transitional zone between the transparent cornea and the opaque sclera.[7] Clinically, the limbus is oval shaped, the longer side in a horizontal position and the sclerocorneal interface wider at the vertical meridian than at the horizontal meridian. In this zone, the corneal epithelium has anatomical ridges called palisades of Vogt. In these structures, the limbal epithelium is different from the epithelium of the bulbar conjunctiva in that it is devoid of goblet cells, and it differs from the corneal epithelium in that it has Langerhans' cells, melanocytes, and underlying blood vessels.[8] We can, therefore, deduce that the anatomical integrity of the corneoscleral limbus is very important because it is necessary for the maintenance of the stem cell reserve for normal corneal epithelial regeneration processes and in maintaining corneal transparency and its important optical function.

In eyes with significant alteration of the corneal epithelial surface and compromised corneoscleral limbus, the conjunctival epithelium cells are responsible for the ability of the corneal epithelium to regenerate, leading to conjunctivalization of the corneal epithelium with the characteristic loss of secondary corneal transparency, accompanied by chronic inflammation, persistent defects in the epithelium, scar formation in the stroma, and neovascularization.[9,10] In these cases, anatomical recovery of the corneoscleral limbus is needed so that the corneal surface can be populated with stem cells, which will then take over the job of corneal epithelial regeneration. In this way, corneal transparency and its optical function can be recovered. Anatomical recovery of the corneoscleral limbus can only be achieved by stem cell transplantation, either with keratoepithelioplasty,[11] limbal transplantation (either associated with AMT or not),[12] or more recently, by transplanting epithelial stem cells cultivated[13] on different media such as amniotic membrane.[14]

CORNEAL EPITHELIAL REGENERATION

The kinetics of corneal epithelial maintenance are characterized by both vertical and horizontal cell movement. Vertical movement has been documented experimentally, observing previously divided basal cells that move due to proliferative pressure in the basal cell layers.[15,16] Horizontal movement of corneal epithelial cells from the peripheral cornea toward the central cornea was observed experimentally in healing processes of the corneal epithelium.[15,16] In keratoplasty in the rabbit, it has also been observed that donor epithelium regenerates, moving centripetally from the peripheral epithelium of the receptor.[17] Observations in humans bear out these theories.[10,18,19]

Therefore, it is deduced that corneal epithelial regeneration requires the processes of division, migration, stratification, and cell maturation.[20] It is impossible to understand the perpetual nature of this cellular regeneration without the existence of stem cells, and renovation (harvesting corneal type epithelium) involves stem cell differentiation.[20] In order for cell mass to be stable, there must be a balance between cell division, maturation, death, and desquamation.[21,22]

Three different theories have sought to explain the way in which corneal epithelium is regenerated:

1. The classical theory set out to explain corneal epithelial renewal as a vertical process in which epithelial surface cells continuously exfoliate and are

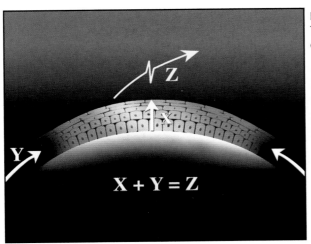

Figure 19-1. Thoft's X, Y, Z theory. This theory tries to explain how corneal epithelium is renewed.

replaced by basal cells. This theory, while verified in multilayered epithelium such as the epidermis, does not apply to corneal epithelium because it does not explain the differences in mitotic activity in different areas of the cornea[23] or the centripetal movement of cells.[24]

2. The cell transdifferentiation theory implies that the corneal epithelium may have a conjunctival origin through a phenomenon known as transdifferentiation. This theory is based on experimental studies[9] that were later effectively refuted,[25] demonstrating that the conjunctival transdifferentiation theory is based on studies conducted in conditions that do not allow for the elimination of any possible regeneration of cells from the corneoscleral limbus.[20]

3. The current stem cell theory underscores the important role of the limbal basal epithelium in maintaining corneal epithelial mass under physiological conditions and its importance in epithelial regeneration of epithelial defects. Davanger and Evensen[26] were the first to speculate that corneal epithelium had its origin in the limbal palisades of Vogt; 15 years later, Schermer, Galvin, and Sun[27] laid the foundations for the hypothesis that the limbus was the origin of corneal epithelium and, more specifically, that limbal basal epithelium contains its stem cells, corroborating Thoft and Friend's X, Y, Z theory[22] on corneal epithelial maintenance: "The exfoliated cells (component Z) are continually replaced not only by dividing basal cells (X), but also by cells that migrate from the periphery (Y)" (Figure 19-1).

The stem cell theory only serves to confirm and emphasize the importance of the limbus based on evidence confirming the movement of cells from the peripheral cornea toward the central cornea[2] and a preferential desquamation of central as opposed to peripheral corneal epithelium[28-30] (Figure 19-2).

It is logical, therefore, to deduce the importance of keeping the corneoscleral limbus intact and preserving the stem cell population in order to maintain the processes of corneal epithelium repair in both physiological and pathological situations. In the latter, when the integrity of the limbus is compromised, anatomical and functional reconstruction is of the outmost importance to maintain a population of stem cells that can ensure corneal epithelial regeneration.

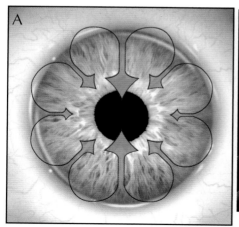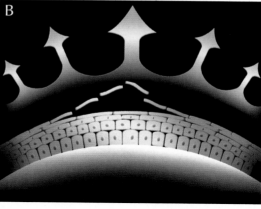

Figure 19-2. Foundations of corneal epithelial regeneration. The stem cell theory is based on the confirmation of centripetal movement of corneal epithelial cells (A) and on preferential desquamation of central corneal epithelium (B).

Ocular Surface Disease

Limbal insufficiency, understood as the failure of the stem cells in an eye to regenerate and maintain a healthy ocular surface, has recently been termed *ocular surface disease*. The term is more general than and not nearly as precise as limbal insufficiency. A number of unrelated disorders can be grouped under ocular surface disease, from dry eye and other autoimmune disorders, to iatrogenic conditions, including problems induced by the use and abuse of contact lenses or medications.

The possible clinical manifestations of the absence or deficit of stem cells have been profusely detailed based on findings from experimental studies.[31,32] In practice, there are clinical clues that can lead us to suspect the possibility of limbal insufficiency, including patient-described symptoms in their varying degrees of impreciseness (loss of vision, foreign body sensation, chronic irritation) and signs (loss of limbal anatomy; superficial and peripheral corneal vascularization; fibrovascular pannus; diffuse staining of the pathologic, irregular, and thinned epithelium; unstable tear film; and a certain degree of scarring or keratinization). In any event, the most characteristic signs are the breakdown of the limbal vascular barrier (Figure 19-3) in more than two-thirds of the limbal circumference; abnormal impregnation of the corneal epithelium with vital dyes; impression cytology, especially if performed at different sites, thus confirming abnormal epithelial patterns; the presence of goblet cells on the corneal epithelium; and the most recent immunohistochemistry techniques, which detect expression of cytokeratins specific to the conjunctiva on the corneal epithelium, demonstrating that the corneal epithelium has conjunctival origin.

Once limbal insufficiency has been verified (Table 19-1), it is essential to determine the amount of functioning limbus and how much functioning limbus is needed to ensure corneal epithelial stability. The presence of limbal insufficiency and the amount of existing limbus can be further clarified when other factors come into play, such as the vascular microenvironment, the condition of the tear film, and inflammation resulting from the surgery itself.

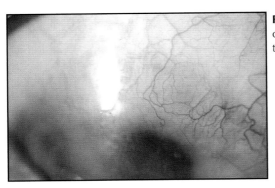

Figure 19-3. Breakdown of the limbal vascular barrier. This is one of the early signs that may be observed in limbal insufficiency.

Table 19-1
PATHOLOGIES WITH POTENTIAL RISK FACTORS FOR LIMBAL INSUFFICIENCY

- Chemical burns.
- Thermal burns.
- Stevens-Johnson syndrome.
- Limbal excisions caused by neoplasia.
- Aniridia.
- OCP.
- Pterygium.
- Irradiation keratopathy.
- Contact lens keratopathy.
- Abuse of topical anesthetics.
- Others.

If we can gain a good understanding of the clinical outcomes deriving from stem cell failure, we will be able to determine which pathologies might benefit from limbal transplantation. The primary pathologies include chemical burn injuries, thermal burns, Stevens-Johnson syndrome, limbal excisions caused by neoplasia, aniridia, OCP, erythema multiforme, pterygium, irradiation keratopathy, and contact lens keratopathy. However, limbal deficiency is only one of the multiple clinical manifestations shown in these pathologies. Whether autoimmune, inflammatory, or otherwise, if these circumstances are not considered on an individual basis and treated previously, they can lead to failure in high-risk transplantation. All of the pathologies listed here, therapeutically oriented from an etiopathogenic perspective, could benefit from techniques involving limbal transplantation, which according to literature,[12,33] is the source of stem cells, and from corneal epithelial cell expansion techniques on different media for subsequent transplantation.[13,14]

Basic Therapeutics in Ocular Surface Disease

It is important to know how to manage eyelid disease and meibomian pathology, inflammatory processes of the conjunctiva and the episclera, palpebral disorders in both secretion and drainage dynamics, and (needless to say) the different forms of keratoconjunctivitis, whether associated with exposure, infection, inflammation, toxins, or a combination of some or all of these forms. It is also essential to know how to use the immune suppressors used in transplantations when considering treatment for ocular surface disorders and improving the prognosis.[34] Techniques aimed at stabilizing the ocular surface should be understood as previous to other reconstructive techniques that involve tissue transplantation so as to improve the prognosis.

We should know the principles of correcting palpebral disorders (cicatricial entropion and ectropion), how to manage dry eye (medical treatment and lacrimal punctum occlusion techniques), control overexposure of the ocular surface (tarsorrhaphies and conjunctival flaps), and prepare keratoplasty surgery (AMT and limbal stem cell transplantation).[34] When considering a reconstructive technique for the ocular surface with clear presence of dry eye, certain adjuvant measures could determine the prognosis. Punctal occlusion[35,36] is useful in patients with dry eye for whom medical treatment (artificial tears, secretagogues, humid environments) is insufficient. This technique is particularly indicated in cases of aqueous deficiency, although it may decrease the need for artificial tears in this circumstance and in other forms of dry eye.[34]

Tarsorrhaphy is still indicated in certain circumstances, especially in the management of certain pathologies of the ocular surface. It may decrease the exposed area of the ocular surface, reduce loss of tears through evaporation, allow for longer contact between tears and the ocular surface, and prevent palpebral friction in particularly sensitive and disturbed areas, all of which can extend the cell cycle of the corneal-conjunctival epithelium by reducing loss via desquamation induced by blinking.[34] Generally speaking, in spite of the introduction of a number of therapeutic alternatives, the conjunctival flap is still useful for solving clinical problems in the acute stages; it can be therapeutic or preliminary to penetrating keratoplasty for optical purposes.[34]

Regeneration of the Ocular Surface: Alternatives

It should be pointed out that as long as there is 25% of functioning limbus, this may be enough to maintain the epithelial mass, either by itself or in association with other techniques such as AMT or sequential epithelial mass sectorial conjunctival epitheliectomy,[37,38] ensuring that the epithelial repair processes guarantee stable epithelium under physiological conditions. In this case, it is vital to take advantage of this potential before deciding on limbal transplantation. The techniques described above may be repeated over several sessions. When these techniques fail to regenerate healthy epithelium on the functioning visual axis, other techniques will have to be implemented.

Limbal Transplantation

José I. Barraquer[39] was the first author to propose limbal epithelial transplantation (ie, taking corneoconjunctival epithelium from the healthy eye to improve the epithelium of the cornea damaged by burn injuries) as a technique performed prior to keratoplasty. During the same period, Strampelli[40] suggested a similar technique.

Conjunctival Transplantation

The conjunctival transplantation procedure proposed by Thoft[41] involved taking conjunctiva obtained from the contralateral eye. It proved effective as a source of epithelial cells in regenerating the corneal epithelium of eyes with persistent epithelial defects, such as those observed in burn injuries. In practice, however, use of this procedure depends on the condition of the contralateral eye, which is often compromised in burn injuries. In these cases, an allogeneic conjunctival transplantation was suggested, either by harvesting grafts from cadaver donors[42] or live donors.[43]

Keratoepithelioplasty

Keratoepithelioplasty was described by Thoft[11] for the treatment of persistent epithelial defects in patients without healthy donor corneoconjunctival epithelium in their fellow eye. The first cases described were performed on patients with ocular burn injuries. This technique should be considered the precursor to limbal transplantation as we know it today.

LIMBAL TRANSPLANTATION

Kenyon and Tseng[12] described the current indications for limbal transplantation. It has been demonstrated both clinically[12,44-47] and experimentally[33] that epithelial regeneration prompted by limbal transplantation improves stromal repair processes, slowing down the development of opacity and corneal neovessels, thus enabling better recovery of corneal transparency.

The following have been considered the classical options for limbal transplantations.

Autograft From the Same Eye or From the Contralateral Eye

The surgical technique[6,12] usually involves the transfer of 2 free grafts of limbal tissue from the uninjured or less injured donor eye to the severely injured recipient eye. First, the injured eye is prepared. The vascularized scar is removed by a conjunctival peritomy. The abnormal epithelium and fibrovascular pannus can be dissected on the corneal surface with a spatula or scaler, or simply peeled using cellulose sponges and tissue forceps. Cleaning can occasionally be done on the stromal surface, but a real lamellar keratectomy is only indicated for chronically scarred corneas.

Kenyon and Tseng[12] prefer obtaining 2 free grafts of limbal tissue from the donor eye, spanning approximately 0.5 mm centrally in the cornea and approximately 2 mm peripherally in the bulbar conjunctiva. Each graft includes 4 clock hours, measuring approximately 3 x 10 mm. It is generally useful to mark the margins beforehand to properly evaluate the size of the graft and to avoid errors when positioning the graft in the recipient bed. The initial incision should be made at the corneal margin using a scaler to prevent poor surgical visualization caused by bleeding that would occur if the dissection were initiated at the conjunctival edge. The donor bed can either be left open or closed. Donor eyes heal quickly with no refractive changes, chronic inflammation, persistent epithelial defects, or corneal neovascularizations during the postoperative period, thus proving to be a safe technique for the donor eye. However, it is important to discount any subclinical pathologies that could be overlooked at the time of donation but that could lead to future complications.

The autografts are then transferred to the recipient eye and attached in the proper anatomical position with 10–0 nylon sutures at the corneal margin and absorbable 8–0 Vicryl sutures at the conjunctiva margin.

Limbal Allograft Transplantation

The procedure is performed following the technique described using cells from a donor.[48] Eyes from donor banks can be used; however, it is better to use donor tissue from a relative, preferably of the same blood group. Although there have been conflicting reports regarding the role of HLA typing, patients can benefit from the HLA matching.

Limbal allograft transplantation is only performed if the fellow eye is impaired or, if for whatever reason, it is not considered wise to harvest tissue from the contralateral eye. In these cases donors should be under the age of 50 to ensure stem cell population. Systemic immunosuppression should be considered essential, thus calling for a thorough study of the recipient's bill of health. The recipient should be informed of the potential benefits of the surgical technique as well as the risks of immunosuppression and the need for middle- to long-term postoperative follow-up.

Initially, the technique used in limbal allograft transplantations was similar to the autograft technique except that by using donor tissue it was possible to perform corneolimbal ring graft techniques using 360x rings. The corneoscleral ring is removed together with the limbus from the cadaver eye. A penetrating annular keratotomy is performed on the cornea with a 9-mm trephine, and if a 13- to 14-mm trephine is available, the sclera is trephined concentrically. If not, dissect the sclera with circular scissors in order to obtain a 360x corneolimbal ring. After obtaining the ring, the sclera and the peripheral cornea are thinned to one-third of their original thickness. The recipient bed is prepared with a 360x conjunctival peritomy and a corneal fibrovascular tissue dissection. The corneoscleral ring is then placed on the recipient bed and sutured with 10–0 nylon sutures on the cornea and 8–0 Vicryl sutures on the episclera.

Holland[49] proposed a change in the limbal allograft transplantation technique that, at least theoretically, would increase the number of available stem cells. Two donor eyes are needed to perform this technique, transplanting 3 120-degree sections of corneoscleral limbus.

When penetrating central corneal and limbal transplantations must be associated, whether sectorial or annular, simultaneous or sequential, the refractive corneal surface presents a large number of sutures that only complicate the surgical technique and postoperative period.

Manual Large Diameter Lamellar Keratoplasty and Stem Cell Transplantation

In an attempt to improve the above-mentioned difficulties, a manual technique of large diameter lamellar keratoplasty including corneoscleral limbus has been suggest-

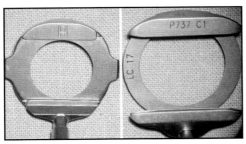

Figure 19-4. Microkeratome rings. ALTK System H ring (Moria, France) and large-diameter ring from the new system (Moria, France).

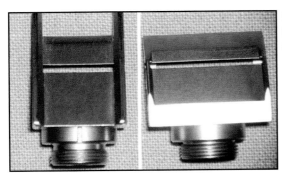

Figure 19-5. Microkeratome heads. ALTK System and head from the new system (Moria, France).

ed.[49] This technique is useful if the deep corneal stroma is transparent; if there is opacification of the deep stroma, lamellar techniques would have to associate simultaneous deep stroma transplantation and large diameter lamellar transplantation or a subsequent penetrating keratoplasty.

Automatic Large Diameter Lamellar Keratoplasty and Stem Cell Transplantation

We[38,50] suggest the possibility of performing a large diameter lamellar transplantation using rings (Figure 19-4) and one of the ALTK microkeratome system heads (Moria, France) (Figure 19-5). The characteristics of the head limit the ability to obtain donor buttons that include limbus with this system, making it virtually impossible to obtain buttons greater than 12 mm; therefore, in our first experiences using this system, we selected donors with white-white corneal diameters measuring less than 12 mm in order to include stem cells. Later a new ring (see Figure 19-4) and head (see Figure 19-5) were designed for the microkeratome system that made it possible to obtain lamellar grafts of 13 to 14 mm for the same purpose: stem cell transplantation.[51,52]

We have been working with this head since 2003. From our experience, we can say the following: 1) corneal flaps of 13 to 14 mm and 100 to 150 μm in thickness can be cut, 2) pressure must be exerted on the donor eye when passing the microkeratome to create the donor button, otherwise loss of suction is likely, thus creating irregular flaps or flaps with buttonholes, and 3) the technique is not reproducible enough to cut the recipient bed and in cases where we have tried, suction is easily lost when the head comes in contact with the globe. Therefore, we have explored other recipient cutting possibilities.

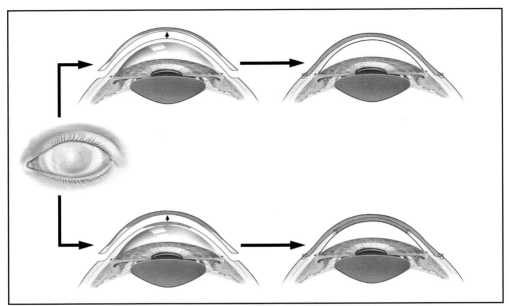

Figure 19-6. Situations associated with limbal dysfunction. Figure on top—limited alteration of superficial corneal stroma. Figure on bottom—with deep corneal stromal opacification.

From our experience over the years in clinical situations, we have seen 2 situations associated with limbal dysfunction (Figure 19-6):
1. Limbal dysfunction with limited alteration of the ocular surface and transparent deep corneal stroma, generally in relatively recent situations and without a great inflammatory component associated.
2. Limbal dysfunction with the entire corneal thickness compromised, generally in situations where ocular surface diseases are serious, with inadequate inflammation management in the original process or very advanced processes.

In the first situation, only the anterior corneal stroma needs to be transplanted. On the contrary, in the second, there is still opacification in the deep stroma after removing the anterior corneal surface, and thus it needs to be replaced (see Figure 19-6).

In either of the 2 cases, the process is as follows:
- Obtain a donor button of 13 to 14 mm with a 100 to 150 μm thickness. After the donor eye is enucleated, a dissection of the perilimbal conjunctiva is performed so that it does not obstruct in the passing of the microkeratome. If the globe is soft, saline solution or BSS can be injected through the optical nerve to achieve the proper tone. The eye is then ready to create the donor button. Although this procedure can be performed directly on the operating table, we prefer to use an experimental surgery globe holder since it reduces the risk of displacement. It is essential to identify the horizontal and vertical axes of the cornea and to mark the vertical meridian (at 6 and 12 o'clock) with a surgical marker. We then position the ring onto the sclera (Figure 19-7), activate the suction pump, and make sure there is adequate suction to secure the eye. The head is inserted onto the guide and the cornea irrigated with saline solution or BSS. The ring is pressed against the globe, the globe against the holder, and the

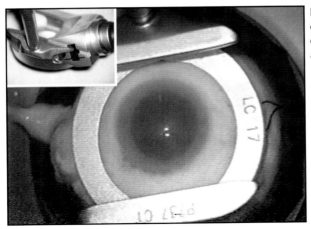

Figure 19-7. Preparing the donor eye. The ring is on the enucleated eye before passing the microkeratome.

microkeratome activated, running it slowly and evenly over the donor cornea. This is how we harvest a donor button with the mentioned characteristics: 13 to 14 mm with a 100 to 150 μm thickness. Once the donor button is obtained and the corneal graft is marked, a silk suture is placed at the 12 o'clock position of the epithelial side of the donor button to prevent the graft from shifting.

- In case the deep stroma is needed, we dissect the deep cornea at the level of the limbus in 360 degrees, using silk suture to identify the 12 o'clock position on the anterior side.
- Both the anterior and deep corneal buttons can be used immediately or stored in the corneal preservation medium if the transplantation is to be delayed for hours or days.
- After adequately anesthetizing the patient, we perform a 360-degree conjunctival peritomy, eliminate any fibrovascular pannus, and coagulate enough to control bleeding and to prevent any scleral ischemia that might compromise the integrity of the graft. Using the standard 130- to 150-μm head of the ALTK System, an 8- to 10-mm central stromal bed is cut in the recipient eye; 250- or 350-μm heads can also be used if corneal stromal opacification compromises more than 150 μm of superficial stroma. We then mark a 13- or 15-mm ring parallel to the limbus with a 13- or 15-mm trephine with a stop device (Moria, France) to avoid penetration. The second surgical step involves connecting the edge of the keratectomy to the scleral bed, cutting it with the proper instrument, our preference being the crescent scalpel by Alcon Laboratories (Fort Worth, Tex). In this way, we have a central corneal bed cut uniformly with the microkeratome mechanical device and a peripheral edge cut manually (Figure 19-8A), which provides security and has little relevance to postoperative visual acuity.

The donor button is sutured onto the recipient bed if the deep stroma is transparent (Figure 19-8B). The donor button must be properly oriented in the recipient bed: the horizontal axis of the donor (larger than vertical axis) should be positioned horizontally in the recipient bed. Although it has little clinical relevance, the aesthetic situation could be striking otherwise. To prevent such risks, the ref-

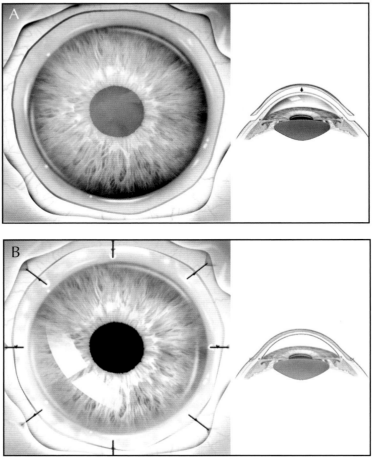

Figure 19-8. Large diameter anterior lamellar keratoplasty. (A) After superficial anterior keratectomy. (B) After suturing the 13- to 14-mm graft, which includes corneoscleral limbus and stem cells.

erence marks recommended in the previous paragraph are very useful. Eight 10–0 nylon sutures with the knots buried are sufficient. The corneal interface is then washed with a BSS and the conjunctiva is secured onto the graft with 8 absorbable 8–0 Vicryl sutures. Surgical recovery in these cases is fast and the long-term refractive situation good since there are no sutures in the central stroma (Figure 19-9).

- Once step 4 is completed (Figure 19-10A), if opacification is observed in the deep corneal stroma, the deep donor button needs to be prepared before trephining the deep recipient stromal bed (Figure 19-10B). Recover the deep corneal bed from the donor cornea and trephine the back side with a 7.5- to 8-mm trephine. This is done as with penetrating keratoplasties, except that the button harvested here will lack the epithelial surface and the anterior stroma, which has been removed previously. Then, the deep donor button is sutured (Figure 19-10C) followed by the superficial cornea (Figure 19-10D). We suture the deep stroma with 4 or 8 10–0 nylon sutures and on top of this, the large

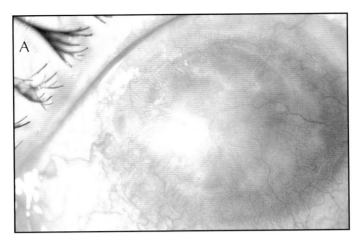

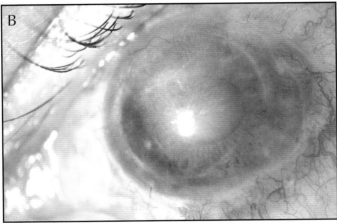

Figure 19-9. Ocular surface disease with limbal insufficiency due to abuse of topical anesthetics. (A) Preoperative situation. (B) At 1 year.

diameter lamellar graft is sutured with 8 10–0 nylon sutures, generally alternating with the 8 deep sutures as described in the previous paragraph. In these cases, the deep sutures are to be left in place, since they can only be removed with a yttrium-aluminum-garnet (YAG) laser (Figure 19-11).

LIMBAL TRANSPLANTATION AND EXPECTED OUTCOMES

Conceptually, the limbal transplantation is highly attractive. According to different authors[6,12] and based on our own experience,[33,38,47,50] we can expect the following outcomes:
- Symptomatic relief from ocular irritation. Rapid healing of the corneal surface brings about symptomatic relief from annoyances generally caused by epithelial instability.

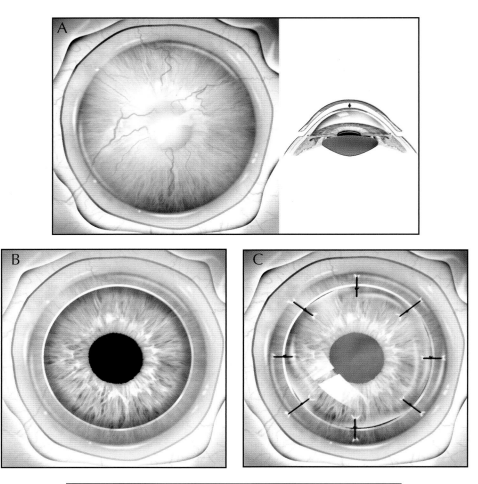

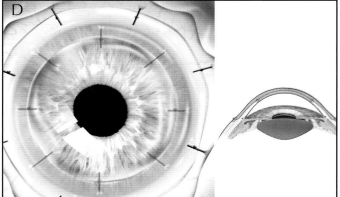

Figure 19-10. Large diameter anterior lamellar keratoplasty followed by keratoplasty. (A) After superficial anterior keratectomy. (B) After trephining the deep bed. (C) After suturing the deep button. (D) After suturing the superficial cornea.

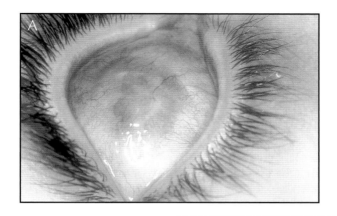

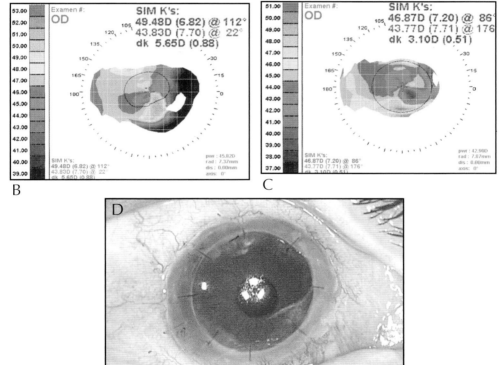

Figure 19-11. Large diameter lamellar keratoplasty for treating severe burns. (A) Preoperative situation. (B) One year after manipulating sutures. (C) One year after selectively cutting deep sutures with YAG laser. (D) Final situation.

- Improved visual acuity. Approximately 50% of patients have a visual acuity of 2/10.[12] This visual improvement, together with better aesthetic results owing to less inflammation, photophobia, and protective ptosis, can eliminate the need for a keratoplasty.
- Rapid healing with a stable surface. Postoperatively, limbal grafts revascularize in 5 days, and the epithelium generally covers the denuded areas of the cornea and conjunctiva in 7 to 21 days.[33]
- Suppression or regression of corneal neovascularization. It begins a few days after corneal re-epithelialization is completed. Reduction and even regression of neovascular activity can occur.[6,12,33,47]
- Greater success of future procedures (penetrating keratoplasty) The development of a stable corneal epithelium surface eliminates one of the causes of keratoplasty failure in chemical or thermal injuries.[38,50]

In addition to the benefits already described from the limbal transplantation technique we propose (large diameter lamellar keratoplasty with microkeratome), there are also further benefits such as:

- Better anterior corneal surface quality. We obtain a uniform, suture-free surface that quickly regains its transparency and does not exert friction on the eyelids when blinking, since there are no irregularities from conventional limbus transplantations or keratoplasties.
- Better refractive results:
    * This is explained by the absence of sutures on the refractive corneal surface and by cutting the donor button and the center of the recipient bed with the microkeratome.
    * The above is based on topographic and refractive studies of patients on whom we have performed these techniques.
    * If there are astigmatisms in the transplantations that require only superficial lamellar keratoplasty, the sutures can be removed very early since a watertight seal has been maintained at all times with the anterior chamber. We prefer to perform a topography-guided suturo-lysis beginning at the third month.
    * When associated deep stromal bed transplantation is required, topography and slit lamp examination help identify the sutures responsible for the astigmatism. If the sutures from the large diameter keratoplasty are responsible for the astigmatism, we proceed as mentioned in the previous paragraph. However, we recommend waiting at least 3 months before taking any further action since, in this case, the watertightness of the anterior chamber was not respected during surgery. YAG laser is used to cut deep sutures if the astigmatism is caused by them (see Figure 19-11) because they can not obviously be removed. The cut sutures will remain in the deep corneal bed but will no longer exert pressure.
- Less risk of infection. It is known that sutures and suture-induced irregularities can promote the adherence of bacteria and thus the risk of infection. Since the corneal surface has no sutures and the peripheral sutures can be removed early, in addition to being protected by conjunctiva, the risk of infection should be lessened, at least theoretically.
- Good harvest of stem cells if for whatever reason a penetrating keratoplasty should be necessary in the future. If penetrating keratoplasty is needed fol-

lowing a superficial large diameter lamellar keratoplasty, there are no difficulties other than those associated with the initial penetrating keratoplasty. If superficial large diameter lamellar keratoplasty is associated with deep keratoplasty, all efforts should be made to ensure a larger diameter for the penetrating keratoplasty to facilitate suturing and prevent leaving behind remnants in the deep stroma.

COMPLICATIONS

Some of the complications observed in large diameter lamellar keratoplasties are intraoperative, while most are postoperative; some are associated with any type of corneal transplantation technique, while others are particular to this technique; some are of little relevance, while others have serious functional repercussions.

The most significant intraoperative complications include:

- Incorrect harvest of donor button. Owing to the potential difficulties in obtaining the right diameter and thickness of donor button, we suggest that our proposed technique be strictly followed, that more than one globe be made available, and to prepare the buttons before transplanting into the recipient.
- Improper identification of horizontal and vertical meridians in the donor eye, which can lead to malposition of the button in the recipient. Correct positioning in the operating theater without the use of marks can be complicated. A complication of this type can require subsequent surgery to reposition the graft in the recipient.
- Perforation of the recipient bed. If care is not taken to measure corneal thicknesses before passing the microkeratome in the recipient, an inadvertent micro- or macroperforation can occur when practicing the keratectomy on the recipient. This can be due to an abnormally thin cornea associated with an underlying pathology (ie, burns) or caused iatrogenically when dissecting fibrovascular pannus that might cover the cornea in limbal insufficiency.

Postoperative complications include:

- Inadvertent malpositioning of meridians during surgery can, as pointed out earlier, require rotation of the graft.
- Bleeding between the layers of the cornea (Figure 19-12). This type of surgery generally involves a lot of blood, and excessive coagulation is not recommended; the presence of blood in the interface is relatively common. An excessive amount may require surgical irrigation, but in our experience, the blood is spontaneously reabsorbed in most cases with no serious clinical repercussions.
- Astigmatisms. Unlike our experience with keratoplasty, the presence of astigmatisms with magnitudes warranting keratotomies is exceptional. Generally speaking, astigmatisms can be controlled by careful removal of sutures following the topography-guided procedure described earlier.
- Trophic epithelial defects. They are common. Other alterations of the ocular surface associated with these cases, such as dry eye and inflammation, and neurotrophic aspects caused by the surgery itself, make the corneal epithelium surface unstable, particularly during the first 6 months. Management of such problems calls for the use of artificial tears and other types of ocular

Figure 19-12. Large diameter anterior lamellar keratoplasty. (A) Preoperative situation. (B) Blood in the interface in the immediate postoperative period. (C) Situation following reabsorption of blood and cataract surgery.

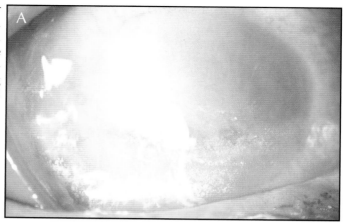

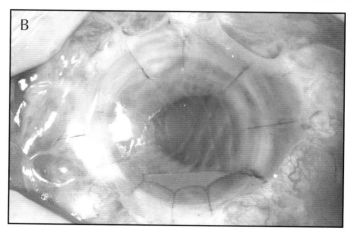

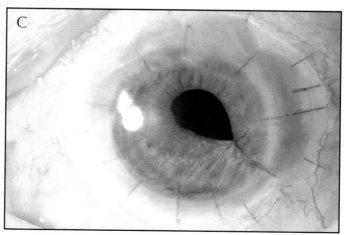

lubrication, therapeutic contact lenses in some instances, and autologous serum; inflammation and risk of rejection must also be properly managed.

- Rejection. Eyes that require limbal transplantation are already at high risk due to their underlying pathology and have less than a 50% chance of maintaining corneal transparency in the midterm.[53] Although these techniques have reached an acceptable degree of standardization and excellence in spite of their complexity, it is unquestionably the risk of rejection that casts the darkest shadow on their prognosis. In limbal allograft transplantations (ie, large diameter lamellar keratoplasty), blood group compatibility and HLA typing will surely improve the prognosis of transplantations of this type, as will the use of immunosuppressant drugs available today.

CONCLUSIONS

In our opinion, large diameter lamellar keratoplasty offers certain advantages in treating limbal insufficiencies associated with corneal opacity, particularly if we compare it with limbal transplantation associated with keratoplasty. Among the advantages is the ability to perform both operations (limbal transplantation and keratoplasty) in a single-stage surgical procedure, thus allowing for early patient rehabilitation. Moreover, the resulting refractive corneal surface is more uniform, with the associated refractive benefits and the possibility of favoring peripheral limbal cell migration on the corneal surface without the barriers imposed by sutures first in the corneoscleral ring and then in the keratoplasty button. In superficial anterior lamellar keratoplasty with no associated endokeratoplasty, the technique is extraocular, reducing the risk not only of intraocular complications but also of endothelial rejection.

Limbal insufficiency and corneal opacity can be resolved in a single surgical procedure using a single donor if superficial anterior lamellar keratoplasty is associated with endokeratoplasty. This avoids the increased risk of corneal rejection more common when performing both techniques (limbal transplantations and keratoplasty) in 2 separate operations, which requires 2 donor corneas. The disadvantage is that the specific technology necessary is not always available or affordable. In either case, much the same as other limbal allograft transplantations, it is important to remember that topical and systemic immunosuppression is essential when considering these techniques.

Key Points

1. The current stem cell theory underscores the important role of the limbal basal epithelium in maintaining corneal epithelial mass under physiological conditions and its importance in epithelial regeneration of epithelial defects.
2. Limbal insufficiency, understood as the failure of the stem cells in an eye to regenerate and maintain a healthy ocular surface, has recently been termed *ocular surface disease.*
3. There are clinical clues that can lead us to suspect the possibility of limbal insufficiency, including patient described symptoms in their varying degrees of impreciseness (loss of vision, foreign body sensation, chronic irritation) and signs (loss of limbal anatomy; superficial and peripheral corneal vascularization; fibrovascular pannus; diffuse staining of the pathologic, irregular, and thinned epithelium; unstable tear film; and a certain degree of scarring or keratinization). In any event, the most characteristic sign is the breakdown of the limbal vascular barrier.
4. One can perform a large diameter lamellar transplantation using rings and one of the ALTK microkeratome system heads.
5. Some of the complications observed in large diameter lamellar keratoplasties are intraoperative, while most are postoperative; some are associated with any type of corneal transplantation technique, while others are particular to this technique; some are of little relevance, while others have serious functional repercussions.

REFERENCES

1. Thoft RA, Friend J. Biochemical transformation of regenerating ocular surface epithelium. *Invest Ophthalmol Vis Sci.* 1977;16:14–20.
2. Thoft RA, Wiley LA, Sundarraj N. The multipotential cells of the limbus. *Eye.* 1989;3:109–113.
3. Hanna C. Proliferation and migration of epithelial cells. *Am J Ophthalmol.* 1966;61:55–62.
4. Schermer A, Galvin S, Sun TT. Differentiation-related expression of a major 64K corneal keratin in vivo and in culture suggests limbal location of corneal epithelial stem cells. *J Cell Biol.* 1986;103:49–62.
5. Kruse FE. Stem cells and corneal epithelial regeneration. *Eye.* 1994;8:170–183.
6. Tseng SCG. Concept and application of limbal stem cells. *Eye.* 1989;3:141–149.
7. Van Buskirk EM. The anatomy of the limbus. *Eye.* 1989;3:101–108.
8. Kinoshita S, Kiorpes TC, Friend J, Thoft RA. Limbal epithelium in ocular surface wound healing. *Invest Ophthalmol Vis Sci.* 1982;23:73–80.
9. Shapiro MS, Friend J, Thoft RA. Corneal re-epithelialization from the conjunctiva. *Invest Ophthalmol Vis Sci.* 1981;21:135–142.
10. Dua HS, Forrester JV. The corneoscleral limbus in human corneal epithelial wound healing. *Am J Ophthalmol.* 1990;110:646–656.
11. Thoft RA. Keratoepithelioplasty. *Am J Ophthalmol.* 1984;97:1–6.

PROGNOSIS

A study of patients with ocular surface disease who had the ocular surface rehabilitated through limbal stem cell grafting with subsequent penetrating keratoplasty for attempted visual rehabilitation[39] showed a 50% success rate in terms of maintenance of clear grafts. This rate represents an improvement in the success in this area, compared with straightforward penetrating keratoplasty without prior rehabilitation of the ocular surface. Causes of loss of corneal clarity included limbal stem cell graft rejection (42% of eyes), keratoplasty rejection (22%), infection (13%), and surface damage from matters such as exposure (7%). This study, though encouraging, also proves[40,41] that ocular surface rehabilitation in patients with the more severe forms of limbal stem cell deficiency and ocular surface disease is an extremely difficult task, the most limited success occurring in patients with the greatest need (eg, Stevens-Johnson syndrome).

FUTURE CONSIDERATIONS

Currently, most limbal stem cell and large diameter anterior lamellar allografts are performed by manually dissecting donor corneoscleral material for transplantation.[42–45] Manual dissection is technically challenging and time intensive, and excessive handling of tissue may decrease the likelihood of obtaining viable limbal stem cells. These mechanical factors, along with problems concerning immune rejection, have prevented limbal stem cell allografts from becoming more widely used. Recently, a microkeratome has been adapted to harvest the entire anterior corneal surface, including limbal stem cells.[46] Preliminary results have been encouraging and give hope that this instrument may prove to be of benefit to patients in the near future.

SPECIALIZED MICROKERATOME FOR ANTERIOR CORNEAL SURFACE AND LIMBAL STEM CELL HARVESTING

A large-sized microkeratome (suction ring diameter = 16 mm) has been adapted to harvest the entire anterior corneolimbal surface from donor globes for keratolimbal allograft surgery[46] (Figure 20-2). A nitrogen gas-powered turbine is used to drive a blade within the microkeratome head at 15,000 oscillations per minute at an orientation of 25 degrees to the cut plane. Using this device, lamellar dissection of a corneoscleral lenticule can be performed easily and quickly in a procedure lasting less than 30 seconds.[47] Scanning electron microscopy has demonstrated that the epithelium of the keratolimbal cap remains intact and that smooth cut edges can be obtained.[46] In addition, the lenticule thickness has been shown to be reproducible, with variability similar to corneal lamellar cuts produced by microkeratomes in use in refractive surgery.[47]

In 2002, a portable version of this microkeratome was developed by substituting a hand pump vacuum device (MityVac, San Antonio, Tex) for the original electricity-powered suction ring[48] (Figure 20-3). The lenticules obtained by this version were shown to be reproducible and similar in quality to the original device in both porcine[48] and human eyes.[49] The ease and portability of this device may add to its applicability and versatility, potentially allowing surgeons to use it in the operating room and eye bank technicians to harvest lenticules in the field.

Figure 20-2. Mechanical limbal harvester. The oversized head of 200-μm—thick plate (A), the enlarged blade (B), and the suction ring (C) allow the cut of a large diameter corneoscleral cap. The nitrogen gas-driven turbine (D) is the same as that used in a commercially available microkeratome.

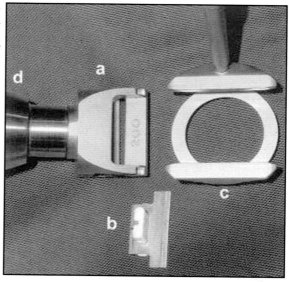

Figure 20-3. Total anterior corneal surface harvesting using a mechanical microkeratome. (A) The globe is placed in a holder, and the suction ring is centered on the cornea. (B) Vacuum is achieved using the hand pump. (C) The keratome head is placed on the tracks and passed from right to left. (D) A lenticule is obtained.

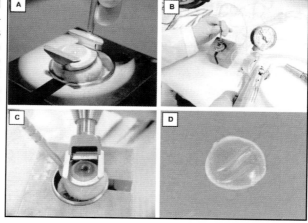

A recent study evaluating limbal epithelium after such anterior lamellar harvesting has demonstrated that a median of 95.0% of limbal basal epithelial cells remain viable after 9 days in 4°C cold organ storage culture.[50] Twenty-two human anterior lenticules were harvested using the portable version of the microkeratome device by first infusing whole human globes with 0.9% normal saline solution through the optic nerve to maintain an IOP between 15 and 25 mmHg (Modular One Pneumotonometer, Mentor O&O, Norwell, Mass). The 16-mm diameter suction ring attached to the hand pump was placed centrally on the cornea, and manual pumping was initiated to achieve a pressure of 65 mmHg. The modified microkeratome with a 170-mm depth head was then passed manually along the parallel guiding track of the suction ring at 15,000 oscillations per minute. The entire anterior lamellar cap was then stored in Optisol GS at 4°C. Using viability staining with calcein AM (CAM) and ethium homodimer 1 (EH-1) (Molecular Probes Inc, Eugene, Ore), in conjunction with fluorescence confocal microscopy (Bio-Rad Laboratories, Hercules, Calif), live and dead cells were detected and counted within multiple randomized areas of multilayered central and limbal epithelia stored in solution for 0, 3, 6, and 9 days.

Basal epithelial layers, which contain the limbal stem cell population, were found to have greater viability than middle epithelial layers. In addition, the limbal basal epithelium viability was significantly greater than central basal epithelium. On day 0, median viabilities of limbal basal versus central basal epithelium were 100% (range 71.7% to 100%) versus 98.4% (range 88.9% to 100%) ($p > 0.05$); 100% (range 64.3% to 100%) versus 63.4% (range 13.6% to 95.5%) at day 3 ($p < 0.0005$); on day 6, median viabilities were 95.0% (range 35.0% to 100.0%) versus 28.0% (range 0% to 92.0%) ($p < 0.0005$); and on day 9, median viabilities were 95.0% (range 3.7% to 100%) versus 68.6% (range 0% to 100%) ($p < 0.0005$).

Optisol GS storage medium is optimally formulated to preserve corneal endothelium because the survival of corneal grafts in penetrating keratoplasty is very much dependent on the health of the endothelium at the time of corneal transplantation. It seems likely that the storage time of limbal basal epithelium may be extended with research and development of a storage medium optimized for limbal epithelium.

Current microkeratome technology obtains lenticules ranging from 152±52, 190±54, 190±59, 155±70, 222±15 mm at the center, superiorly, inferiorly, and at both the beginning and the end of the pass, respectively.[48] Since the limbal epithelium is 90 to 100 mm thick,[50–54] inclusion of the limbal stem cell region in the basal limbal epithelium can be guaranteed in nearly every microkeratome cut, but the stromal carrier can be thick in some instances. To achieve a thinner cut inclusive of a higher percentage of epithelium in the thickness of the achieved anterior lenticule, a modified femtosecond laser microkeratome with an accuracy of ±5 mm is being explored.

FEMTOSECOND TECHNOLOGY

Currently, femtosecond lasers are being used in a small proportion of the 1.5 million LASIK cases performed in the United States each year. However, avoidance of microkeratome flap complications and improved precision in cutting of the corneal flap in LASIK will likely increase its availability and usage in refractive surgery.

Current Eye Bank Association of America regulations permit only one recipient for each donor tissue. Given the issue of tissue shortages and the fact that the vast majority of the 35,000 penetrating keratoplasties performed in the United States each year are performed to replace either the anterior corneal surface or the endothelium, it appears that changing these regulations to allow multiple recipients to benefit from one donor may be necessary in the future. Modifying femtosecond laser technology would make these anterior and posterior lamellar corneal harvesting and transplantation procedures much easier to do and may potentially increase the number of transplantation procedures that may be performed.

The potential number of lamellar procedures that may be performed by femtosecond laser may never quite approximate that of refractive surgery. However, modification of the femtosecond laser for lamellar transplantation would allow those procedures to be more widely performed as the availability of the femtosecond laser grows. This expansion of the versatility of the femtosecond laser machine may provide an impetus for each community to have access to this technology in order to offer this

Figure 20-4. Eyes of patients that have undergone transplantation of sheets of tissue-engineered autologous oral mucosal epithelial cells. Photos on the right show the eyes 13 to 15 months post-transplantation.

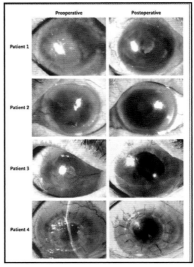

surgical option to their patients. In addition to being a faster and easier way to obtain lamellar grafts, femtosecond laser technology may provide mechanical advantages as well. Greater precision and accuracy of the femtosecond laser system may allow lamellae of varying thicknesses to be precisely harvested. For example, a major improvement in total anterior corneal surface and limbal stem cell transplantation would be to use the femtosecond laser to create a corneoscleral lenticule that is of sufficient thickness to include the limbal basal epithelium, but does not include extraneous tissue that is not of use. Using current surgical techniques, the limbal stem cell allograft is often bulky and of varying thickness, since the dissection is performed manually. A thinner graft may allow better tissue apposition to the host, resulting in better wound healing, and allow a more regular anterior surface.

Ex Vivo Tissue Culture

With the development of new strategies for immunosuppression, surgical manipulation, and the refinements in screening for donor tissue compatibility, allograft procedures for limbal stem cell transplantation have become more common in the last few years.[55–59] Even more exciting is the recently proposed treatment for severe ocular surface disease that either utilizes cultivated corneal[60,61] or oral mucosal epithelial[62,63] transplantation. These emerging ocular surface corneal transplantation techniques, involve expansion of a few harvested epithelial cells *in vitro* before grafting. This method has allowed full coverage of the ocular surface with clear, somewhat long-lasting epithelium.

Research has focused on expanding limbal stem cells in tissue culture. Moreover, not only have limbal stem cells from the contralateral eye been grown outside of the body and replaced onto the damaged ocular surface, but autologous oral mucosal epithelial cells[63] have also recently been used to replace the ocular surface with clinical success (Figure 20-4). Because these newer techniques have been in existence for only the past couple of years, we look forward to validating their long-term clinical success and their introduction into mainstream clinical ocular surface reconstruction.

Perhaps the last frontier in the progress of these epithelial surface transplantation techniques will be the development of a universal donor pool especially important for those who do not have readily available autologous cell replacement sources (eg, Stevens-Johnson syndrome with advanced mucosal disease). Considering the rate of advancement of stem cell replacement science, it would not be unrealistic to expect development of universal donor cell populations besides epithelium from other parts of the body (eg, bone marrow mesenchymal stem cells).

SUMMARY

Research into improving the outcome of penetrating keratoplasty in patients with ocular surface disorders is progressing rapidly. Limbal stem cell transplantation is a promising technique with many opportunities for improvement through technological innovation. Implementation of microkeratome technology would certainly make these procedures much easier to perform and likely make them more available to patients. In addition to decreasing procedure time, microkeratomes give the surgeon an idea of the actual thickness achieved with the procedure, a feature not realized in manual techniques. Although the modified mechanical microkeratome for anterior corneal surface and limbal stem cell harvesting has been shown to be successful and reproducible in the laboratory as discussed here, it is currently not yet in clinical use. Since the market for this device is likely to remain relatively small, clinical implementation may prove to be a difficult challenge. Perhaps a more feasible and promising option lies in adaptation of the femtosecond laser microkeratome. This would involve re-programming the laser for the particular use of lamellar corneal and limbal stem cell harvesting and may be more economically feasible, since it is already being used for other applications. Preliminary studies indicate that the femtosecond laser is more precise and accurate than mechanical microkeratomes. In any case, these emerging technologies should help the field of limbal stem cell transplantation move forward, ensuring greater access to more patients who may potentially be helped by these innovative procedures. Perhaps most exciting is the possibility of *ex vivo* tissue culture expansion and subsequent cell layer grafting. It is certainly an exciting time in corneal transplantation science.

Key Points

1. A keratoplasty in patients with ocular surface disorders, whether lamellar or penetrating, is generally not successful because the host's corneal epithelium is only temporarily replaced and the limbal function continues to remain poor.
2. Ocular surface disorders increase the chances of vascularization, scarring, recurrent or persistent epithelial defects, melting and perforation of the graft, infectious keratitis, rejection, and failure of the graft.
3. Preoperatively, all patients should be evaluated for eyelid anatomy and function, tear dynamics, dry eye syndromes, limbal ischemia, limbal stem cell deficiency, signs of chronic inflammation, scarring and keratinization of the conjunctiva, punctate epithelial staining, pannus formation, vascularization and scarring, and recurrent or persistent epithelial defects of the cornea. Treatment should be directed toward correction of all these factors.
4. A keratoplasty may be combined with limbal stem cell transplantation or done at a later sitting, although it is preferable to do it later, once the ocular surface is restored to as near normalcy as possible.
5. Recently, a microkeratome has been adapted to harvest the entire anterior corneal surface, including limbal stem cells.
6. Modifying femtosecond laser technology would make anterior and posterior lamellar corneal harvesting and transplantation procedures much easier to do and may potentially increase the number of transplantation procedures that may be performed.
7. Emerging ocular surface corneal transplantation techniques involve expansion of a few harvested epithelial cells *in vitro* before grafting.

REFERENCES

1. Tseng SCG, Maumenee AE, Stark WJ, et al. Topical retinoid treatment for various dry-eye disorders. *Ophthalmology.* 1985;92:717.
2. Kinoshita S, Kiorpes TC, Friend J, et al. Goblet cell density in ocular surface disease: a better indicator than tear mucin. *Arch Ophthalmol.* 1983;101:1284.
3. Foster CS. Cicatricial pemphigoid. *Trans Am Ophthalmol Soc.* 1986;84:527.
4. Mondino BJ, Brown SI. Ocular cicatricial pemphigoid. *Ophthalmology.* 1981;88:95.
5. Shapiro MS, Friend J, Thoft RA. Corneal re-epithelialization from the conjunctiva. *Invest Ophthalmol Vis Sci.* 1981;21:135.
6. Thoft RA, Friend J. Biochemical transformation of regenerating ocular surface epithelium. *Invest Ophthalmol Vis Sci.* 1977;16:14.
7. Brown SI, Bloomfield SE, Pearce DB. Follow-up report on transplantation of the alkali burned cornea. *Am J Ophthalmol.* 1974;77:538–542.
8. Abel R Jr, Binder PS, Pilack FM, et al. The results of penetrating keratoplasty after chemical burns. *Trans Am Acad Ophthalmol Otolaryngol.* 1975;79:584–595.
9. Ben Ezra D, Pe'er J, Brodsky M, et al. Cyclosporine eye drops for the treatment of severe vernal keratoconjunctivitis. *Am J Ophthalmol.* 1986;101:278.

10. Ben Ezra D, Matamoros N, Cohen E. Treatment of severe keratoconjunctivitis with cyclosporin A eyedrops. *Transplant Proc.* 1988;20(suppl 2):644.

11. Kruit PJ, Van Balen AThM, Stilma JS. Cyclosporin A: treatment in two cases of corneal peripheral melting syndrome. *Doc Ophthalmol.* 1985;59:33.

12. Nussenblatt RB, Palestine AG. Cyclosporine: immunology, pharmacology and therapeutic uses. *Surv Ophthalmol.* 1986;31:159.

13. Newsome DA, Gross J. Prevention by medroxyprogesterone of perforation in the alkali-burned rabbit cornea: inhibition of collagenolytic activity. *Invest Ophthalmol Vis Sci.* 1977;16:21.

14. Abelson MB, Butrus SI, Kliman GH, et al. Topical arachidonic acid: a model for screening anti-inflammatory agents. *J Ocul Pharmacol.* 1987;3:63.

15. Nishida T, Nakagawa S, Awata T, et al. Fibronectin promotes epithelial migration of cultured rabbit cornea in situ. *J Cell Biol.* 1983;97:1653.

16. Nishida T, Ohashi Y, Awata T, el al. Fibronectin. *Arch Ophthalmol.* 1983;101:1046.

17. Nishida T, Yagi J, Fukuda M, et al. Spontaneous persistent epithelial defects after cataract surgery. *Cornea.* 1987;6:32.

18. Fujikawa LS, Foster CS, Harrist TJ, Lanigan JM, Colvin RB. Fibronectin in healing rabbit corneal wounds. *Lab Invest.* 1981;45:120.

19. Nelson JD, Gordon JF, Chiron KCS. Study group: topical fibronectin in the treatment of keratoconjunctivitis sicca (KCS). *Am J Ophthalmol.* 1992;114:441.

20. Soong HK, Hassan T, Varani J, et al. Fibronectin does not enhance epidermal growth factor-mediated acceleration of corneal epithelial wound closure. *Arch Ophthalmol.* 1989;107:1052.

21. Tseng SCG, Maumenee AE, Stark WJ, et al. Topical retinoid treatment of various dry-eye disorders. *Ophthalmology.* 1985;92:717.

22. Soong HK, Martin NF, Wagoner MD, et al. Topical retinoid therapy for squamous metaplasia of various ocular surface disorders. *Ophthalmology.* 1988;95;1442.

23. Ubels JI, Edelhauser HF, Austin KH. Healing of experimental corneal wounds treated with topically applied retinoids. *Am J Ophthalmol.* 1983;95:353.

24. Castor CW, Cabral AR. Growth factors in human disease. The realities, pitfalls, and promise. *Semin Arthritis Rheum.* 1985;15:33.

25. Savage CR Jr, Cohen S. Proliferation of corneal epithelium induced by epidermal growth factor. *Exp Eye Res.* 1973;15:361.

26. Brightwell JR, Riddle, SL, Eiferman RA, et al. Biosynthetic human EGF accelerates healing of neodecadron-treated primate corneas. *Invest Ophthalmol Vis Sci.* 1985;26:105.

27. Petroutsos G, Courty J, Guimaraes R, et al. Comparison of the effects of EGF, pEGF, and EDGF on corneal epithelium wound healing. *Curr Eye Res.* 1984;3:593.

28. Daniele S, Frati L, Fiore C, et al. The effect of epidermal growth factor (EGF) on the corneal epithelium in humans. *Graefes Arch Clin Exp Ophthalmol.* 1979;210:159.

29. Soong HK, McClenic B, Varani J, et al. EGF does not enhance corneal epithelial cell motility. *Invest Ophthalmol Vis Sci.* 1989;30:1808.

30. Dua HS, Azuara-Blanco A. Autologous limbal transplantation in patients with unilateral corneal stem cell deficiency. *Br J Ophthalmol.* 2000;84:273–278.

31. Azuara-Blanco A, Pillai CT, Dua HS. Amniotic membrane transplantation for ocular surface reconstruction. *Br J Ophthalmol.* 1999;83:399–402.

32. Dua HS, Azuara-Blanco A. Amniotic membrane transplantation. *Br J Ophthalmol.* 1999;83:748–752.

33. Pellegrini G, Traverso CE, Franzi AT, Zingirian M. Long-term restoration of damaged corneal surface with autologous cultivated corneal epithelium. *Lancet.* 1997;349:990–993.

34. Schwab IR. Cultured corneal epithelia for ocular surface disease. *Trans Am Ophthalmol Soc.* 1999;97:891–986.

35. Schwab IR, Isseroff RR. Bioengineered corneas—the promise and the challenge. *N Engl J Med.* 2000;343:136–138.

36. Schwab IR, Reyes M, Isseroff RR. Successful transplantation of bioengineered tissue replacements in patients with ocular surface disease. *Cornea.* 2000;19:421–426.

37. Tsai RJ, Li LM, Chen JK. Reconstruction of damaged corneas by transplantation of autologous limbal epithelial cells. *N Engl J Med.* 2000;343:86–93.

38. Soong HK. Penetrating keratoplasty in ocular surface disease. In: Krachmer JH, Mannis MJ, eds. *Cornea.* Vol 3. St. Louis, Mo: Mosby Year Book; 2004:1781–1788.

39. Nordland ML, Derby E, Schwartz GS, Holland EJ. Success of subsequent penetrating keratoplasty in patients with severe ocular surface disease treated with stem cell transplantation. Program and abstracts of the Association for Research in Vision and Ophthalmology 2004 Annual Meeting; April 25-29, 2004; Fort Lauderdale, Fla. Abstract 608.

40. Samson CM, Nduaguba C, Baltatzis S, Foster CS. Limbal stem cell transplantation in chronic inflammatory eye disease. *Ophthalmology.* 2002;109:862–868.

41. Shimazaki J, Aiba M, Goto E, et al. Transplantation of human limbal epithelium cultivated on amniotic membrane for the treatment of severe ocular surface disorders. *Ophthalmology.* 2002;109:1285–1290.

42. Sundmacher R, Reinhard T. Homologe lamellare zentrale limbokeratoplastik bei schwerer limbusstammzellinsuffizienz. *Klin Monatsbl Augenkeilkd.* 1998;213:254–255.

43. Melles GR, Remeijer L, Geerards AJ, Beekhuis WH. The future of lamellar keratoplasty. *Curr Opin Ophthalmol.* 1999;10:253–259.

44. Vajpayee RB, Thomas S, Sharma N, Dada T, Tabin GC. Large-diameter lamellar keratoplasty in severe ocular alkali burns. A technique of stem cell transplantation. *Ophthalmology.* 2000;107:1765–1768.

45. Shimmura S, Ando M, Shimazaki J, Tsubota K. Complications with one piece lamellar keratolimbal grafts for simultaneous limbal and corneal pathologies. *Cornea.* 2000;19:439–442.

46. Chuck RS, Behrens A, McDonnell PJ. Microkeratome-based limbal harvester for limbal stem cell transplantation: preliminary studies. *Am J Ophthalmol.* 2001;131:377–378.

47. Behrens A, Shah SB, Li L, et al. Evaluation of a microkeratome based limbal harvester device for limbal stem cell transplantation. *Cornea.* 2002;21:51–55.

48. Sarayba MA, Li L, Sweet PM, Chuck RS. A portable microkeratome-based anterior corneal surface harvesting device. *Cornea.* 2002;21:589–591.

49. Sarayba M, Tungsiripat T, Sweet PM, Chuck RS. A portable microkeratome for harvesting the human anterior corneal surface. *Cornea.* 2004;23:443–446.

50. Tungsiripat T, Sarayba MA, Taban M, Sweet PM, Osann KE, Chuck RS. Viability of limbal epithelium after anterior lamellar harvesting using a microkeratome. *Ophthalmology.* 2004;111:469–475.

51. Hayes W, ed. *Principles and Methods of Toxicology.* 3rd ed. New York: Raven Press; 1994.

52. Poole CA, Brookes NH, Clover GM. Keratocyte networks visualized in the living cornea using vital dyes. *J Cell Sci.* 1993;106:685–691.

53. Lau KR, Evans RL, Case RM. Intracelluar Cl-concentration in striated intralobular ducts from rabbit mandibular salivary glands. *Pflugers Arch.* 1994;427:24–32.

54. Means TL, Geroski DH, L'Hernault N, et al. The corneal epithelium after Optisol-GS storage. *Cornea.* 1996;15:599–605.

55. Terry MA. The evolution of lamellar grafting techniques over twenty-five years. *Cornea.* 2000;19:611–616.

56. Shimazaki J. The evolution of lamellar keratoplasty. *Curr Opin Ophthalmol.* 2000;11:217–223.

57. Shimazaki J, Kaido M, Shinozaki N, et al. Evidence of long-term survival of donor-derived cells after limbal allograft transplantation. *Invest Ophthalmol Vis Sci.* 1999;4:1664–1668.

58. Tsai RJ, Tseng SC. Human allograft limbal transplantation for corneal surface reconstruction. *Cornea.* 1994;13:389–400.

59. Tsubota K, Satake Y, Kaido M, et al. Treatment of severe ocular-surface disorders with corneal epithelial stem-cell transplantation. *N Engl J Med.* 1999;340:1697–1703.

60. Schwab IR, Reyes M, Isseroff RR. Successful transplantation of bioengineered tissue replacements in patients with ocular surface disease. *Cornea.* 2000;19:421-426.

61. Koizumi N, Inatomi T, Suzuki T, Sotozono C, Kinoshita S. Cultivated corneal epithelial stem cell transplantation in ocular surface disorders. *Ophthalmology.* 2001;108:1569–1574.

62. Nakamura T, Inatomi T, Sotozono C, Amemiya T, Kanamura N, Kinoshita S. Transplantation of cultivated autologous oral mucosal epithelial cells in patients with severe ocular surface disorders. *Br J Ophthalmol.* 2004;88:1280–1284.

63. Nishida K, Yamato M, Hayashida Y, et al. Corneal reconstruction with tissue-engineered cell sheets composed of autologous oral mucosal epithelium. *N Engl J Med.* 2004;351:1187–1196.

21

Keratolimbal Allografting

Daniel Böhringer, MD;
Rainer Sundmacher, MD, FRCOphth; and
Thomas Reinhard, MD

INTRODUCTION

Regeneration of the corneal epithelium depends on continuous renewal of cells originating from basal stem cells of the corneal limbus.[1] Substantial stem cell loss in over 60% to 70% of the limbal circumference results in functional insufficiency of the limbus. Opacification of the central cornea from superficial conjunctivalization is the primary clinical sign of this condition. Additionally, scarring of deeper layers of the central corneal stroma, mostly from complicating central ulcerations, is commonly observed.

Common causes of limbal stem cell insufficiency are stem cell destruction due to direct trauma or to chronic limbal inflammation. Rarely, limbal insufficiency is due to inborn dysgenesis of the limbal stem cells, a condition that is associated with further severe ocular abnormalities. Further rare causes of limbal insufficiency are degeneration of stem cells due to nutritional factors or contact lens wear. Table 21-1 lists causes of limbal stem cell insufficiency.

GENERAL CONSIDERATIONS

Early graft failure from conjunctivalization or recurrent graft ulceration is inevitable in patients with severe limbal stem cell insufficiency following conventional penetrating keratoplasty because the graft epithelium mostly does not survive for longer than 6 to 12 months.[2]

Table 21-1

CAUSES OF LIMBAL STEM CELL DEFICIENCY

Condition	Symmetry	Remark
Congenital		
Sclerocornea	Bilateral	Poor visual prognosis due to amblyopia
Congenital aniridia	Bilateral	Lamellar homologous limbo-keratoplasty is an option, poor visual prognosis due to amblyopia, nystagmus, and hypoplasia of the macula and optic nerve
Traumatic		
Chemical/thermal burns	Uni-/bilateral	Autologous stem cell transplantation is an option in unilateral cases
Immunologic		
OCP	Bilateral	Underlying immunologic disease has to be properly treated
Trachoma	Bilateral	
Stevens-Johnson syndrome/erythema multiforme	Bilateral	Underlying skin disease has to be properly treated
Atopic condition	Bilateral	Underlying skin disease has to be properly treated
Blepharokeratoconjunctivitis	Bilateral	Blepharitis causes chronic limbal inflammation and marginal keratitis. Lid margins should be treated consequently, combined with long-term topical immunosuppression, when appropriate
Nutritional		
Xerophthalmia	Bilateral	Nutritional defects have to be sufficiently treated
Improper contact lens wear	Uni-/bilateral	Discontinuation of contact lens wear

Thus, in severe limbal stem cell insufficiency, restoration of the optic axis is only possible with transplantation of viable limbal stem cells either simultaneously or prior to penetrating keratoplasty.

Autologous transplantation is generally preferable from immunologic considerations (see the following paragraphs) and taking into consideration the potential for transmission of infection from allogeneic grafts, the appropriate surgical approach thus primarily depends on availability of stem cells for autologous transplantation.

Applicability of autologous transplantation is thus limited to the minority of unilaterally affected patients, where enough viable stem cells for repopulating at least 40% of the limbal circumference can be safely harvested from the other eye. This can potentially be achieved rather atraumatically via transplantation of *ex vivo* expanded autologous limbal stem cells (Figure 21–1A). Long-term results for this approach are, however, currently unavailable.[3] The established lamellar en-bloc transplantation (Figure 21-1B) is technically challenging, but yields good long-term results.[4] However, this technique can potentially induce limbal stem cell insufficiency in the donor eye.

For the majority of bilaterally affected patients, autotransplantation is not an option. In these patients, the surgical approach primarily depends on the depth and extent of central corneal scarring. Superficial corneal opacification can commonly be addressed with restoration of limbal stem cell function alone (see Figure 21-1A and B), whereas penetrating procedures are required for deep central corneal opacification.

In patients with deep central corneal opacification, a one-stage procedure (see Figure 21-1B, C, and D) may be preferable because such patients commonly suffer from legal blindness. Instant improvement of vision is preferable for socioeconomic and practical reasons. Additionally, stem cells and the corneal graft should originate from the same donor (see Figure 21-1C and D) due to immunologic considerations (see the following paragraphs) and for reducing the risk of transmittable disease. Thus, homologous central limbokeratoplasty[5] (see Figure 21-1D) can currently be considered the first line procedure for cases of bilateral limbal stem cell insufficiency combined with deep central corneal opacification, such as in Figure 21–2.

Preoperative Management

Comorbidity such as severe tear insufficiency should be addressed by punctal occlusion. Other pathophysiologic changes such as severe cicatricial symblepharon or eyelid pathologies should accordingly be corrected in advance. Immunosuppression and HLA matching both reliably increase the chances of graft survival and survival of the transplanted stem cells.

Histocompatibility Matching

Histocompatibility matching is an adjunct to immunosuppression, yielding a permanent reduction in the risk of immunologic graft rejection without exerting any side effects. A multitude of recent studies demonstrated the beneficial effect of matching the most important loci of the HLA system in significantly reducing graft rejections in conventional keratoplasty for normal and high-risk situations.[6] Older studies, failing to demonstrate the HLA effect, suffered from poor statistical power, mostly due to poor HLA typing accuracy.[7] Accordingly, long-term results after allogeneic penetrating limbo-keratoplasty are only encouraging if grafts have been matched at the HLA loci A, B, and DR.

Fortunately, it has been demonstrated, contrary to common belief, that the majority of patients can be served with an HLA compatible graft at loci A, B, and DR within well below a year, even on a monocenter waiting list.[8,9] Waiting time for a histocompatible graft can be predicted and discussed with each patient in advance.[8] This prediction helps in reducing the percentage of patients waiting in vain for a histocompatible donor. The

Description	Remark	Schematic
(A) The use of ex vivo expanded limbal stem cells placed on amniotic membrane or other layers. Cells can be harvested from either living or cadaveric donors.[3]	Living donors can either be autologous (other eye) or homologous (relative).[10] The procedure has to be followed by penetrating keratoplasty in case of deep corneal scars. Long-term results are currently not available.[3] No immunologic threat in autologous situation.	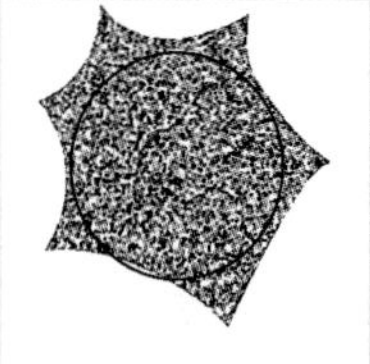
(B) The use of en-bloc lamellar limbal grafts, either from living or cadaveric donors.	Living donors can either be autologous (other eye) or homologous homologous (relative). Penetrating keratoplasty has to be performed in case of deep corneal scars either simultaneously or as separate procedure. Long-term results are promising.[4] No immunologic threat in autologous situation.	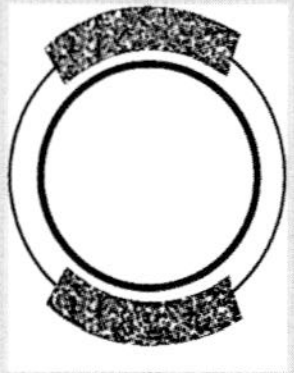
(C) The use of oversized grafts from a cadaveric donor.	Penetrating procedures may be associated with severe glaucoma from destruction of the trabecular meshwork. Lamellar procedures have recently been described.[11] Long-term data for the latter procedure are currently missing. The immunologic threat is high.	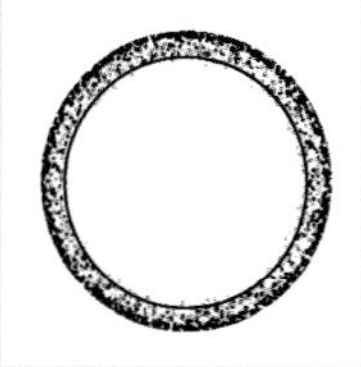
(D) The use of an eccentrically trephined keratolimbal graft from a cadaveric donor.[5]	This easily performable approach allows for simultaneous transplantation of limbal stem cells in around 40% to 50% of the graft circumference. Immunologic threat is higher than in conventional penetrating keratoplasty.	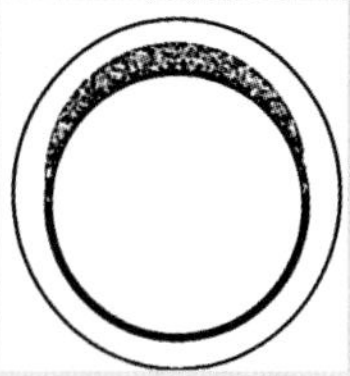

Figure 21-1. Four possibilities of transplantation of limbal stem cells prior to or together with penetrating keratoplasty.

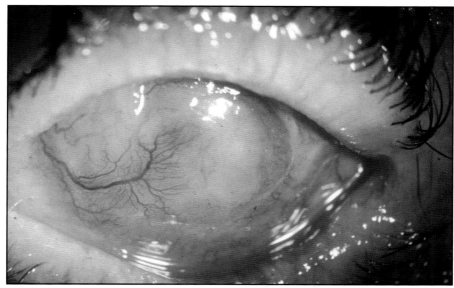

Figure 21-2. An eye with complete corneal conjunctivalization due to insufficiency of the limbal stem cells following severe, bilateral chemical burn. Note the deep corneal scarring requiring penetrating keratoplasty.

HLA matchmaker algorithm can balance waiting time and histocompatibility for these problematic patients with rare (homozygotic) HLA phenotype.[9]

SURGICAL PROCEDURE

Keratolimbal allografting can be performed under retrobulbar or general anesthesia. Ocular compression with 30 mmHg for 20 to 30 minutes and intravenous administration of 500 mg acetazolamide to reduce vitreous pressure following retrobulbar injection are advisable.

The graft button is trephined eccentrically from the endothelial side so that limbus tissue is present in 40% of the graft's circumference (see Figure 21-1D). The graft diameter can be varied according to individual requirements, mostly from 8.2 to 8.7 mm. The recipient cornea is trephined from the epithelial side with a 0.2 mm smaller trephine.

From this point, the procedure is similar to conventional penetrating keratoplasty. Unless the recipient corneal bed is unsuitably thin, a double-running cross-stitched suture according to Hoffmann[12] should be performed to fix the graft. The crescent shaped donor limbus should be positioned close to the region with the severest damage to the host limbus (Figure 21-3), or if there is no such preferable position, rotated to the 12 o'clock position, where limbus is covered by the eyelid in primary gaze position.

Figure 21-3. The same eye as in Figure 21-2 immediately after homologous penetrating limbokeratoplasty. Note the crescent shaped white graft limbus at the 6 o'clock position.

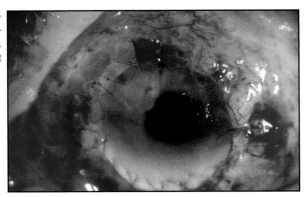

Figure 21-4. Immunological destruction of the transplanted limbal stem cells with dilated vessels in the graft limbus and surface disorders. The edematous appearance of the graft is suggestive of a concurrent endothelial graft rejection.

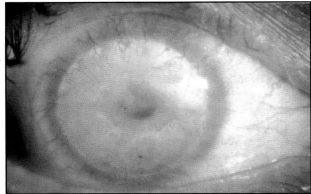

COMPLICATIONS

Immunologic Rejection

Immunologic rejection of either the limbal stem cells or the corneal graft poses the primary threat to clear graft survival after limbokeratoplasty (Figure 21-4). Resulting failure or insufficiency of the transplanted limbal stem cells results in surface disorders, conjunctivalization and recurrent central ulceration of the graft, eventually involving the perilimbal area as well. There is currently no direct diagnostic aid in demonstrating ongoing rejection of limbal stem cells. Immunologic rejection of the graft endothelium, however, is readily observable from edematous graft swelling and endothelial leukocyte precipitates. This condition eventually results in bullous graft edema.

When diagnosed early, intense topical and systemic treatment with corticosteroids and intracameral injection of corticosteroids can sometimes revert the graft failure. The rate of endothelial immune reactions after limbokeratoplasty is increased as compared to conventional high-risk keratoplasty.[4] An explanation for this high risk of graft rejections in limbokeratoplasty would be antigen-presenting Langerhans' cells that are possibly located in the grafted donor limbus.

Table 21-2 COMPLICATIONS FOLLOWING HOMOLOGOUS LIMBOKERATOPLASTY		
Condition	*Cause*	*Treatment*
Graft conjunctivalization	• Failure of the transplanted limbal stem cells	• Repeat limbokerato-plasty
Graft ulceration	• Failure of the transplanted limbal stem cells • Dry eye condition • Secondary microbial infection	• Intense lubrication with unpreserved hyaluronidate preparations • Repeat limbo-keratoplasty if graft center is concerned
Failure of the graft endothelium	• Immunologic rejection • Chronic endothelial cell loss • Secondary glaucoma	• Repeat limbokerato-plasty • Glaucoma surgery if intraocular pressure is elevated

Degeneration of the Graft Stem Cells Due to Malnutrition and Improper Local Milieu

Long-term survival of the stem cells is limited even in "normal risk" limbokeratoplasty for lattice and granular dystrophy.[13] There are no additional risk factors for immune reactions besides the presence of limbal tissue as discussed above.

It is currently presumed that the unphysiological position of the transplanted stem cells inside the avascular clear cornea predisposes for stem cell degeneration. The absence of blood vessels close to the transplanted limbus might especially result in poor stem cell performance due to malnutrition. Thus, vascularization of the graft limbus may be of benefit because this condition might be associated with prolonged survival of the transplanted stem cells.

Additionally, tear film insufficiency as in dry eye conditions limits external nutrition. Table 21-2 lists complications following homologous limbokeratoplasty.

POSTOPERATIVE MANAGEMENT

Prophylactic Immunosuppression

Despite the fact that the graft can directly be reached with steroids in extremely high concentrations via topical application, this treatment is insufficient in limbokeratoplasty. Clonal expansion of activated alloreactive T cells occurs in lymphoid organs such as the spleen. These specific T cells eventually destroy the graft tissue. It is therefore crucial to employ immunosuppressive substances systemically along with prophylactic application of topical steroids in limbokeratoplasty. In addition to reducing the risk of graft rejections,

Table 21-3
IMMUNOSUPPRESSIVES IN LIMBOKERATOPLASTY
(C12: BLOOD LEVEL 12 HOURS AFTER LAST ADMINISTRATION)

	Duration and Dosage	*Remark*
Topical corticosteroids	Initially 5 drops per day, tapered over 3 months Three drops daily indefinitely	Discontinuation upon severe surface disorder and steroid response glaucoma
Topical FK506 (Tacrolimus)	FK506 0.06% 3 times per day	Data only available for normal-risk keratoplasty, topical side effects[14]
Systemic CSA	Blood level adapted dosage (C12: 120 to 150 ng/mL)	Regular workups to exclude contraindications
Systemic MMF	Two times 1 g for at least 1 year, either in addition to CsA or as monotherapy in patients with contra-indications against CsA	Regular workups to exclude contraindications advisable. Side effects less frequent and less severe than with CsA[15]
Systemic rapamycine	Blood level adapted dosage (C12: 4 to 10 ng/mL)	Clinical data promising regarding efficacy, high risk of side effects
Systemic FK506 (Tacrolimus)	Blood level adapted dosage (C12: 5 to 10 ng/mL)	Promising option in limbo-keratoplasty[16]
Basiliximab	Perioperative intravenous application	Promising short term data from pilot study in addition to systemic CsA[17]

systemic immunosuppression is of benefit in most causative inflammatory skin disease (Table 21-3).

Whenever possible, systemic immunosuppression should be sustained for at least 1 year to promote graft survival. The main goal of this timely limited systemic immuno-suppression is prevention of acute rejection episodes. A second goal is interference with the initial graft-host interaction in a way that graft-protective factors are promoted to improve the long-term graft survival with topical immunosuppression alone. Unfortunately, the latter goal has not been clearly demonstrated yet, and systemic immunosuppression cannot be sustained indefinitely due to systemic side effects such as nephrotoxicity, hepatotoxicity, potential carcinogenicity, and—last but not least—for socioeconomic reasons due to the costs of the regimen. Thus, upon discontinuation of the regimen, the risk of immune reactions may increase back to the original level, limiting long-term prognosis in most cases.

In general, prior to any systemic immunosuppression, a thorough medical workup is advisable to exclude general and specific contraindications.

CYCLOSPORINE A

It is the most established systemic immunosuppressant in high-risk penetrating keratoplasty that has been successfully administered for over 10 years.[4] The main disadvantage of systemic CsA is the narrow therapeutic range due to nephrotoxicity and induction of high blood pressure. The dosage has to be initially adapted from blood levels of CsA that have to be continuously monitored throughout administration, at least monthly, after a steady state in blood levels is reached. Levels of 120 to 150 ng/mL (EDTA-blood samples collected exactly 12 hours after prior administration) should be aimed for. Measurements should be performed using commercially available immunoassay kits such as the Tdx or AxSYM assays (Abbott Laboratories, Inc, Abbott Park, Ill).

MYCOPHENOLATE MOFETIL

It is another established immunosuppressant. Serious side effects are less frequent and less severe as compared to CsA. Common dosage is 1 g twice daily. For immunosuppression with MMF, usually no dosage monitoring is required due to wide therapeutic range.

Unlike conventional high-risk penetrating keratoplasty, a monotherapy with either CsA or MMF yields insufficient protection against immunologic rejection of the transplanted stem cells, respectively.[12]

Whenever possible, a combination of systemic CsA and MMF for prophylaxis of graft rejection is recommended, together with topical corticosteroids. Frequency of topical corticosteroids should initially be 5 drops daily upon epithelial closure, tapered on a monthly basis down to 3 drops a day over the first 3 months. This dosage should be sustained as long as possible unless steroidal side effects such as glaucoma and destabilization of the graft epithelium develop.

Treatment of Coexisting Morbidity

Schirmer's test should be performed to diagnose aqueous tear deficiency. Punctum occlusion may be performed accordingly. Topical lubrication with commercially available hyaluronic acid preparations should be performed in all patients, regardless of aqueous tear deficiency. This regimen increases tear film stability. It is important to avoid toxicity from preservatives by strictly refraining from preserved lubricants. Wet chamber occlusion overnight may be necessary to prevent lagophthalmic ulcerations of the graft.

Concomitant chronic blepharokeratoconjunctivitis predisposes to an inflammatory milieu in the tear film, potentially exerting toxicity toward the limbal stem cells. Thus, it is important to instruct the patient to chronically clean the lower eyelid margins whenever possible. Additionally, topical antibiotic agents for 10 days may help in reducing bacterial load initially.

One should keep in mind, however, that severe surface disorders might result due to an immune reaction against the transplanted limbal stem cells. High dose topical steroids may be of use in such a situation.

Trials

The authors recently published 5-year data on a series of 48 homologous limbokeratoplasties for patients suffering from total limbal stem cell deficiency.[13] This analysis demonstrated long-term survival of transplanted limbal stem cells as well as importance of HLA matching for long-term clear graft survival.

All patients received systemic CsA and/or MMF in the postoperative course for around 1 year. Thirteen patients received grafts with 0 to 1 HLA mismatches at the HLA-A, HLA-B, and HLA-DR loci; 13 received grafts with 2 to 6 mismatches; and in the remainder of 22 patients, no HLA typing had been performed. Five years postoperatively, 65% of the grafts with 0 to 1 mismatch, 41% of the grafts with 2 to 6 mismatches, and only 14% of the untyped remainder maintained clarity using the Kaplan-Meier method. This difference turned out statistically significant from log rank test ($p = 0.03$).

Molecular genetic analysis on epithelial cells harvested from the central graft could be performed successfully in 7 patients and revealed donor DNA in 5 of these 7 cases (71%) up to 56 months postoperatively.

Prognosis

Long-term survival of donor epithelium and the central graft clarity is possible, especially for the majority of HLA-matched limbokeratoplasties. However, further improvement of long-term prognosis is still desirable. This can most likely be achieved by further reducing the risk of graft rejections.

Thus, further improvement of the immunosuppressive regimen is required. An ideal immunosuppressant improving long-term graft survival would be a topical agent not exerting serious topical or systemic side effects. FK506 might be such a candidate.[10]

Additionally, identification and matching of further transplantation antigens such as the minor transplantation antigens might bring long-term prognosis nearer to the excellent prognosis of autologous transplantation in the future.

Future Considerations

Newer Immunosuppressives

Tacrolimus (FK506) and rapamycine: Few data are available for these substances (see Table 21-3).

Newer Adjunctive Biologicals

The same is true for these, which include humanized monoclonal antibodies targeting interleukin receptors (basiliximab [see Table 21-3]).

Matching of Minor Transplantation Antigens

Further antigen systems are likely to be involved in graft rejection because even patients with optimal match for the HLA loci A, B, and DR still experience graft rejections. Ongoing research points to an important role of minor transplantation antigens so that eventually, graft survival following homologous methods might approach the excellent prognosis of autologous transplantation.

SUMMARY

Prognosis of penetrating limbokeratoplasty in patients suffering from severe limbal stem cell insufficiency may be poor because the graft and the limbal stem cells are constantly challenged by a multitude of potential postoperative complications (see Table 21-2).

Key Points

1. In severe limbal stem cell insufficiency, restoration of the optic axis is only possible with transplantation of viable limbal stem cells either simultaneously or prior to penetrating keratoplasty.
2. At present, applicability of autologous transplantation is limited to the minority of unilaterally affected patients where enough viable stem cells for repopulating at least 40% of the limbal circumference can be safely harvested from the other eye.
3. Homologous central limbokeratoplasty can currently be considered the first line procedure for cases of bilateral limbal stem cell insufficiency combined with deep central corneal opacification.
4. Long-term results after allogeneic penetrating limbokeratoplasty are only encouraging if grafts have been matched at the HLA loci A, B, and DR.
5. Whenever possible, a combination of systemic CsA and MMF for prophylaxis of graft rejection is recommended, together with topical corticosteroids.
6. Long-term survival of donor epithelium and the central graft clarity is possible, especially for the majority of HLA matched limbokeratoplasties. However, further improvement of long-term prognosis is still desirable.

REFERENCES

1. Chen JJ, Tseng SC. Corneal epithelial wound healing in partial limbal deficiency. *Invest Ophthalmol Vis Sci.* 1990;31:1301–1314.
2. Hanna C. The fate of cells in the transplant. *Surv Ophthalmol.* 1966;11:405–414.
3. Sangwan VS, Matalia HP, Vemuganti GK, et al. Early results of penetrating keratoplasty after cultivated limbal epithelium transplantation. *Arch Ophthalmol.* 2005;123:334–340.
4. Solomon A, Ellies P, Anderson DF, et al. Long-term outcome of keratolimbal allograft with or without penetrating keratoplasty for total limbal stem cell deficiency. *Ophthalmology.* 2002;109:1159–1166.
5. Sundmacher R, Reinhard T. Central corneolimbal transplantation under systemic cyclosporin A cover for severe limbal stem cell insufficiency. *Graefes Arch Clin Exp Ophthalmol.* 1996;234 (Suppl 1):S122–S125.

6. Reinhard T, Spelsberg H, Henke L, et al. Long-term results of allogeneic penetrating limboker-atoplasty in total limbal stem cell deficiency. *Ophthalmology.* 2004;111:775–782.

7. Volker-Dieben HJ, Claas FH, Schreuder GM, et al. Beneficial effect of HLA-DR matching on the survival of corneal allografts. *Transplantation.* 2000;70:640–648.

8. Böhringer D, Reinhard T, Böhringer S, Enczmann J, Godehard E, Sundmacher R. Predicting time on the waiting list for HLA matched corneal grafts. *Tissue Antigens.* 2002;59:407–411.

9. Böhringer D, Reinhard T, Duquesnoy RJ, et al. Beneficial effect of matching at the HLA-A and -B amino-acid triplet level on rejection-free clear graft survival in penetrating keratoplasty. *Transplantation.* 2004;77:417–421.

10. Lam DS, Young AL, Leung AT, Fan DS, Wong AK. Limbal stem cell allografting from related live donors for corneal surface reconstruction. *Ophthalmology.* 2000;107:411–412.

11. Sundmacher R, Reinhard T. Homologous lamellar central limbokeratoplasty in severe limbal stem cell deficiency. *Klin Monatsbl Augenheilkd.* 1998;213:254–255.

12. Hoffmann F. Nahttechnik bei perforierender Keratoplastik. *Klin Monatsbl Augenheilkd.* 1976;169:584–590.

13. Spelsberg H, Reinhard T, Henke L, Berschick P, Sundmacher R. Penetrating limbo-keratoplasty for granular and lattice corneal dystrophy: survival of donor limbal stem cells and intermediate-term clinical results. *Ophthalmology.* 2004;111:1528–1533.

14. Reinhard T, Mayweg S, Reis A, Sundmacher R. Topical FK506 as immunoprophylaxis after allogeneic penetrating normal-risk keratoplasty: a randomized clinical pilot study. *Transpl Int.* 2005; 18:193–197.

15. Reinhard T, Reis A, Böhringer D, et al. Systemic mycophenolate mofetil in comparison with systemic cyclosporin A in high-risk keratoplasty patients: 3 years' results of a randomized prospective clinical trial. *Graefes Arch Clin Exp Ophthalmol.* 2001;239:367–372.

16. Sloper CM, Powell RJ, Dua HS. Tacrolimus (FK506) in the management of high-risk corneal and limbal grafts. *Ophthalmology.* 2001;108:1838–1844.

17. Schmitz K, Hitzer S, Behrens-Baumann W. Immune suppression with a combination of basiliximab and cyclosporin in high-risk keratoplasty. A pilot study. *Ophthalmologe.* 2002;99(1):38–45.

22

Keratoprosthesis

*M. Emilia Mulet, MD, PhD and
Jorge L. Alio, MD, PhD*

INTRODUCTION

Corneal diseases remain a major cause of blindness throughout the world, with more than 10 million patients suffering from corneal blindness. Corneal opacity can be successfully treated by corneal transplant. However, a number of these patients requiring corneal transplant surgery are considered at high risk of corneal graft failure. The original idea of replacing an opaque cornea with glass was created by Pellier of Quengsy in 1771,[1] and in 1853, Nussbaum[2] performed the first implant in an animal model. Later, in 1855, Weber[3] performed the same surgery in a human eye. Following that, many trials were performed in the same field. There were multiple and varied keratoprosthesis designs (monoblock,[3–5] two pieces[6–10]) and many biomaterials were used. In 1945, plastic derivatives such as PMMA were introduced as an optic center for good optic quality and biotolerance. Haptic materials used include gold, glass, tantalio,[3] titanium,[11] ceramic,[12] and platinum.[13] Eye fixation has also changed over time, but at present intracorneal anchoring is used or (according to Strampelli) osteoodontokeratoprosthesis, which has been performed since 1967.[14]

INDICATION

Patients with bilateral corneal blindness cannot be treated by repeated standard penetrating keratoplasty.[15] Restoration of visual acuity can often only be achieved by a keratoprosthesis in patients with dry eye, like pemphigoid, Fuchs' dystrophy, Stevens-Johnson syndrome, and xerophthalmia; eyes with severe vascularization of the cornea due to severe burns; in a leukoma adherens; or following recurrent transplant rejections as well as in cloudy corneas of silicone-filled eyes. In these cases, an intact posterior segment and retinal function are required as well as uncorrected visual acuity of less than 20/200.

Figure 22-1. An optical cylinder supported by an osteoodonto lamina from a tooth. (Courtesy of Dr. Temprano.)

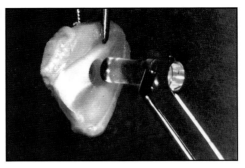

Figure 22-2. Osteoodontokeratoprosthesis. (Courtesy of Dr. Temprano.)

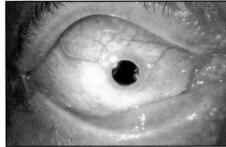

Indications for keratoprosthesis have changed over the years. Many alkali burns and practically all aphakic bullous keratopathy have been eliminated from the indications.[16]

KERATOPROSTHESIS TYPES

All devices consist of a transparent center. Currently, all devices have a PMMA optic and microporous skirt-haptic support of biocolonizable and biodegradable materials such as nylon, dacron, teflon, silastic, silicone, proplast, hydrophilic plastics, or aluminum oxide ceramique.

Biological Origin

- The materials used for the haptic are autologous tissue such as tooth,[14] ear cartilage, or tibia bone.[17]
- Osteoodontokeraprosthesis: It is a 2-stage procedure. The surface of the cornea is removed and covered with a graft of buccal mucosa. An optical cylinder supported by an osteoodonto lamina planed from a tooth is then inserted into the mucosa to act as a lens (Figures 22-1 and 22-2).

Nonbiological Origin

- PMMA-PTFE (expanded polytetrafluoroethylene [FCI [18-20]], Rantigy, France).
- PHEMA (Chirila-AlphaCor Kpro, CooperVision Surgical, Perth, Australia),[21,22] Archen Seoul type (Seoul, Korea),[23,24] and champagne cork.[25]
- Titanium haptic (MICOF) (Moscow, Russia),[26] silicone,[27] and others. There are phakic and aphakic models[28] (Figure 22-3).

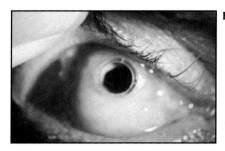

Figure 22-3. PMMA-PTFE keratoprosthesis (FCI).

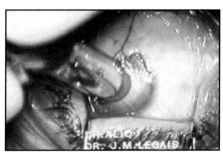

Figure 22-4. Surgical technique: cornea trephination.

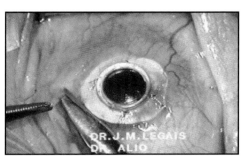

Figure 22-5. Surgical technique: keratoprosthesis implant into intralamellar stromal pocket.

SURGICAL TECHNIQUE

Keratoprosthesis implantation is by means of an intralamellar technique, with a conjunctival flap in most cases.[29] The cornea is trephined 4.5 or 5.5 mm (Figure 22-4). Then a 360-degree intralamellar stroma corneal pocket is created. Implantation of the keratoprosthesis haptic in a lamellar pocket is then done (Figure 22-5). The optic is then positioned through a hole trephined in the central cornea.

KERATOPROSTHESIS LIMITS

- Restricted visual field (30 to 40 degrees).[30,31]
- Impossible to measure IOP (Aachen Kpro [Germany] allows measurement of IOP due to its flexible optical part with a modified Schiøtz tonometer, but measurements with the Goldmann tonometer [HAAG-STREIT USA Inc, Mason, Ohio] and Tono-Pen [Medtronic Xomed Ophthalmics, Inc, Jacksonville, Fla] are not possible).[23]
- Poor visual prognosis: In the majority of cases, the visual acuity achieved is at least 20/200 vision due to pre-existing retinal or optic damage.[16]

Prognosis

Prognosis can be ranked according to the degree of vision achieved and retained as follows:[16]

- Graft failure in eyes without past inflammation (corneal edema, etc).
- Graft failure in eyes with past inflammation (herpes simplex or zoster, uveitis, etc).
- Pemphigoid (susceptible to retroprosthetic membrane formation).
- Chemical burns (susceptible to glaucoma and retinal detachment).
- Stevens-Johnson syndrome (poor prognosis and high risk of endophthalmitis).

The prognosis of keratoprosthesis surgery varies markedly according to the preoperative diagnosis. Graft failures in noncicatrizing conditions are most favorable, whereas Stevens-Johnson syndrome has the worst prognosis. OCP and chemical burns occupy the middle ground. The difference between the groups seems to correlate with the degree of past preoperative inflammation. Patients with immune-related corneal surface diseases can exhibit marked inflammatory responses, leading to necrosis, stromal melting, and the formation of an epithelial fistula. In contrast, patients without autoimmune corneal diseases demonstrate a remarkably noninflamed cornea with intact keratocytes and without epithelial ingrowth, commensurate with their clinical appearance.[32,33]

Results

The visual results in some cases have been gratifying and heartbreaking. The degree of improvement usually depends on the pre-existing damage to the eye. Visual results varied from 20/20 to counting fingers.[3,16,22,34]

Fifty-seven percent of cases had a visual acuity of 20/200 or better.[16] Thirty percent of the patients attained 20/15 to 20/40 visual acuity; however, with long-term follow up[3,19,26,34-37] or a large series of cases, there is a loss of initial good visual acuity due to the numerous and severe complications that lead to patients requiring close observation and aggressive early treatment of inflammatory conditions affecting the lids or cornea. Sometimes, visual acuity improved to a good level and then gradually deteriorated to hand movements or light perception because disastrous complications can occur many years after surgery.[16] Only 13%[3] to 16%[34] maintained this level of acuity over a long-term period. The operation had to be repeated in 30% of the cases.[19,34] The patients who failed to achieve a visual acuity of 20/200 after keratoprosthesis surgery (57%), despite an uneventful operative course, had preexisting conditions that limited their visual prognosis (age-related macular degeneration , retinal detachment, cataract, glaucoma) and were not recognized before the keratoprosthesis surgery.[16,22]

The most common complications encountered in the course of follow up were glaucoma in 49% of the cases[3,16,34] followed by retroprosthesis membrane with an average of 37%[3,16,19,34] and in 45.5% of the eyes the membrane recurred,[19] and endophthalmitis[32,35] was the third most frequent complication in 36.4 % of the cases.[19] The number of complications has been reduced by the use of the new biomaterials. The implantation technique is not complicated and initial results are usually good. The multiple complications, however, make it necessary for these cases to be followed by a surgeon who is familiar with the management of complications.

Despite their use being limited to only some forms of keratopathy, keratoprostheses seem to offer a solution in cases where no other treatment is available.

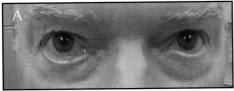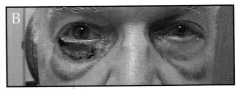

Figure 23-5. (A) Patient with cicatricial ectropion of both lower lids. (B) One week postoperative after bilateral lateral canthoplasties and full thickness retroauricular skin graft to right lower lid.

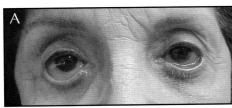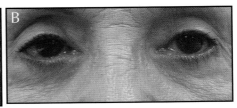

Figure 23-6. (A) Preoperative photo of cicatricial ectropion after a lower lid blepharoplasty. (B) Postoperative photo of repair of cicatricial ectropion with lower eyelid tightening by lateral tarsal strips.

subtype is determined, the mass or malar bags should be excised. If a cicatricial ectropion has occurred in association with trauma, burns, or previous surgical intervention, then a skin graft may be necessary (Figures 23-5 and 23-6). The contralateral upper eyelid is the preferred donor site, but retroauricular, supraclavicular, or skin from the inner arm can be utilized. If the ectropion is a result of topical glaucoma medications, the offending drug should be discontinued. Early surgical intervention may be required if the sensitivity to topical drops is widespread. Lower eyelid retraction is more challenging than upper eyelid retraction because gravity works against surgical repair. If horizontal laxity is present, a lateral tarsal strip procedure is helpful, but release of the lower eyelid retractors and placement of a spacer graft is often required.[9,10] Spacer graft options include tarsal transplant, hard palate, auricular cartilage, Enduragen (collagen implant) (Porex Surgical, College Park, Ga), and Alloderm (acellular dermis) (LifeCell Corp, Woodlands, Tex).

Lagophthalmos

Lagophthalmos is defined as an inability to completely close the eye and is most commonly seen in patients with seventh nerve palsy. A lateral tarsorrhaphy is helpful in the acute setting of corneal decompensation secondary to exposure. However, the procedure can be cosmetically unsatisfying and alternatives are present. A gold weight implant is a successful operation on patients who present with lagophthalmos (Figure 23-7). Prior to placement, measurements are made to choose an implant that will allow the eyelid to remain open but will help close the lid completely on closure and sleep. The weight is placed in the pretarsal space, sutured securely with 5–0 Vicryl stitches, and the orbicularis and overlying skin are closed securely to prevent extrusion.

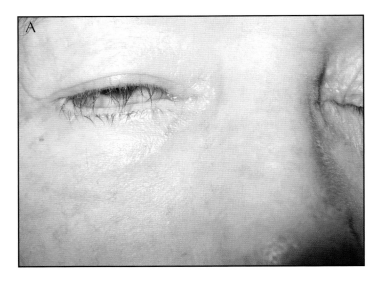

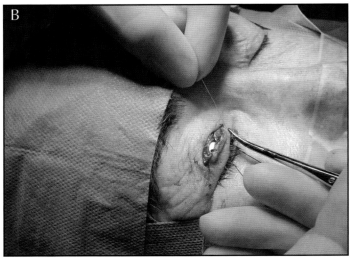

Figure 23–7. (A) Preoperative photo of patient with right lagoph-thalmos and exposure keratopathy from seventh nerve palsy. (B) Intraoperative photo of gold weight placement into the pretarsal area with closure of the overlying orbicularis muscle.

SPECIAL SURGICAL CONSIDERATIONS IN DRY EYE PATIENTS

An evaluation for dry eyes is imperative on any patient interested in having ptosis repair or blepharoplasty of both the upper and/or lower lids. Determination of the proper surgical technique rests on knowledge of a history of dry eyes.[11] A levator tuck or advance-ment is a useful procedure in patients with dry eyes who require ptosis repair (Figure 23-8). By not excising any levator, a revision can be performed if symptoms of dry eyes are

Section IV

Special Situations

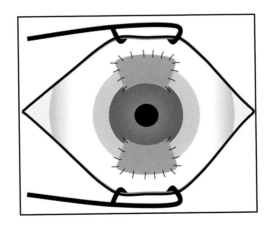

24

Contact Lens-Induced Dry Eye

Kenneth Daniels, OD, FAAO

INTRODUCTION

The introduction of a contact lens onto the ocular surface is a simple form of insult that will justifiably cause a reaction by the eye, leading to the change in its natural physiology and metabolism. The normal tear environment is always under attack from the natural environment. If a contact lens is introduced to the eye, the tear film can be dramatically changed. It is generally thought that initially there is an increase in tear production that will occur with the introduction of the contact lens or a stimulant drop onto the eye. However, tear production will "fatigue" over time, decreasing the efforts of the lacrimal system and increasing the potential for contact lens deposits, microbial infection, corneal infiltration and edema, and ultimately patient dissatisfaction with contact lenses. With the use of ocular lubricants as a supplement or stimulant, the eye becomes "subjectively comfortable" but little is known in regards to their long-term effect on the various tear film structures and corneal physiology. With respect to supplement interaction with the material and the material's interaction with the eye, the contact lens design and material are the key long-term comfort and physiological balance in the potential success of the contact lens patient.

CONTACT LENS-INDUCED DRY EYE

Contact lens intolerance can be a key essential symptom of dry eye. A patient with mild to moderate dry eye may not experience symptoms until contact lenses are fitted. When the lens is placed on this subclinical marginal dry eye patient, he or she becomes symptomatic, leading to a phase of contact lens-induced dry eye (CLIDE).[1-13]

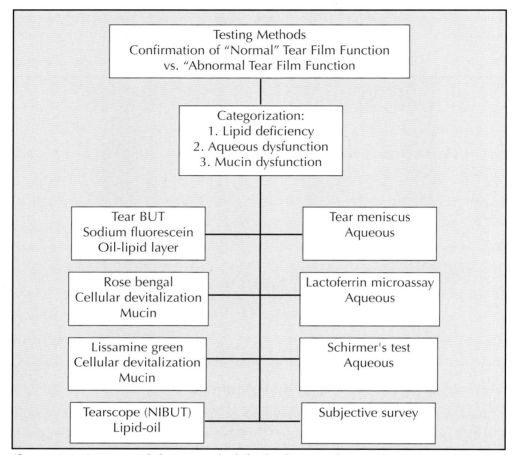

Figure 24-1. Recommended testing methods for the dry eye and contact lens patient.

The placement of a contact lens can upset the delicate balance of tear film production and distribution, leading to lens intolerance. The CLIDE patient subjectively and objectively demonstrates lens discomfort or intolerance in association to a rapid evaporation of the tears from the eye, causing irritation, protein deposits, infection, and pain.

TESTING METHODS

There are various objective and subjective testing methods (Figure 24-1) utilized to determine the potential success of a contact lens patient and the possible relationship of tear film and dry eye issues that may ultimately dissuade the patient away from contacts.

Some of these tests (Table 24-1) can be easily modified to enhance the testing of the contact lens patient's tolerance to lenses and appreciation for lens-induced dryness. For example, the Schirmer's test can be performed with and without contact lenses to differentiate the tear volume reduction with the lens inserted and will allow the clinician to determine the competitive effect the contact lens has for the supportive tear

Table 24-1
TEAR TESTING METHODS

Tear Function Test	Reason	Method
Schirmer's test without and with anesthesia (basal/reflexive secretion)	Lacrimal gland function (aqueous production)	Placement of #41 millipore filter paper onto the lid margin on the temporal angle: the paper will absorb aqueous and flow down the paper via capillary action over a measured 5-minute period. Performed without anesthetic (Schirmer's 1 defines reflexive) and with anesthetic (Schirmer's 2, basal) Normal >10 mm/5 min
Schirmer's test without anesthesia and with contact lens inserted	Lacrimal function with completion of the contact lens	Placement of #41 millipore filter paper onto the lid margin on the temporal canthal angle: the paper will absorb aqueous and flow down the paper via capillary action over a measured 5-minute period. Performed without anesthetic (Schirmer's 1 defines reflexive) with the habitual contact lens in places. Differentiation of lacrimal-aqueous challenge induced by the contact lens.
Tear BUT	Meibomian gland function (oil layer production tear film stability)	Instill sodium fluorescein (NaFl) onto the conjunctiva. Observe the NaFl on the cornea for staining and disruption to the spread of the dye. Ask the patient to gently close his or her eyes then open and refrain from blinking. Count the number of seconds till the NaFl starts to dissipate, which is observed as black areas or negative staining. Normal <15 seconds Average <10 to 15 seconds Below normal <9 seconds.
Noninvasive BUT (NIBUT)	Meibomian gland function (oil layer production tear film stability)	Tear film is observed in a similar method as the tear BUT using either a keratometer or adapted raster grid projection. The patient is asked to close his or her eyes, open, then refrain from blinking while the keratometric mires or raster grid is projected onto the tear film and observed. The examiner will time tear break up based upon the first appearance of mire or grid pattern distortion. *(continued)*

Table 24-1
TEAR TESTING METHODS (CONTINUED)

Tear Function Test	*Reason*	*Method*
		Normal <30 seconds Below normal <20 seconds
NIBUT tearscope	Meibomian gland function (oil layer production tear film stability)	Utilizes specular reflectance to characterize the POTF.
Hamano phenol red	Lacrimal gland function (aqueous production)	Similar to Schirmer's test, this test is less invasive. The thread is impregnated with phenol red, which changes color over a 30-sec time period. Normal >17 mm/30 sec Average: 9 mm to 17 mm Below normal <9 mm
Tear meniscus	Lacrimal function/ aqueous volume	Fifty percent of the tear volume will be located in the tear meniscus or tear lake observed aligning the inferior lid margin. The meniscus is measured in millimeters. Normal 0.3 to 0.4 mm Average 0.2 mm Below normal < 0.1 mm
Tearscope slit lamp specular reflection topography	Integrity of the lipid layer	Baseline evaluation of the lipid layer spread over the entirety of the ocular surface. Should appear as a multiple "rainbow" coloration or "oil slick."
Lactoferrin assay	Quantitative measure of the lacrimal function: measures the lactoferrin component of the tear film	An ability to measure a "component" of the tear film tear film is considered to be much more reliable than the previously mentioned procedures. This is an ELISA test that requires the collection of a 0.5-ul sample of tears. The sample of tear fluid is collected with a microcapillary tube and mixed with a 0.5-ul sample of diluent. A 2-ul sample of diluted tear fluid is then transferred to a millipore filter card after which a drop of a conjugate, wash, and substrate are administered sequentially over a 5-min period. The card is placed into a desktop keyboard-spectrophotometer.

(continued)

Tear Function Test	Reason	Methods
		Normal >1.5 Average 1.0 to 1.5 Below normal <.9
Punctal patency	Indication of the punctal–canaliculi function	Noted as a positive or negative regurgitation of aqueous from the orifice of the punctum.
Lid closure	Indication of possible lagophthalmos	Patient is asked to close his or her eyes. The examiner observes the lid closure through the slit lamp to document if a gap exists between the upper and lower lid margins.
Blink rate	Efficiency of tear film spread and exposure and prevention of tear evaporation	Observation of the frequency of complete blink. Normal: 7 blinks per minute
Lid tension	Interaction between lid and lens	Measured on a 0-to-4 scale based upon the difficulty level when inverting the lid to observe the superior palpebral conjunctiva.
Fischer-Schweitzer mosaic	Integrity of the epithelium	Upon closing the eye, lightly rub the superior lid. Upon opening, observe the cornea with cobalt blue and NaFl. + mosaic: wavy distortion across the corneal surface
Digital expression of meibomian glands	Integrity of the secretory function	Subtle digital compression of the lid margin to express or pump a trace of oil out of the orifice.
Jones punctal patency test	Patency of the lacrimal drainage system Determination of obstruction of canaliculus	Jones 1. Instill ample amount of NaFl for 5 minutes; blow nose (each nostril separately). Jones 2. Irrigate the inferior canaliculus; blow nose. Jones 3. Option: retrieve NaFl by introducing a sterile applicator into the nostril. Analysis: Observable NaFl in tissue or applicator
Rose bengal or lissamine green	Mucin and conjunctival goblet cell function	Instillation of this vital stain to determine the amount of cellular devitalization. *(continued)*

Table 24-1
TEAR TESTING METHODS (CONTINUED)

Table 24-1 TEAR TESTING METHODS (CONTINUED)		
Tear Function Text	*Reason*	*Methods*
Impression cytology	Goblet cell function	Microscopic technique that captures goblets cells. The cells are stained after which the stain is absorbed by the cell nucleus. The vitality of the cell is determined by the characterization, via stain absorbance, of the nucleus.
Keratometry corneal topography wavefront aberrometry	NIBUT and dynamic observation of tear film	Both instruments utilize cold light rather than a hot lamp used by the biomicroscope that enhances tear BUT. NIBUT will be based on the time to the first observation of mire distortion on keratometry and/or first blink. Topography and wavefront aberrometry are observations of the lipid layer of the tear film and the potential dry spots or "missed data" on the image acquisition.

film. Additionally, it will assist in the determination of the requirements for substitutive support to maintain the lens and ocular surface physiology.

THE PRE- AND POSTOCULAR LENS TEAR FILM

The preocular tear film (POTF) is viewed as a thin, mostly aqueous film covering a hydrophilic ocular surface with an inferior and superior margin meniscus or reservoir for added support. The aqueous layer is coated by an even thinner lipid layer, creating a homogenous coverage and protection of the ocular surface. Gravity has a negligible effect on the tear film. Hydraulic flow of tears can only occur in the meniscus. The instability of the preocular tear film, which can be caused by several factors, appears to be characteristic of all dry eye states irrespective of etiology.

A stable precorneal tear film (PCTF) is necessary to sustain contact lens wear.[1-3] Several iatrogenic changes occur to the PCTF and adnexa with the introduction of a contact lens to the ocular surface. Initially, a thinning of the PCTF (ie, lipid layer disruption) occurs. The disruption to the lipid layer leads to the lack of tear spreading and increases the risk of tear evaporative processes. This will in turn lead back to an aberrance in the blink rate and potentially increase the mucous discharge into the tear film due to the irregularity of the blink reflex.[2] If the lipid layer is in depletion or is not confluent, the subsequent effect is an unstable tear film that cannot properly support the ocular surface and most certainly would be unable to support a contact lens. In this situation, the tear film would have a 4-fold increase in evaporation.[3]

The dynamics of the tear film defines the ability of the lipid layer to be spread over the ocular surface. As the upper lid moves downward, the accumulated lipid layer is compressed and thickens, yielding an interference color similar to that of oil on top of water on a hot road surface. The lipid layer is then spread as a single layer over the lens surface upon lid closure and reopening. If the lid movement becomes deviated or dysfunctional, then the lipid layer spread will become amorphic, leading to variant exposures or dry spots across the lens–ocular surface.

The lack of continuity of the lipid layer then leads to variant areas of evaporation and enhanced dryness and a decrease in the available tear meniscus. The tear meniscus acts as the reservoir of aqueous required to support not only the hydration of the ocular surface but also, via capillary dynamics, the hydration of the hydrogel lens and acts as a cushion and optical support for gas permeable lenses.[1]

The integrity of the PCTF is directly proportional to the ability to maintain proper contact lens wettability and lens surface hydration. If the lipid layer is poor, the evaporative process increases, leading to a greater loss of aqueous and the induction of a forward osmotic draw across the contact lens surface, leading to lens dehydration. With lens dehydration, the hydrophilic lens will steepen mechanically, pulling on a weakened epithelial surface and allowing for corneal compromise visualized as corneal epithelial desiccation.

When the ocular surface becomes "unprotected," there is the development of neuronal hyposensitivity as well as the barrier effect created by the contact lens interface. As the contact lens develops a substantial dehydration, it will tend to vault away from the ocular surface, leaving an exposed gap between the postlens surface and the corneal surface. The gap, however, is not fluid filled and leaves the ocular surface unprotected, leading to compromise of the epithelium and aberration to neural regulation and biofeedback to the lid structure.

As the contact lens starts to dehydrate and there is an induced dryness, oxygen transmissibility of the lens is reduced, a reduction in the dk/l (oxygen coefficient over thickness), which in turn increases the hypoxic stress on the cornea and reduces its sensitivity. This leads to a reduced reflex tearing and subsequently an even drier eye. It is also assumed that in this process there is an increased tear osmolarity that dehydrates the lens and the cornea, resulting in an increased dehydration of the ocular surface and contact lens.[4,5] As the epithelium becomes compromised, so does the underlying subbasal neural plexus.

As in LASIK, the dry eye symptomatology is thought to be related to the severance and disruption of the neural signal due to the microkeratome cutting of the neurons. CLIDE may have a similar basis. It can be assumed that the hypoxia deadens the neurons, leading to a lesser degree of biofeedback in the neuronal loop. The disruption of this loop not only affects the stimulus to produce the proper amounts of aqueous, mucins, and oils, but also deleteriously diminishes the feedback for a full and complete blink reflex.

The contact lens is a true disruptor to the tear film, dividing it into the POTF and the postocular tear film (POLTF). Upon the evaporation of the POTF, a hydrophilic contact lens will start to dehydrate. Due to the loss of the POTF aqueous, the contact lens in turn relies on the POLTF, leading to an increased absorbance of the posterior aqueous tear film in order to maintain its proper hydration. It is assumed that lenses of a greater thickness with a low water content would have a lesser percentage of dehydration while thinner lenses with a high water content would have a greater level of dehydration.

Evaporative water loss at the anterior lens surface is a most probable cause of contact lens dehydration and of POLTF depletion. There is a direct correlation to subjective discomfort, dryness, and lens adhesion or binding. It has been reported that within 1 hour of hydrophilic lens wear, there is a substantial reduction in the POLTF as observed via specular reflection of the lens-corneal surface. The decrease in the aqueous component of the POLTF allows for the accumulation of debris and particulates that can yield microtrauma and epithelial compromise due to the inhibition of the tear flow and exchange.[6]

COMPLICATIONS ASSOCIATED WITH CONTACT LENS-INDUCED DRY EYE

Approximately 1 out of every 20 contact lens wearers develops a contact lens-related complication each year, particularly amongst extended wear patients.[7,8] The majority of concerns range from a self-limiting to sight-threatening clinical problem that will require an immediate diagnosis and subsequent treatment. Lens dehydration that directly relates to the imbibement of surface and intramatrix protein accumulation decreases the oxygen transmissibility of the lens but also acts as a nutritional source for bacterium. As the contact lens loses its water while wearing the lens with a decrease in the dK, there is an increase in the hypoxic stress on the cornea and reduction in sensitivity and loss of structural integrity.[9] Contributing to this process is an increased tear osmolarity that dehydrates the lens and the cornea, resulting in a dry lens-eye state.

Hypoxic-related complications associated with CLIDE are the major root causes for the majority of complications. Lens dehydration and the effects on the cornea and the ocular surface simply add to the risk. In essence, all complications are caused by hypoxia (deprivation of oxygen) to the cornea, leading to hypercapnia and acidosis.

The lack of cleanliness or the increase in mucoprotein film due to the dehydration of the contact lens and the inability to cleanse the lens surface due to aberrance in the blink reflex leads to the process of protein denaturation. The cascade will lead to an increased potential for more serious ocular reactions such as giant papillary conjunctivitis (GPC) and superior limbic keratoconjunctivitis (SLK).

If one relates the characteristics of the patient (eg, the properties of the tear film, blink pattern, wear schedule, method of cleaning, tear pH, diet, and medications) and how they relate to the polymer (eg, the ionicity, water content, base chemistry (silicone, HEMA, GMA-HEMA) and wetting angle, then one will find a direct correlate to observe pathology and subjective complaints. These pathologies and complaints would manifest as visual disturbance (specific or vague), dry eye complaints, punctuate keratopathy, microbial keratitis, blink abnormalities, ocular surface keratinization, xerosis, hemorrhage, and inflammation.

Poor visual quality and acuity with contact lenses occurring during the tear break-up is subjectively described as foggy or steamy and clears temporally with a blink. The tear film break-up (TFBU) develops as a surface irregularity, causing light scatter and optical aberrations. The scatter creates the appearance of viewing objects through a "fogginess or shadowing" similar to "coma aberration." With a blink, the tear film is spread more evenly over the lens surface, thereby improving vision during the short time interval until TFBU starts to occur again.

Lid abnormalities can either induce, exacerbate, or be exacerbated by contact lens and dry eye conditions. The lid, based on the neural loop, is negatively affected when a lens is introduced to the eye. If the eye is borderline dry and the contact lens interrupts the blink mechanism, any lid anomaly will be amplified thus amplifying the underlying disruption to proper tear production and balance of the lens-tear-ocular surface relationship. Other lid conditions, summarized in Table 24-2, will also adversely effect lens wear.

TIGHT CONTACT LENS SYNDROME

Tight contact lens syndrome (TCLS) occurs when a contact lens fits poorly due to an aberrantly steep base curve or sagittal depth in relation to the flat keratometric measures or in combination to lens dehydration. Evaporative tear film deficiency with secondary steepening lens curvature as related to the corneal curvature is the underlying cause for a tight contact lens syndrome even if the lens is initially fit well.[11]

The patient usually complains that the contact lens is generally comfortable yet starts to develop a lesser tolerance for the lens after a few hours of wear to the point that he or she feels the lens must be removed or has a difficult time in lens removal. Upon lens removal, the eye is red, such that the patient feels that he or she must rigorously rub his or her eyes to generate comfort. Some patients may present with a subsequent subconjunctival hemorrhage. The symptoms usually resolve within a few hours after discontinuance of contact lens wear.

TCLS is easily observed later in the day during biomicroscopic exam. The lens will have poor translation or movement, particularly in the vertical meridian, and will demonstrate a conjunctival impression or intralimbal epithelial split (Figure 24-2).[11] Resolution of the problem entails fitting a contact lens with a flatter base curve or smaller diameter. In essence, the lens must fit more loosely on the eye, allowing the tear film better access to the cornea beneath the contact lens.

The more important concerns with a TCLS is the overall compromise to the cornea and the loss of the epithelial barriers and protection from pathogens via a depleted tear film support. The weakened cornea is highly susceptible to abrasion and microbial infiltration.

SUBCONJUNCTIVAL HEMORRHAGE

Subconjunctival hemorrhages are common events in patients who wear contacts and have a "dryness" to the conjunctival surface. It usually presents as a focal, bright red, completely painless lesion that obscures the underlying white of the sclera. It will primarily occur after somewhat aggressive removal of the contact lens from the eye. The contact lens, which has dehydrated throughout the day, is adherent to the eye surface and causes a form of trauma upon removal. As the lens is forcefully grasped by the patient, the superficial conjunctival surface is distended, causing a small petechial hemorrhage.

Treatment requires palliative care only and patient reassurance. The patient should be instructed to avoid any form of anticoagulant such as aspirin, ginkgo biloba, erectile dysfunction preparations, and any other form of blood thinning or blood flow enhancement agent. He or she should also be advised to avoid vasoconstrictive agents because these may initially constrict the blood vessels yet upon dissolution of the agent, a rebound dilation of the vessels occurs, manifesting a more profound bleed. Contact lens use should be limited until there is a moderate resolution of the hemor-

Table 24-2
LID ABNORMALITIES AFFECTING CONTACT LENS AND DRY EYE PATIENTS

Condition	Description	Symptoms and Treatment
Cellulitis	An inflammation or an infection of the tissues	Preseptal cellulitis Generally treated with oral antibiotics
Orbital cellulitis	Orbital cellulitis when the infection extends to the deeper tissues	Oral and intravenous antibiotics, possible hospitalization with orbital imaging surveillance
Chalazion	Sterile inflammation of the meibomian glands described as localized pain, redness, and tenderness	Hot compresses and lid massage, topical antibiotic-steroid combination, steroid injection, or surgical intervention
Dacryoadenitis	Inflammation of the lacrimal gland	Oral and topical antibiotics with systemic analgesic (if needed)
Dacryocystitis canaliculitis	Inflammation or an infection of the lacrimal sac or canaliculus	Symptoms include pain, redness, and swelling of the side of the nose. Other symptoms may include tearing, with a mucous-like discharge. Hot compresses, massage, and antibiotics usually control the situation. Rule out occlusion neoplastic disorder or mechanical occlusion by punctal plug.
Ectropion	A turning outward of the upper and/or lower eyelid margin. As a result of the space between the eyelid and eyeball, the tear fluid will have a tendency to spill on the cheek rather than lubricate the eye	Artificial tears, warm compresses, and/or topical antibiotic ointment or surgical reconstruction
Entropion	An inward turning of the upper and/or lower eyelid margin toward the eyeball. This irritation is caused by the rubbing of the lashes on the corneal surface	Topical antibiotic ointments are recommended. Definitive treatment requires surgery.
Growths or lesions	Abnormal growth such as a neoplasm, cystoid formation, eyelash anomaly, redundant benign tissue growth	Neoplasm: enlargement, bleeding, or changing color of the lesion requires a biopsy.

(continued)

Table 24-2

LID ABNORMALITIES AFFECTING CONTACT LENS AND DRY EYE PATIENTS (CONTINUED)

Condition	Description	Symptoms and Treatment
		Cystoid growths such as retention cysts, pyogenic granulomas, or sebaceous cyst can be monitored or removed surgically with palliative antibiotic care. Eyelash anomalies such as trichiasis (inward turning of the lashes) or distichiasis (abnormal row of lashes) require simple excision of the irritant cilia. Forceps removal, cryotherapy (focal freezing treatments), or electrolysis.
Floppy eyelid syndrome (FES)	Tear film abnormality is prevalent in patients with FES and is characterized by lipid tear deficiency, leading to rapid tear evaporation. The FES lid skin is also characterized by high temperature, high water evaporation rate, and hyperpigmentation. Linkage of lid changes and meibomian gland dysfunction.	Treatment includes lubricants, antibiotics, taping of the lids at night. Rarely, eyelid surgery is necessary.
Hordeolum	Bacterial infection of the sebaceous glands of the eyelid. External hordeolum: base of the hair follicles versus an internal hordeolum, which results from a similar bacterial infection of the meibomian glands.	Pain or tenderness usually results when the area is touched. An eyelid scrub procedure and/or hot compresses are generally needed. Usually a topical antibiotic/steroid ointment.
Lagophthalmos (also associated with Bell's or fifth nerve palsy)	Incomplete eyelid closure, leaving the ocular surfaces exposed and causing front surface drying and potential scarring.	Sandy, gritty feeling accompanied by increased tearing of the eyes. Treatment may include artificial tears, lubricating ointment, and occasionally taping the eyelid or

(continued)

Condition	Description	Symptoms and Treatment
		patching at bedtime. If medical therapy fails, surgically closing with lid tarsorrhaphy or the implantation of gold weights.

Table 24-2
**LID ABNORMALITIES AFFECTING CONTACT LENS AND DRY EYE PATIENTS
(CONTINUED)**

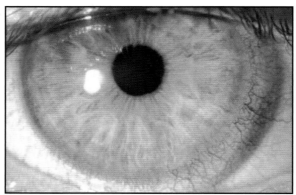

Figure 24-2. Tight contact lens syndrome.

rhage. Upon future lens removal, the patient should be instructed to moisturize the lens prior to removal as well as instructed to lightly lift the lens from the ocular surface rather than aggressively grasping the lens.

CORNEAL WARPAGE

Induced corneal deformity by a contact lens is very often associated with lens dehydration causing a pseudocentral island or distortion coincident with the corneal and visual axis. This is called induced corneal warpage. It can be seen with both rigid gas-permeable or soft contact lenses. The cornea is literally "molded" by the contact lens into a distorted shape. Warpage is best diagnosed by patient history of subjective visual distortion with an associated inability to achieve the prefit level of visual acuity and quality as well as frequent lens power changes, and in some cases, an irritated red eye and pseudo-dry eye symptomatology. In conjunction with the subjective issues, objective measures of topography, aberrometry, and pachymetry; decrease in contrast sensitivity; and poor low contrast logmar acuity will be evidenced.[12]

Prolonged contact lens wear may produce gradual and unpredictable changes in the contour of the cornea-corneal warpage. The astigmatism or the general steepness may be either increased or decreased. Typically, corneal warpage produces an irregular astigmatism, which reduces the best spectacle correction. Corneal warpage commonly is seen with hard lenses but can also occur with soft contact lens wear. Corneas usually regain a stable and regular shape after discontinuation of the contact lenses, but it may take weeks or even months.

TREATMENT OF CONTACT LENS-INDUCED DRY EYE

If the tear film is insufficient to support the cornea, then it is most certainly insufficient to support a combination of a lens cornea system. The treatment for dry eye and CLIDE is to relieve the underlying problem by first identifying the portion of the tear film that is dysfunctional. Once identified, the treatment should be biased to complement the lens with minimal complexity to the patient.

Always consider RGP lenses first for borderline dry eye patients. A deficient or unstable tear film requires high oxygen permeability and a lens with low surface reactivity that moves adequately to minimize the risk of complications. Silicone hydrogel materials may be appropriate for oxygen enhancement but are not promising when treating a CLIDE patient. Silicone hydrogels would be highly desirable once the CLIDE patient has been treated and the eye has resumed a feasible level of comfort and proper tear film balance.

In order to achieve the proper tear film balance, the CLIDE patient must be treated as a normal "dry eye" patient. Following a flow chart of treatment, such as proper tear and nutritional supplementation, is the first step. The selection of supplementation and/or medicine is critical. The author prefers to define medicinal care by the determination of dry eye as a "white" or "red" dry eye. If the patient presents symptomatically and objectively as a dry eye yet has a "white" noninflamed conjunctiva, the use of goblet cell-mucin enhancers in conjunctival with lacrimal gland stimulus (ie, cyclosporine) would be considered appropriate. If the patient appears with a "red" inflamed dry eye, then the intervention with steroids would be deemed more appropriate. At the same time, a clinical decision must be made to refrain from contact lens use or limit it during the initial stages of therapy.

Once the inflammatory response is subdued and the patient is achieving a level of comfort, preservation of the tear film without complexity is mandatory. Thus punctal occlusion needs to be considered in a staged manner. When staging a punctal occlusion for a contact lens patient, it is best to start with a unilateral upper and lower collagen occlusion without contact lenses. This is done as a contralateral trial against the effectiveness and requirements for supplementation. A question regarding convenience and proper maintenance by the patient needs to be determined. Once this is determined and if punctal occlusion is deemed as an improvement by the patient, a bilateral trial with the lower puncta of both eyes should be performed with collagen plugs while introducing the appropriate lens material back onto the eye. If the patient finds that the lenses are now more tolerable and that lens wear has improved, the introduction of silicone (punctal orifice fixed—Freeman style or intracanalicular Von Herrick style) plugs should be placed into the lower punctum. To best determine the true needs of the patient, after a 1 or 2 week period, challenge a potential increase in tear film preservation by introducing a trial collagen plug into the upper punctum of both eyes.

If this benefits the patient without causing epiphora, then a silicone-based plug should be placed into the upper punctum.

SUMMARY

CLIDE is an everyday common event with the contact lens patient that presents from a subclinical finding to a mild to the most extreme complaint and complications. The avoidance of CLIDE and related contact lens drop-out or discontinuance starts with a practitioner who is attentive to the history of the patient. Based on proper survey and questioning, prior to or after lenses have been fit, the proper material and care products can be selected. As a commentary, selecting the "standard" lens or "marketed" lens is not always in the best interest of the patient nor the clinician. When addressing the long-term care of the dry eye patient and/or the CLIDE patient, do not be afraid to readdress the fit. A rechallenge of newer materials and care products may be of great benefit in extending a patient's success with contact lens wear and assist in the avoidance of CLIDE.

ACKNOWLEDGMENTS

Many thanks to Joe Vehige, OD and Peter Simmons, PhD (Allergan, Inc), Dave Sattler and Chuck Marshall, PhD (Alcon Labs), Nikki Iravanni, OD and Rose Britton (CooperVision), Patrick Benz, PhD and Jose Ors, PhD (Benz R&D), and Sally Dillehay, OD and Rick Weisbarth, OD (Ciba Vision) for their assistance in providing informative product and educational support.

Key Points

1. Contact lens intolerance can be a key essential symptom of dry eye. A patient with mild to moderate dry eye may not experience symptoms until contact lenses are fitted.
2. The placement of a contact lens can upset the delicate balance of tear film production and distribution, leading to lens intolerance.
3. The CLIDE patient subjectively and objectively demonstrates lens discomfort or intolerance in association to a rapid evaporation of the tears from the eye, causing irritation, protein deposits, infection, and pain.
4. Approximately 1 out of every 20 contact lens wearers develops a contact lens-related complication each year, particularly amongst extended wear patients.
5. TCLS occurs when a contact lens fits poorly due to an aberrantly steep base curve or sagittal depth in relation to the flat keratometric measures or in combination to lens dehydration.
6. Always consider RGP lenses first for borderline dry eye patients. A deficient or unstable tear film requires high oxygen permeability and a lens with low surface reactivity that moves adequately to minimize the risk of complications.

REFERENCES

1. Tomlinson A. Contact lens-induced dry eye. In: Tomlinson A, ed. *Complications of Contact Lens Wear.* St. Louis, Mo: Mosby; 1992.
2. Snyder C. Preocular tear film anomalies and lens-related dryness. In: Silbert J, ed. *Anterior Segment Complications of Contact Lens Wear.* 2nd ed. Boston: Butterworth-Heinemann; 2000: 3-21.
3. Bron AJ. Understanding dry eye disease: an update on etiology, diagnosis and treatment. *Surv Ophthalmol.* 2001;45:Supplement 2.
4. Craig JP, Tomlinson A. Importance of the lipid layer in human tear film stability and evaporation. *Optom Vis Sci.* 1994;74(1):8-13.
5. Larke JP. The eye in contact lens wear. In: *Tears and Lens Deposits.* Boston: Butterworth; 1986:24.
6. Xu KP, Yagi Y,Tsubota K. Decrease in corneal sensitivity and change in tear function in dry eye. *Cornea.* 1996;15(3):235-239.
7. Gilbard JP, Gray KL, Rossi SR. A proposed mechanism for increased tear-film osmolarity in contact lens wearers. *Am J Ophthalmol.* 1986;102(4):505-507.
8. Bruce AS, Brennan NA. Clinical observations of the post tear film during the first hour of hydrogel lens wear. *ICLC.* 1988;15(10):304-309.
9. Schein OD, Glynn RJ, Poggio EC. The relative risk of ulcerative keratitis among daily wear and extended wear soft contact lenses: a case control study: Microbila Keratitis Study Group. *N Eng J Med.* 1989;321:773-778.
10. Poggio, EC, Abelson, M. Complications and symptoms in disposable extended wear lenses compared with conventional soft daily wear and soft extended wear lenses. *CLAO J.* 1993;19:31-39.
11. Liu DT, Di Pascuale MA, Sawai J, Gao YY, Tseng SC. Tear film dynamics in floppy eyelid syndrome. *Invest Ophthalmol Vis Sci.* 2005;46:1188-1194.
12. Netland PA. Tight lens syndrome with extended wear contact lenses. *CLAO J.* 1990;16(4):308.

13. Hine H, Back A, Holden BA. Etiology of arcuate epithelial lesions induced by hydrogels. *Trans Br Cont Lens Assoc Conf.* 1987;48-50.

14. Daniels KM. With gas permeable lens patients, always question the previous fit. *Ocular Surgery News.* 2005;23(2):86-88.

Disclaimer of financial interest: The author has no financial interest in any companies mentioned in the text, but does hold common stock in Johnson and Johnson, Inc.

25

Cataract Surgery in the Dry Eye Patient

Suresh K. Pandey, MD;
Brighu N. Swamy, MBBS (Hons), M Med (Clin Epi);
and Amar Agarwal, MS, FRCS, FRCOphth

INTRODUCTION

Patients with dry eyes who have cataract surgery are reported to have a relatively less favorable outcome. Patients with an age-related decrease in tear flow and deficient tear surfacing are also prone to complications. Complications such as superficial punctuate keratitis, recurrent filamentary keratitis, secondary infections including conjunctivitis and infectious keratitis, persistent or recurrent epithelial defects, stromal keratolysis, and corneal ulceration have been reported in patients after conventional extracapsular cataract extraction (ECCE). In conventional cataract surgery, a large incision is made at the limbus, denerving the superior half of the cornea. This leads to corneal desensitization with subsequent complications. This, combined with the presence of sutures and prolonged use of topical steroids and antibiotics postoperatively, often precipitates these complications, sometimes with a devastating outcome.[1]

ETIOLOGY AND PATHOGENESIS

There is a multifactorial etiology for the less favorable outcome postcataract surgery in patients with dry eyes. It is reported that the loss of corneal sensitivity after cataract surgery often persists for more than 2 years and can be permanent. The sensory denervation interferes with the normal physiology of the corneal epithelium and decreases epithelial cell mitosis and causes delayed wound healing. The inability of the epithelium to re-establish the continuity of the corneal surface also triggers cell biologic and biochemical mechanisms. The deficiency in the aqueous layer and an unstable tear film make the cornea susceptible to epithelial cell breakdown, leading to superficial punctuate keratopathy, erosions, or ulceration of the cornea.

There is an increased risk of infection in dry eyes with staphylococcus and strepto-coccus, the most common causes. Dry eyes have impaired ocular immunological defense mechanisms as a result of decreased quantities of various protective enzymes, lactoferrin, b-lysins, and immunoglobulins.

The use of topical steroids and poor compliance with dry eye treatment have also been identified as risk factors for postoperative complications and poor visual outcome.

SURGICAL METHOD OF CHOICE IN PATIENTS WITH DRY EYES

The tremendous advancement in cataract surgical techniques, implants, and other adjuncts (Table 25-1) during the past several years was helpful to enhance safety of cataract surgery in routine cases and to increase visual outcome in cataract associated with dry eye. Previously, extracapsular extraction was the first choice for patients with cataracts and dry eye syndrome or other ocular comorbidities. However, with the currently preferred surgical technique, such as phacoemulsification (Figure 25-1), IOL implantation, and evolving techniques of ultra-small incision cataract surgery using phakonit and microphakonit, the situation has changed.[2,3] It is now regarded that phacoemulsification and other techniques of microincision cataract surgery[4–25] may be associated with minimal complications in patients with dry eye. An air pump (Figure 25-2) (gas-forced infusion) helps prevent shallowing of the anterior chamber. However, these patients must be counseled on the possible postoperative complications. Phacoemulsification and other techniques of microincision cataract surgery offer advantages over conventional ECCE in patients with dry eye, including:

- A much smaller incision, which causes less corneal desensitization.
- Minimal tear-film surfacing problems.
- Smaller risk of infection as no sutures are used.
- Faster visual rehabilitation of patients permits rapid tapering of topical drops.

Cataract surgery can worsen pre-existing dry eye symptoms or surgically induce dry eyes. The management of cataract surgery in dry eyes involves preoperative management, surgical procedure, as well as postoperative management.[2]

Preoperative Management

Diagnosis of dry eye syndrome is essential. If dry eyes are suspected, then a series of investigations including TFBUT and fluorescein staining of the corneal epithelium should be done prior to surgery. If superficial punctuate keratitis exists, artificial drops should be prescribed or eye drops containing hyaluronic acid should be prescribed. Preservative-containing eye drops should be avoided.

Surgical Procedure

Topical anesthetic application to the cornea should be minimized in patients with dry eyes. Anesthetic techniques for cataract surgery have advanced significantly. Table 25-2 presents evolution of anesthetic techniques for cataract surgery. Currently, topical anesthesia is preferred in cataract surgery using phacoemulsification using eye drops application, sponge anesthesia, eye drops plus intracameral injection, and most recently a combination of viscoelastic and anesthetic agent termed *viscoanesthesia*. Recent

Table 25-1

EVOLUTION OF TECHNIQUES FOR CATARACT SURGERY

Technique	Year	Author
Couching	800 BC	Susutra
ECCE* (inferior incision)	1745	J. Daviel
ECCE (superior incision)	1860	von Graefe
ICCE** (tumbling)	1880	H. Smith
ECCE with PC-IOL***	1949	Sir H. Ridley
ECCE with AC-IOL****	1951	B. Strampelli
Phacoemulsification	1967	C. D. Kelman
Foldable IOLs	1984	T. Mazzocco
CCC	1988	H. V. Gimbel/T. Neuhann
Hydrodissection	1992	I. H. Fine
In-the-bag fixation	1992	D. J. Apple/E. I. Assia
Accommodating IOLs	1997	S. Cummings/Kamman
Phakonit (bimanual phaco)	1998	A. Agarwal
Air pump to prevent surge (gas-forced infusion)	1999	S. Agarwal
FAVIT technique	1999	A. Agarwal
MICS terminology	2000	J. Alio
Microphaco terminology and using a 0.8-mm phaco needle	2000	R. Olson
Dye-enhanced cataract surgery	2000	S. K. Pandey/L. Werner/ D. J. Apple
Sealed capsule irrigation	2001	A. J. Maloof
Factors for PCO prevention	2002 to 2004	D. J. Apple/L. Werner/ S. K. Pandey
Microcoaxial phaco and sub-2 mm AcrySof IOL implantation	2004 to 2005	T. Akahoshi
Microphakonit cataract surgery with a 0.7-mm tip	2005	A. Agarwal

*ECCE: extracapsular cataract extraction
**ICCE: intracapsular cataract extraction
***PC-IOL: posterior chamber intraocular lens
****AC-IOL: anterior chamber intraocular lens

Figure 25-1. Phacoemulsification being performed.

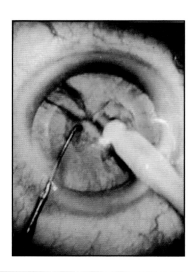

Figure 25-2. Air pump used to prevent surge in phaco and phakonit. In the air pump system, a locally manufactured automated device used in fish tanks (aquariums) to supply oxygen is utilized to forcefully pump air into the irrigation bottle. It has an electromagnetic motor that moves a lever attached to a collapsible rubber cap. There is an inlet with a valve that sucks in atmospheric air as the cap expands. On collapsing, the valve closes and the air is pushed into an intravenous line connected to the infusion bottle. The lever vibrates at a frequency of approximately 10 oscillations per second. The electromagnetic motor is weak enough to stop once the pressure in the closed system (ie, the AC) reaches about 50 or 100 mmHg. The rubber cap ceases to expand at this pressure level. A micropore air filter is used between the air pump and the infusion bottle so that the air pumped into the bottle is clean of particulate matter. In phaco, one should use 50 mmHg of pressure and in microphakonit (0.7 m cataract surgical set), 100 mmHg.

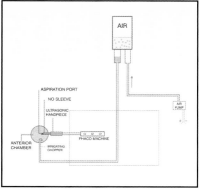

reports indicate performing phacoemulsification by a highly experienced, skilled surgeon without causing an unacceptable level of pain using no-anesthesia cataract surgery as first shown by Dr. Amar Agarwal.

The exposure of the operating microscope to the light source should be kept to a minimum as well. TFBUT can be increased for up to 1-month postsurgery. The nature of the surgical incision does not seem to be an important factor for phacoemulsification. Cataract surgery in patients of dry eye can be challenging, necessitating several tools and techniques. Most of the surgeons are familiar with conventional cataract surgical procedure using small incision cataract surgery. We believe it will be pertinent to provide brief details of ultra-small incision cataract surgery. Ultra-small incision cataract surgery techniques are currently evolving, and experience in cataract surgery in dry eye cases is limited at present. Nevertheless, as we gain more experience, it is clear that

Table 25-2		
EVOLUTION OF ANESTHETIC TECHNIQUES FOR CATARACT SURGERY		
Technique	*Year*	*Author*
General anesthesia	1846	—
Topical cocaine	1881	Koller
Injectable cocaine	1884	Knapp
Orbicularis akinesia	1914	Van Lint, O'Briens, Atkinson
Hyaluridinase	1948	Atkinson
Retrobulbar (4% cocaine)	1984	Knapp
Posterior peribulbar	1985	Davis and Mandel
Limbal	1990	Furata et al
Anterior peribulbar	1991	Bloomberg
Pinpoint anesthesia	1992	Fukasawa
Topical	1992	Fichman
Topical plus intracameral	1995	Gills
No anesthesia	1998	Agarwal
Cryoanalgesia	1999	Gutierrez-Carmona
Xylocaine jelly	1999	Koch and Assia
Hypothesis, no anesthesia	2001	Pandey and Agarwal
Viscoanesthesia	2001	Werner, Pandey, Apple, et al

these minimally invasive surgical methods will be helpful to enhance visual outcome following cataract surgery in dry eye cases.

Ultra-small incision cataract surgery, termed *phakonit, bimanual microphacoemulsification,* or *microincision cataract surgery*, allows removal of cataract using sub 1.4-mm incision. In phakonit (Figure 25-3), the phaco needle is used without a sleeve and an irrigating chopper is used in the other hand. The acronym phakonit has been proposed as bimanual phacoemulsification (phaco) being done with a needle (N) opening via an incision (I) and with the phaco tip (T). In other words, it is phaco with a needle incision biology (phakonit). Once the nucleus is removed, bimanual cortical aspiration is done. The only limitation to realizing the goal of astigmatism neutral cataract surgery was the size of the foldable IOL because the wound had to be extended for implantation of the currently available foldable IOLs. With the advent of the rollable IOLs (Acritec lenses were invented by Christine Kreiner from Germany and Thinoptx lenses by Wayne Callahan from the United States), the advantage of the phakonit incision could be realized because the ultra-small incision lenses could pass through a 1.5-mm incision.

In 1998, Dr. Amar Agarwal performed 1-mm cataract surgery. Dr. Jorge Alio coined the term *microincision cataract surgery* (MICS) for all surgeries including laser cataract surgery and phakonit. Dr. Randall Olson first used a 0.8-mm phaco needle and a 21-gauge irrigating chopper and called it microphaco. On May 21, 2005, a 0.7-mm phaco needle tip with a 0.7-mm irrigating chopper was used by Dr. Agarwal for the first time

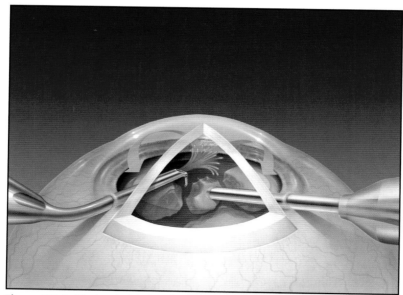

Figure 25-3. Phakonit. Notice the irrigating chopper with an end opening. (Courtesy of Larry Laks, Microsurgical Technology.)

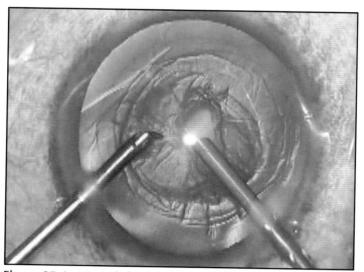

Figure 25-4. Microphakonit being performed with a 0.7-mm irrigating chopper and a 0.7-mm sleeveless phaco needle.

to remove cataracts through the smallest incision possible as of the time of this writing. This is called microphakonit (Figure 25-4). The 22-gauge (0.7-mm) irrigating chopper connected to the infusion line with foot pedal on position. The phaco probe is connected to the aspiration line and the 0.7-mm phaco tip without an infusion sleeve is introduced through the clear corneal incision. Using the phaco tip with moderate ultrasound power, the center of the nucleus is directly embedded starting from the superi-

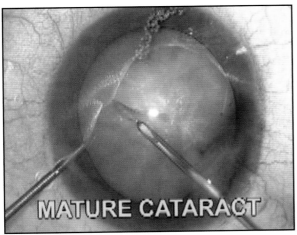

Figure 25-5. Mature cataract. It is difficult to visualize the rhexis in such cases, so we need to stain the anterior capsule with a dye (trypan blue). The rhexis is started with the needle. Note a straight rod in the left hand to stabilize the eye.

or edge of rhexis with the phaco probe directed obliquely downward toward the vitreous. The settings at this stage are 50% phaco power, flow rate 24 mL/min, and 110 mmHg vacuum. Using the karate chop technique, the nucleus is chopped. Thus, the whole nucleus is removed. Cortical washup is then done with the bimanual irrigation aspiration (0.7 mm set) technique. During the microphakonit procedure, gas-forced infusion is used. The instruments are made by Larry Laks from Microsurgical Technology (Redmond, Wash). At the time of this writing, this is the smallest one can use for cataract surgery. With time, one would be able to go smaller with better instruments and devices. The problem at present is the IOL. We have to get good quality IOLs going through sub 1-mm cataract surgical incisions so that the real benefit of microphakonit can be given to the patient.

It is important to remember that cataract surgery in dry eye cases may be associated with suboptimal visibility intraoperatively and, therefore, the surgeon should use the familiar surgical technique to help overcome intraoperative difficulties and to minimize complications. Trypan blue is an indispensable tool to enhance vision when white cataract is combined with corneal opacity (Figure 25-5). The dye-staining combined with frequent regrasping allowed capsulorrhexis to be successfully performed. Work on dye-enhanced cataract surgery was done extensively by Pandey et al.[26] The blue-stained rim aided in confining phacoemulsification maneuvers to the posterior plane. Implementing the soft-shell technique partitioned the anterior chamber into a viscoelastic-occupied space and a surgical zone protecting the delicate endothelial cells fluid turbulence.

Postoperative Management

Eye drops containing preservatives tend to cause epithelial disturbances. Nonsteroidal anti-inflammatory drugs such as diclofenac sodium can cause corneal epithelial breaches. For patients already diagnosed with dry eyes, only an antibiotic and steroid regimen is used. Additional use of artificial eye drops will increase the stability of the tear film. If SPK is severe, then consider stopping all eye drops except the artificial eye drops. In treatment-resistant cases, autologous serum eye drops may be prescribed. Finally, intracanalicular plugs can be used to prevent drainage of tears and provide a stable and moist corneal surface postoperatively. Rarely, severe cases of dry eye associated with an autoimmune disorder (eg, Stevens-Johnson syndrome) may require additional procedure such as AMT, stem cell transplantation, or PK.

Key Points

1. Patients with dry eyes who have cataract surgery are reported to have a relatively less favorable outcome. Patients with an age-related decrease in tear flow and deficient tear surfacing are also prone to complications.
2. It is reported that the loss of corneal sensitivity after cataract surgery often persists for more than 2 years and can be permanent. The sensory denervation interferes with the normal physiology of the corneal epithelium and decreases epithelial cell mitosis, delaying wound healing.
3. If dry eyes are suspected, then a series of investigations including TFBU and fluorescein staining of the corneal epithelium should be done prior to surgery. If superficial punctuate keratitis exists, artificial drops or eye drops containing hyaluronic acid should be prescribed. Preservative-containing eye drops should be avoided.
4. Topic anesthetic application to the cornea should be minimized in patients with dry eyes.
5. Previously, extracapsular extraction was the first choice for patients with cataracts and dry eye syndrome or other ocular comorbidities. However with the development of modern technique, such as phacoemulsification, phakonit, and microphakonit, the situation has changed.

REFERENCES

1. Ram J, Gupta A, Brar G, Kaushik S. Outcomes of phacoemulsification in patients with dry eye. *J Cataract Refract Surg.* 2002;28:1386–1389.
2. Bissen-Miyajima H. Cataract surgery in the presence of other ocular co-morbidities. In: Steinert RF, ed. *Cataract Surgery.* Philadelphia: CV Mosby; 2004:369–373.
3. Agarwal A, Agarwal S, Agarwal AT. No anesthesia cataract surgery. In: Agarwal A, et al, eds. *Phacoemulsification: Laser Cataract Surgery and Foldable IOL's.* 1st ed. India: Jaypee Brothers Medical Publishers Ltd; 1998:144–154.
4. Pandey SK, Werner L, Agarwal A, Agarwal S, Agarwal AT, Apple DJ. No anesthesia cataract surgery. *J Cataract Refract Surg.* 2001;28:1710.
5. Agarwal A, Agarwal S, Agarwal AT. Phakonit. A new technique of removing cataracts through a 0.9 mm incision. In: Agarwal A, et al, eds. *Phacoemulsification: Laser Cataract Surgery and Foldable IOL's.* 1st ed. India: Jaypee Brothers Medical Publishers Ltd; 1998:139–143.
6. Agarwal A, Agarwal S, Agarwal AT. Phakonit and laser phakonit: lens surgery through a 0.9 mm incision. In: Agarwal et al, eds. *Phacoemulsification, Laser Cataract Surgery and Foldable IOL's.* 2nd ed. India: Jaypee Brothers Medical Publishers Ltd; 2000:204–216.
7. Agarwal A, Agarwal S, Agarwal AT. Phakonit. In: Agarwal A, et al, eds. *Phacoemulsification, Laser Cataract Surgery and Foldable IOLs.* 3rd ed. India: Jaypee Brothers Medical Publishers Ltd; 2003:317–329.

8. Agarwal A, Agarwal S, Agarwal AT. Phakonit and laser phakonit. In: Boyd B, Agarwal A, eds. *LASIK and Beyond LASIK*. Panama: Highlights of Ophthalmology; 2000:463–468.

9. Agarwal A, Agarwal S, Agarwal AT. Phakonit and laser phakonit—cataract surgery through a 0.9 mm incision. In: Boyd B, Agarwal A, et al, eds. *Phako, Phakonit and Laser Phako*. Panama: Highlights of Ophthalmology; 2000:327–334.

10. Agarwal A, Agarwal S, Agarwal AT. The phakonit Thinoptx IOL. In: Agarwal A, ed. *Presbyopia: A Surgical Textbook*. Thorofare, NJ: SLACK Incorporated; 2002:187–194.

11. Agarwal A, Agarwal S, Agarwal AT. Antichamber collapse. *J Cataract Refract Surg.* 2002;28:1085.

12. Pandey SK, Wener L, Agarwal A, Agarwal S, Agarwal AT, Hoyos J. Phakonit: cataract removal through a sub 1.0 mm incision with implantation of the Thinoptx rollable IOL. *J Cataract Refract Surg.* 2002;28:1710.

13. Agarwal A, Agarwal S, Agarwal AT. Phakonit. phacoemulsification through a 0.9 mm incision. *J Cataract Refract Surg.* 2001;27:1548–1552.

14. Agarwal A, Agarwal S, Agarwal AT. Phakonit with an Acritec IOL. *J Cataract Refract Surg.* 2003;29:854–855.

15. Agarwal S, Agarwal A, Agarwal AT. *Phakonit With Acritec IOL*. Panama: Highlights of Ophthalmology; 2000.

16. Shearing S, Relyea R, Loaiza A, Shearing R. Routine phacoemulsification through a 1.0 mm non-sutured incision. *Cataract.* 1985;6–8.

17. Hara T, Hara T. Clinical results of phacoemulsification and complete in the bag fixation. *J Cataract Refract Surg.* 1987;13:279–286.

18. Tseunoka H, Shiba T, Takahashi Y. Feasibility of ultrasound cataract surgery with a 1.4 mm incision. *J Cataract Refract Surg.* 2001;27:934–940.

19. Tseunoka H, Shiba T, Takahashi Y. Feasibility of ultrasound cataract surgery with a 1.4 mm incision—clinical results. *J Cataract Refract Surg.* 2002;28:81–86.

20. Jorge Alio. What does MICS require? In: Alio J, ed. *MICS*. Panama: Highlights of Ophthalmology; 2004:1–4.

21. Soscia W, Howard JG, Olson RJ. Microphacoemulsification with Whitestar. A wound-temperature study. *J Cataract Refract Surg.* 2002;28:1044–1046.

22. Soscia W, Howard JG, Olson RJ. Bimanual phacoemulsification through two stab incisions. A wound-temperature study. *J Cataract Refract Surg.* 2002;28:1039–1043.

23. Olson R. Microphaco chop. In: Chang D, ed. *Phaco Chop: Mastering Techniques, Optimizing Technology, and Avoiding Complications*. Thorofare, NJ: SLACK Incorporated; 2004:227–237.

24. Chang D. Bimanual phaco chop. In: Chang D, ed. *Phaco Chop: Mastering Techniques, Optimizing Technology, and Avoiding Complications*. Thorofare, NJ: SLACK Incorporated; 2004:239–250.

25. Kanellopoulos AJ. New laser system points way to ultrasmall incision cataract surgery. *Eurotimes.* 2000.

26. Pandey SK, Werner L, Escobar-Gomez M, et al. Dye-enhanced cataract surgery. Part I. Anterior capsule staining for capsulorrhexis in advanced/white cataracts. *J Cataract Refract Surg.* 2000; 26:1052.

Disclaimer of financial interest: The authors have no financial or proprietary interest in any product mentioned in this chapter. Presented in Part at the Royal Australian and New Zealand College of Ophthalmologists meeting; Hobart; November, 2005. Supported in part by an unrestricted grant from Research to Prevent Blindness, Inc, New York, NY.

26

Refractive Surgery and the Dry Eye Patient

*Ahmad M. Fahmy, OD, FAAO and
David R. Hardten, MD, FACS*

INTRODUCTION

In order to develop and implement the most appropriate treatment plan for the post-refractive surgery dry eye patient, a good understanding of pathogenesis of chronic dry eye is the key. The pre- and postoperative evaluation and treatment of the refractive surgery patient with dry eye should be approached with a similar strategy as used in treating chronically dry eyes. Comparing the physiologic changes postoperatively to eyes without prior surgery can help us better understand and anticipate iatrogenic pathology or exacerbation of existing pathology. Patients suffering from ocular irritation caused by tear film instability are very difficult to manage successfully. An estimated 10 million people in the United States comprise this group of patients suffering from dry eye syndromes.[1] Chronic dry eye is much more prevalent in females than males, and more advanced in postmenopausal women using HRT. Patients developing chronic dry eye after LASIK are also more likely to be female, as demonstrated by a more frequent appearance of corneal punctate epitheliopathy after LASIK.

DEFINITION AND CLASSIFICATION

Dry eye researchers have historically struggled to produce a concise definition and classification of dry eye conditions. As defined by the NEI, dry eye, or KCS, is a "disorder of the tear film due to tear deficiency or excessive evaporation that causes damage to the intrapalpebral ocular surface and is associated with symptoms of discomfort."[2] This classification of dry eye is further delineated into patients with aqueous tear deficiency and those with increased evaporative loss. Deficient aqueous production is

Table 26-1		
PERTINENT MEDICAL HISTORY		
Systemic Pathology	*Medications*	*Symptoms*
Acne rosacea	Antidepressants	Foreign body sensation
OCP	Antihistamines	Redness
Sjögren's syndrome	Antihypertensives	Fluctuation of vision
Stevens-Johnson syndrome		Contact lens intolerance
Rheumatoid arthritis		
Sarcoidosis		
Environmental allergies		
Neurological pathology		
Menopause		
Systemic lupus erythematosus		

a hallmark finding in patients with Sjögren's syndrome and other autoimmune diseases. Evaporative loss can be exacerbated by meibomian gland disease or other surface abnormalities such as excessive exposure or evaporation due to lid abnormalities.

PATIENT SELECTION AND EDUCATION

Patients interested in decreasing their dependence on contact lenses by undergoing refractive surgery who also report dry eye symptoms should be approached carefully. Patient education regarding postoperative visual acuity fluctuation and irritation should be thorough due to the typical increased dryness, especially in the early phase of recovery. For most patients, increased dryness after LASIK is tolerable and not visually significant. Therefore, chronic dry eye is not a definite contraindication to refractive surgery. However, patients with ocular surface disease prior to refractive surgery must be treated aggressively and counseled regarding the likelihood of exacerbation of symptoms postoperatively. Systemic pathology and medications used by the patient can contribute to a dry ocular surface (Table 26-1). The most common symptoms are chronic irritation and uncomfortable foreign body sensation.

Just as it is important to identify systemic causes of dry eye, there are many clinical findings that can help the careful clinician identify ocular surface pathology (Table 26-2). Improving surface lubrication and controlling a concomitant inflammatory component such as blepharitis if present will improve objective and subjective success post-operatively. Postrefractive surgery patients with a markedly compromised tear film due to a combined mechanism etiology can experience significant fluctuations in visual acuity. Most patients report this fluctuation improves just after a blink or instillation of artificial tears. It has been reported that the surface regularity index (SRI) does not significantly change just after instillation of artificial tears in healthy, nonoperative eyes.[3] It is reasonable to attribute some visual acuity fluctuation to poor tear spread over the newly contoured central depression in myopic LASIK cases and the resultant increased

Table 26-2	
PREOPERATIVE CLINICAL EVALUATION	
Ocular Surface	*Systemic*
Tear meniscus/Schirmer's	Rhinophyma
Tear BUT	Dental and gum disease (Sjögren's)
Punctate epithelial keratopathy	
Palpebral fissure	
Exposure/ectropion	
Meibomian gland inspissation	
Conjunctival tylosis	
Conjunctival pleating	
Eyelid collarette formation and telangiectasia	

Table 26-3
SIGNIFICANT FACTORS AFFECTING CHRONIC DRY EYE AND REGRESSION

- Female.
- Smoker.
- Moderate to high refractive error/ablation depth.
- Decreased corneal sensation.
- Ocular surface disease.
- Subjective reports of dry eye symptoms.
- Dry working environment.
- Prolonged computer use.

dioptric power of the precorneal tear film. Intermittent blur after blinking and irritation are bothersome symptoms that can disappoint refractive surgery patients because the expectations of visual outcome continue to increase with progressive improvements in refractive surgery technology. With improved surgical technique and increased experience of the surgeon, LASIK may still be the procedure of choice for mild to moderate levels of myopia in healthy eyes, as well as those with mild to moderate dry eye.[4]

It is important to carefully look for evaporative as well as inflammatory causes of dry eye because many patients will present with both a tear production deficiency and an evaporative component (Table 26-3). In a survey conducted in 2001, the most common "complication" of LASIK was dry eye.[2] Once chronic dry eye has been identified and treated aggressively, evidence shows that regression after LASIK is also reduced.[5] It is always best to proceed with refractive surgery after a smooth, well-lubricated ocular surface has been achieved. In conductive keratoplasty (Figure 26-1), one should also carefully evaluate the ocular surface.

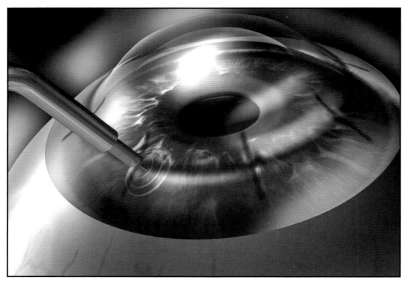

Figure 26-1. Conductive keratoplasty. (Reprinted with permission from Agarwal A. *Presbyopia: A Surgical Textbook.* Thorofare, NJ: SLACK Incorporated; 2002.)

POSTLASER IN SITU KERATOMILEUSIS TEAR PRODUCTION, CLEARANCE, AND SENSITIVITY

The ocular surface and the lacrimal gland work together as a functional unit to stimulate lacrimal tear production. Sensory nerves in the corneal epithelium and stroma trigger the blink mechanism to spread tears uniformly and clear tears from the ocular surface by pumping used tears into the nasolacrimal ducts. Eyelid inflammation, surgical severing of corneal nerves, and laser ablation result in disruption of this important feedback loop, obstructing neural sensory input to the lacrimal gland. As a result, tear production, clearance, and ocular surface sensitivity to touch, including the conjunctiva, decrease. It has been reported that depressed conjunctival sensation postoperatively is caused by placement of the microkeratome suction ring on perilimbal conjunctival nerves.[4] On the question of clearance, it has been suggested that a decreased blink rate caused by corneal denervation and the resultant increased tear film evaporation are important altered tear dynamic factors postoperatively.[4] Decreased tear clearance exacerbates dry eye conditions because pooling of inflammatory constituents damage the ocular surface. Precorneal tear film dysfunction is especially prominent in eyes that have undergone procedures prior to LASIK, such as photorefractive keratectomy (PRK) and radial keratotomy (RK) because the irregular corneal surface limits sustained, even corneal lubrication.[4]

NEUROTROPHIC EPITHELIOPATHY

It is well documented that a temporarily neurotrophic cornea results from creation of the flap during LASIK.[6] Nerve bundles course through the corneal tissue to carry neural input through the stroma and the epithelium centrally. This corneal denervation effect is more prominent in higher refractive corrections and deeper ablations for myopic, as well as hyperopic cases. Disruption of corneal innervation induces anesthesia and hypoesthesia that result in significant punctate epithelial erosions. Ablation results in depression of corneal sensation of surface dryness and results in decreased feedback and stimulation of the lacrimal gland, putting in motion a cycle of events adversely affecting ocular lubrication. The incidence of symptomatic neurotrophic epitheliopathy has been reported to be approximately 4% at 1 to 3 months.[6]

Most patients present early postoperatively without discomfort when the clinical presentation of epithelial erosion is significant due to early hypoesthesia. Many notice the blur in vision but not discomfort. It has been demonstrated that the number of stromal nerve fiber bundles decreases by nearly 90% early after LASIK.[7] The regeneration of these nerve fiber bundles takes place slowly. At 1 year postoperatively, some reports measure that the number of nerve fiber bundles remains less than 50% of that just prior to LASIK, although most studies demonstrate corneal sensation returns back to normal preoperative levels at approximately the 6-month period.[4,6] Nasally-hinged flaps tend to sever less of these nerve fiber bundles and therefore dry eye symptoms postoperatively can be limited by creating a nasally-hinged flap during LASIK.[7] Enhancement is also likely to cause a return of symptoms and clinical evidence of neurotrophic epitheliopathy, because lifting the flap once again interrupts reinnervation. Patients have been thought not to develop a clinically significant degree of epithelial neuropathy, even though corneal sensation is reduced for approximately 3 months postoperatively. Yet in our experience, PRK can still be associated with relatively long periods of epitheliopathy in some patients.

REGRESSION

Sustained dysfunction of the precorneal tear film after LASIK exacerbated by the wound healing response has been reported to contribute significantly to regression of the refractive result. Albietz and colleagues demonstrated an incidence of 27% myopic regression in chronic dry eye patients after LASIK compared to 7% without chronic dry eye in a group of 565 eyes studied retrospectively.[5]

There are several proposed mechanisms of regression. One proposed by Albietz and colleagues involves epithelial hyperplasia due to increased release of epidermal growth factor. It is reasonable to consider that repeated mechanical trauma during blinking of the dry ocular surface postoperatively increases the release of epidermal growth factor, leading to epithelial hyperplasia and regression.[5]

A second reasonable mechanism to consider involves keratocyte apoptosis. It has been suggested that dry eye after LASIK is related to apoptosis of stromal keratocytes induced by inflammatory cytokines. Autoimmune disorders direct cytotoxic reactions in which antibodies and lymphocytes damage surrounding tissue. The most common inflammatory disorder encountered is blepharitis, but as discussed earlier, many patients suffer from a variety of autoimmune conditions that cause similar inflammatory cellular damage. When antibodies to specific cells affix to their corresponding antigen and activate complement on their cell surface to accomplish cytolysis, they are referred to as cytotoxic antibodies. When the cells are foreign, cytolysis is protective; when the cells are self, autoimmune disease occurs. Cells containing mediators are activated by stimuli other than an antigen-antibody union on their surface. Neural, chemical, and physical stimuli also induce mediator release, initiating symptoms that resemble allergic reactions, even though no allergen exposure has taken place. Even in the case of the perfectly healthy postoperative eye, during the wound healing inflammatory cascade, infiltration of the ocular surface with T cells causes tissue damage that leads to apoptosis of stromal keratocytes, underscoring the importance of anti-inflammatory medical treatment.

TREATMENT

Tear Film Supplements

There has been a significant increase in our understanding of the pathogenesis of dry eye syndrome and how to successfully treat it. Traditionally, a very common treatment of dry eyes has been supplementing the tear film with artificial tears (see Chapter 11). Although artificial tear film supplements in solution and ointment form provide immediate lubrication of the ocular surface and patient comfort, it has been shown that use of artificial tear solutions preserved with benzalkonium chloride (BAK) causes significant epithelial toxicity.[1] Nonpreserved formulations provide the added benefit of avoiding increased irritation and are indicated for patients that are increasingly symptomatic shortly after using preserved formulations. Precorneal tear film supplements can alleviate symptoms temporarily and provide an excellent additional treatment, but patients typically achieve long-term relief by addressing the inflammatory component along with decreased tear production. Chronic inflammation of the ocular surface exacerbates early dissipation of the precorneal tear film.

In addition to replenishing the tear film, the addition of nutrients and fatty acid-enriched formulations containing eicosapentaenoic acid (EPA) has also been proven to be very helpful in decreasing inflammation, stimulating aqueous tear production, and augmenting the tear film oil layer.[8,9]

Oral administration of essential fatty acids that contain sufficient amounts of gamma-linolenic-acid (GLA) stimulate the natural production of anti-inflammatory series one prostaglandins (PGE1).[10] These prostaglandins reduce ocular surface inflammation and reduce the inflammatory process associated with meibomitis. The nutrient cofactors vitamin A, vitamin C, vitamin B_6, and magnesium act to facilitate this conversion and are functionally disrupted by alcohol, aging, smoking, elevated cholesterol levels, and other environmental factors.[9] Vitamin E also plays an anti-inflammatory role by stabilizing the essential fatty acids and preventing oxidation. It also works to inhibit cyclooxygenase-2 (COX-2) enzyme activity that promotes the inflammatory response.[11] Vitamin C also enhances the production of immunoglobulin E (IgE) concentrates in tears, which is the first line of basophil and mast cell defense against invading pathogens and allergens that frequently exacerbate dry eye symptoms.[12] These nutrient cofactors also work to modulate goblet cell production.

Autologous Serum

Another approach aimed at prolonging surface lubrication is the addition of topically applied autologous serum, which incorporates growth factors naturally present in the tear film.[13] Autologous serum application has been proven to significantly decrease

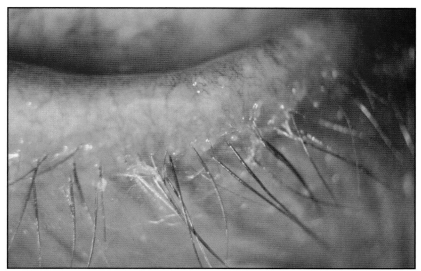

Figure 26-2. Blepharitis. (Reproduced with permission from Agarwal A. *Handbook of Ophthalmology*. Thorofare, NJ: SLACK Incorporated; 2005.)

staining and improve symptoms of ocular surface dysfunction associated with dry eye (see Chapter 12). This has been especially observed in patients with Sjögren's syndrome.[14] Although patients subjectively report autologous serum eye drops are superior to artificial tears in relieving signs and symptoms of dry eye disease, it is not widely used due to limitations including required special preparation and increased risk of infection.[13]

Eyelid Hygiene

In staphylococcal blepharitis (Figure 26-2), inspissation of the meibomian glands may lead to early evaporation of the tear film and the classic punctate keratopathy that is consistent with symptomatic dry eye. The most effective treatment aimed at improving meibomian gland function and the oily contribution to the tear film is the application of warm compresses to both the upper and lower eyelid, followed by eyelid massage with warm water and a mild soap. During the application of warm compresses, we find it helpful to use heat-absorbing substances rather than repeatedly reheating a clean face towel. We typically advise patients to perform the warm compresses and lid hygiene routine for approximately 5 to 10 minutes BID. If the severity of blepharitis is marked, we recommend more sessions (4 times) each day. It is also important to remind the patient to be careful not to use a high concentration of soap, which may irritate the eye and break down the tear film further. Meibomitis is significantly improved with diligent application of warm compresses and massage in most patients.

Ocular Rosacea

The addition of doxycycline to the treatment regimen may be indicated in many patients with rosacea. Tetracycline (and its derivatives) has been observed to decrease bacterial lipase activity in vitro.[15] Interestingly, in addition to its bacteriostatic effect, its proposed anti-inflammatory effects play a significant role in reducing meibomitis. The acceptance of anti-inflammatory aspects of doxycycline and other antibodies was advocated by gastrointestinal disease experts who pondered why antibiotics helped many patients with Crohn's disease despite no clinical evidence of infection. Studies suggest that the clinical anti-inflammatory effect of doxycycline is due in part to its antioxidant effects.[16] Free fatty acid concentrations in the meibum from acne rosacea patients have been shown to decrease with oral minocycline treatment. Adding 100 mg of doxycycline PO BID reduces meibomitis. This dosage is titrated according to severity and tolerance. Patients using doxycycline should be counseled regarding birth control and possible photosensitivity, nausea, and vaginal candidiasis.

Eyelid involvement can also be limited by topically treating the periocular skin and scalp of rosacea patients. Metronidazole (0.75% topical gel) application BID and ketoconazole (2.0% shampoo diluted as a lather) QID are common treatments. With oral and topical skin treatment, 70% to 80% of rosacea patients reported significant improvements in facial redness, papules, pustules, and telangiectasia.[15] In our practice, we typically instruct the patient to avoid applying the metronidazole topical gel close to the eyelid margin, drawing a clear distinction between an eyelid ointment to be applied to the lid margin and a topical gel that is to be applied to the skin around the eye. Rosacea patients are also advised to avoid sunlight because it is the single-most common factor triggering exacerbation of rosacea.

Cyclosporin A

In addition to using warm compresses and lid massage, using eyedrops that have an anti-inflammatory effect can improve tear film quality. It has been shown that 0.05% CsA, an immunomodulator, significantly decreases the concentration of the inflammatory cytokine interleukin-6 (IL-6) in the conjunctival epithelium of moderate to severe dry eye patient.[17] This decrease in IL-6 concentration was not different from baseline at the 3-month interval; however, showed a significant decrease from baseline at 6 months. When adding topical ophthalmic cyclosporine emulsion to the chronic dry eye treatment, the clinician should remind the patient that immediate results are not expected, and consistency in compliance past the 3-month interval is important (see Chapter 13).

Corticosteroids

When a symptomatic patient presents with significant dry eyes, blepharitis, and conjunctival inflammation that is not improved sufficiently with lid hygiene and artificial tear supplements, waiting 3 to 6 months for relief is not reasonable. In this case, it may be helpful to use an anti-inflammatory medication such as lotoprednol etabonate 0.2% or 0.5% and CsA in combination. Studies demonstrate that dry eye patients treated with lotoprednol etabonate showed statistically significant improvement in signs and symptoms, especially those presenting with advanced dry eye and corneal staining. A combined approach could limit further inflammatory damage to the ocular surface by adding a site-specific corticosteroid while CsA begins to deplete cytokine concentrations. As the inflammation and symptoms improve, the regimen can be altered by tapering lotoprednol etabonate while continuing to use CsA for prophylactically.

Nonsteroidal Anti-Inflammatories

Diflunisal (250- to 500-mg tablets) is used to treat mild to moderate pain and relieve inflammation and swelling associated with rheumatoid arthritis. As a nonsteroidal anti-inflammatory, it inhibits prostaglandin synthesis and has been proven to be effective as an added treatment in patients with chronic dry eye symptoms exacerbated by autoimmune inflammation.

Allergies

If there is an allergic component to the ocular inflammation, targeting the allergic cascade with antiallergy medications is essential. We typically use olopatadine hydrochloride 0.1% (Patanol, Alcon Laboratories, Fort Worth, Tex) and epinastine hydrochloride 0.05% (Elestat, Allergan, Irvine, Calif) BID to limit allergic conjunctival inflammation. Patients suffering from chronic environmental allergies will often already be taking a systemic antiallergy medication such as cetrizine hydrochloride (Zyrtec, Pfizer, Manhattan, NY).

Although its exact mechanism of action has not been identified, an immunomodulator, tacrolimus, also was shown to inhibit T cell activation.[18,19] Pimecrolimus 1% cream and tacrolimus 0.03% or 1.0% ointment (Fujisawa Healthcare, Inc, Deerfield, Ill) used in the treatment of a common allergic condition affecting the skin have also been shown to be especially effective in treating steroid-induced rosacea.

Investigational Treatments

Rebamipide 1.0% and 2.0% ophthalmic suspension (Otsuka Maryland Research Institute, Rockville, Md), currently in a phase 3 investigational study, is a quinoline derivative. The oral form was developed and marketed as a new therapy for gastric ulcers. It causes mucin to cover the internal surface of the stomach, providing a protective coating. It is the increased mucus-producing effect of Rebamipide that is spurring the investigation into its use as a promising dry eye treatment.

Punctal Occlusion

Conservation of the tear film by punctual occlusion is one of the most useful treatments available for dry eye patients. Having the option of placing punctal plugs in the lower eyelid, the upper eyelid, or both enables the clinician to titrate the amount of tear film conservation needed precisely. While the main therapeutic mechanism of punctual occlusion is simply increasing retention of the tear film, doing so may exacerbate ocular surface dysfunction if inflammatory blepharitis is a factor. Since punctal occlusion also decreases tear clearance by limiting outflow, keeping inflammatory mediators on the ocular surface longer can worsen the condition. In contrast to punctal cautery, reversible occlusion offers needed flexibility because tear production volume fluctuates over time. Cautery is generally a more permanent solution, although we sometimes see cauterized puncta reopen spontaneously. Punctal occlusion has been reported to improve Schirmer's test scores, reduce punctate staining, and, therefore, improve patient comfort.[20]

Temporary collagen punctal occlusion lasting approximately 4 to 7 days can be used to ascertain if punctal occlusion is effective. If improvement is noted clinically or subjectively, then permanent silicone punctal plugs are implanted. Silicone punctal plugs are permanent in that they do not dissolve; however, they can be removed.

Smart Plug (Medennium, Inc. Irvine, California), is a temperature-sensitive punctal occlusive device. It is made from a thermodynamic acrylic polymer. At room temperature, the device is a thin rigid rod 10.0 mm long and 0.4 mm in diameter. As it is inserted into the puncta, it begins to shorten and expand, forming a soft, gel-like glue that conforms to form fit the punctal space. Unlike traditional plugs, no part of the Smart Plug lies above the surface of the eyelid after insertion, offering added comfort to patients.

Tarsorrhaphy

Conservation of the tear film can also be accomplished by limiting exposure and evaporation. In severe cases in which other treatments have not been successful, this can be achieved surgically. In the case of the patient who has developed severe epitheliopathy, persistent non-healing epithelial defects, or sterile corneal ulceration, tarsorrhaphy is indicated. As with punctal occlusion, this can be done permanently or temporarily. Tarsorrhaphy has been proven to be very effective in healing the compromised cornea after chronic corneal tissue damage from dry eye.[1,13]

Hormone Therapy

Several studies strongly suggest that the low incidence of Sjögren's syndrome in males is due to the protective effects of androgenic hormones such as testosterone and that patients suffering from Sjögren's syndrome are significantly androgen deficient.[21,22] Repeatable findings have demonstrated that the meibomian gland is an androgen target organ that becomes dysfunctional with androgen deficiency, and that androgens regulate lipid production of sebaceous glands throughout the body. Acinar cells in sebaceous glands respond to these androgens by producing proteins that increase both the synthesis and secretion of lipids that, in turn, contribute to tear film stability. Androgens also act to attenuate autoimmune reactions, whereas estrogens tend to contribute to many autoimmune disorders. The immunosuppressive effects of androgens are due in part to the stimulation of TGF-β, a potent immunomodulator and anti-inflammatory cytokine.[21]

SUMMARY

Dry eye is a very important issue to be considered in patients contemplating refractive surgery and during the postoperative management of refractive surgery patients. Postsurgical management is very similar to management in patients without refractive surgery, including careful attention to concomitant lid abnormalities, lid hygiene, artificial tear replacement, and medical therapy. In most patients, there is a temporary exacerbation of symptoms and signs for 3 to 6 months with eventual return to the preoperative state. By implementing these controlling measures, most patients can actually be more comfortable with their eyes in the long run than they were in their contact lenses.

Key Points

1. As defined by the NEI, dry eye, or KCS is a "disorder of the tear film due to tear deficiency or excessive evaporation that causes damage to the intrapalpebral ocular surface and is associated with symptoms of discomfort."
2. For most patients, increased dryness after LASIK is tolerable and not visually significant. Therefore, chronic dry eye is not a definite contraindication to refractive surgery. However, patients with ocular surface disease prior to refractive surgery must be treated aggressively and counseled regarding the likelihood of exacerbation of symptoms postoperatively.
3. Improving surface lubrication and, if present, controlling a concomitant inflammatory component such as blepharitis will improve objective and subjective success postoperatively.
4. Postrefractive surgery patients with a markedly compromised tear film due to a combined mechanism etiology can experience significant fluctuations in visual acuity.
5. Sensory nerves in the corneal epithelium and stroma trigger the blink mechanism to spread tears uniformly and clear tears from the ocular surface by pumping used tears into the nasolacrimal ducts. Eyelid inflammation, surgical severing of corneal nerves, and laser ablation results in disruption of this important feedback loop, obstructing neural sensory input to the lacrimal gland.
6. It is well documented that a temporarily neurotrophic cornea results from creation of the flap during LASIK.
7. Sustained dysfunction of the precorneal tear film after LASIK exacerbated by the wound healing response has been reported to contribute significantly to regression of the refractive result.

REFERENCES

1. Krachmer JH, Mannis MJ, Holland JE. Dry eye. In: Krachmer JH, Mannis MJ, Holland JE, eds. *Cornea: Fundamentals, Diagnosis, and Management.* 2nd ed. London: Elsevier; 2005:521–540.
2. Solomon KD, Holzer MP, Sandoval HP. Refractive surgery survey 2001. *J Cataract Refract Surg.* 2002;28:346–355.
3. Nichols KK, Mitchell LG, Zadnik K. Repeatability of clinical measurements of dry eye. *Cornea.* 2004;23:272–285.
4. Battat L, Marci A, Dursun D, et al. Effects of laser in situ keratomileusis on tear production, clearance, and the ocular surface. *Ophthalmology.* 2001;108:1230–1235.
5. Albietz JM, Lenton LM, McLennan SG. Chronic dry eye and regression after laser in situ keratomileusis for myopia. *J Cataract Refract Surg.* 2004;30:675–684.
6. Wilson SE. Laser in situ keratomileusis-induced (presumed) neurotrophic epitheliopathy. *Ophthalmology.* 2001;108:1082–1087.
7. Toda I, Asano-Kato N, Komai-Hori Y, et al. Laser-assisted in situ keratomileusis for patients with dry eye. *Arch Ophthalmol.* 2002;120:1024–1028.

8. Barham JB, Edens MB, Fonteh AN, et al. Addition of eicosapentaenoic acid to gamma-linolenic acid-supplemented diets prevents serum arachadonic acid accumulation in humans. *J Nut.* 2000;130(8):1925–1931.

9. Wu D, Meydani M, Leka LS, et al. Effect of dietary supplementation with black currant seed oil on the immune response of healthy elderly subjects. *Am J Clin Nutr.* 1999;70:536–543.

10. Barabino S, Ronaldo M, Camicione P. Systemic linoleic and g-linolenic acid therapy in dry eye syndrome with an inflammatory component. *Cornea.* 2003:22(2):97–101.

11. Fujikawa A, Gong H, Amemiya T, et al. Vitamin E prevents changes in the cornea and conjunctiva due to vitamin A deficiency. *Graefe's Arch Clin Exp Ophthalmol.* 2003;241:287–297.

12. McEven AR, Blewell SA. The inhibition of mast cell activation by neutrophil lactoferrin: uptake by mast cells and interaction with tryptase, chymase and cathepsin G. *Biochem Pharmacol.* 2003;65(6):1007–1015.

13. Alm, AA, Anderson DR, Berson, EL. The lacrimal apparatus. In: Hart WM, ed. *Physiology of the Eye: Clinical Application.* 9th ed. London: Mosby Year Book; 1992:18–27.

14. Poon CA, Geerling G, Dart JK. Autologous serum eyedrops for dry eyes and epithelial defects: clinical and in vitro toxicity studies. *Br J Ophthalmol.* 2001;85:1188–1197.

15. Stone DU, Chodosh J. Oral tetracycline for ocular rosacea: an evidence-based review of the literature. *Cornea.* 2004;23:106–109.

16. D'Agostino P, Arocoleo F, Barbera C, et al. Tetracycline inhibits the nitric oxide synthase activity induced by endotoxin in cultured murine macrophages. *Eur J Pharmacol.* 1998;346:283–290.

17. Sall K, Stevenson DO, Mundorf TK, et al. Two multicenter, randomized studies of the efficacy and safety of cyclosporine ophthalmic emulsion in moderate to severe dry eye disease. *Ophthalmology.* 2000;107:631–639.

18. Ashcroft DM, Dimmock P, Garside R, et al. Efficacy and tolerability of topical pimecrolimus and tacrolimus in the treatment of atopic dermatitis: meta-analysis of randomized controlled trials. *BMJ.* 2005;330(7490):516–525.

19. Nghiem P, Pearson G, Langley RG. Tacrolimus and pimecrolimus: from clever prokaryotes to inhibiting calcineurin and treating atopic dermatitis. *J Am Acad Dermatol.* 2002;46:228–241.

20. Yen MT, Pflugfelder SC, Feuer WJ. The effect of punctal occlusion on tear production, tear clearance, and ocular surface sensation in normal subjects. *Am J Ophthalmol.* 2001;131:314–323.

21. Schaumberg DA, Buring JE, Sullivan DA, et al. Hormone replacement therapy and dry eye syndrome. *JAMA.* 2001;286:2114–2119.

22. Sullivan DA, Wickam LA, Rocha EM, et al. Androgens and dry eye in Sjögren's syndrome. *Ann N Y Acad Sci.* 1999;876:312–324.

27

Computer Vision Syndrome

Suresh K. Pandey, MD and
Brighu N. Swamy, MBBS (Hons), M Med (Clin Epi)

INTRODUCTION

According to the American Optometric Association (AOA), computer vision syndrome (CVS)[1-12] is "the complex of eye and vision problems related to near work which are experienced during or related to computer use." CVS doesn't just cause personal discomfort; it can have significant effects on workplace productivity.

INCIDENCE

On average, more than 50% of the workforce now uses a computer on the job. It is estimated that over 100 million workers suffer from computer eyestrain in the United States alone. Approximately 54 million children connect to the Internet each day either at home or in school. Anyone who spends more than 2 hours each day in front of a computer screen is likely to experience some symptoms of CVS.

ETIOLOGY

Vision Problems

People who are already nearsighted, farsighted, or have astigmatism are more likely to develop computer vision syndrome. Multifocal lenses, such as bifocals, make it even more difficult because the screen is higher and further away than the visual field meant for these lenses. If the person has multifocal lenses, it will be helpful to get a separate pair of glasses designed for computer work. According to a recent survey, people who wear glasses are more prone to CVS. It is estimated that almost 71% of those reporting CVS symptoms wore glasses.

Computer Glare and Reflection

Glare from surrounding lamps and lights can lead to eyestrain. Removing direct light sources; moving the computer station; or installing blinds, screens, or shades can reduce glare. In addition, reflections also make it difficult to focus and cause eye strain. This can easily be eliminated by using an antireflective computer screen.

Improper Workstation Design

One of the most common problems in workstation set-up is that the monitor of the computer is placed too high. The top of the screen should be at eye level. This is because the ideal gaze angle is 10 to 20 degrees below the eye. A screen that is too high can lead to dry, irritated eyes because it forces the user to constantly keep his or her eyes wide open and blink less frequently. A screen that is too high can also cause headaches and neck and upper back pain because the head is tilted back to see.

Dry Environment and Dehydration

These 2 very common occurrences in the workplace and home office can worsen irritated, dry eyes. The air quality is poor in many offices.

Reading New, Unfamiliar Material at Work

When the person strains to catch hold of unfamiliar information and has to do it on a tight deadline, the mind can become stressed and agitated. When there is mental agitation or stress, this is transmitted to the whole upper body—the arms, shoulders, neck, and head. Mental states can interfere with normal vision. Most people don't have control over the amount of material they have to read or the mental stress. Taking walks in a park where you only need a light gaze can help provide balance. The practice of yoga can also help.

PATHOGENESIS

Anyone who spends 2 or more hours a day working on a computer is at risk for developing CVS. The reason is simple: human vision is not suited for staring at a computer screen. Computer images are made up of tiny dots, known as pixels. Letters on a video display terminal (VDT) screen consists of round pixels of light forming letters, which are not sharply defined on the edges, instead of solid lines as in normal print. This can create difficulty for the brain to accurately control focusing effort, resulting in blurred vision. Since your eye cannot focus on images, you must constantly refocus to keep them sharp. Eventually, the person gets repetitive stress of the eye muscles. Additionally, after prolonged computer use, the frequency of blinking is decreased and eyes dry out and become sore. As a result, the ability to focus diminishes and vision may blur, resulting in headaches. Because of the elevated gaze, computer users frequently dip their heads, resulting in poor posture and neck pain.

The eyes respond well to most printed material, which is characterized by its dense black characters with well-defined edges, which contrast markedly from their light background. Healthy eyes can easily maintain focus on the printed page. Characters on a computer screen, however, don't have this contrast or well-defined edges. These characters are brightest at their centers and diminish in intensity toward their edges. The eyes are unable to maintain focus and remain on plane with these images. They instead drift out to a point called the resting point of accommodation (RPA). The eyes constantly move to the RPA and then strain to regain focus on the screen. This continuous flexing of the eyes' focusing muscles creates fatigue and tired eyes.

The other key differences between looking at a printed page and a computer screen are as follows:

- A monitor is a dynamic signal, in that the screen is constantly being "redrawn."
- A monitor creates images on the basis of varying light intensity through a fixed set of red, green, and blue points. This results in less distinct edges, and lower contrast.

The illumination profile of points on a monitor is not sharp (bright to dark) but is somewhat rounded, again reducing contrast.

CLINICAL FEATURES

Symptoms of CVS include the following:
- Headaches and ocular ache
- Loss of focus
- Burning eyes
- Ocular fatigue (tired eyes)
- Double vision
- Blurred vision
- Neck and shoulder pains
- Eyestrain
- Sore eyes
- Dry eyes
- Red eyes
- Burning eyes
- Contact lens discomfort
- Changes in color perception
- Glare sensitivity
- Excessive tearing

DIAGNOSIS AND MANAGEMENT

Once computer vision problems are diagnosed using a diagnostic instrument (eg, the PRIO vision tester, PRIO Corp, Beaverton, Ore) that simulates a computer screen, it's a simple matter to produce computer eyeglasses that will allow working comfortably and productively at a computer.

Standard reading glasses in most cases are not enough. Because eyes react differently to the stimulus of a computer, 70% to 75% of the computer users need computer eyeglasses.

Prevention is the best cure. There are certain preventive measures the computer user can take to reduce eyestrain when working at a computer.

Eye Exam

According to the National Institute of Occupational Safety and Health (NIOSH), computer users should have an eye exam before they start working on a computer and once per year thereafter.

Lighting and Glare

Lighting in most offices is too bright for comfortable computer use. If you can reduce the lighting some it will help. It is important to watch for glare from doors, windows, or reflected glare from surfaces. Relocate any lamps that cast a glare on the screen and cover windows with blinds or drapes. Glare reduction filters and hoods also help. If the computer user wears glasses when working on the computer, the glasses should have an antiglare or antireflective coating on them. Glare screen filters may help for some people, but for the most part, they will not solve your computer vision problems because they only affect glare from the computer screen—not the problems related to the constant refocusing our eyes endure when working at a computer. Only when eyes can clearly focus at the plane of the computer screen one can experience relief from the fatiguing effects of CVS. When using computers, lighting should be about half that used in most offices. Reduce lighting by using fewer light bulbs or florescent tubes or lower the intensity of bulbs and tubes.

Regular Breaks

Full time computer users should take a 10-minute break every hour to reduce eyestrain problems according to experts. Part-time users should take frequent breaks after sitting in front of their display for more than 1 hour.

Refocus the Eyes

The computer user should look away from his or her computer screen every 10 to 15 minutes and focus for 5 to 10 seconds on a distant object outside or down the hallway. This prevents the fixed gaze common among computer users. It also lets the eyes blink, which wets the corneal surface.

Frequent Blinking

When staring at a computer, the computer user blinks less frequently—about 5 times less than normal. Tears coating the eye evaporate more rapidly during long nonblinking phases and cause dry eyes. Office buildings may have excessively dry environments that also reduce tearing. In many offices, the air is dry due to air conditioning and heaters. To make matters worse, our rate of blinking reduces when we stare at a computer, allowing the eye to become dry. This can cause a "dry eye" problem that makes the vision blur or the eyes tear. Lubricant eye drops and tear substitutes often help.

Exercise When Sitting

Anyone in a sedentary job, especially those using computers, should also stand up, move about, or exercise frequently. NIOSH recommends several sitting, stretching, and joint rotating exercises for computer users.

Match the Computer Screen to the Brightness of the Environment

Closely match the brightness of the environment with that of the computer screen. The contrast between the background and on-screen characters should be high.

Magnification Lens

The computer user might also consider getting a PC magnifier, which is essentially a lens that is placed in front of the computer screen, creating a larger, more distant image that demands less focusing power, reducing the eye strain associated with computer use.

Ergonomics

To minimize strain and eyestrain, the computer user should sit at a 90-degree angle, with arms reaching to the keyboard at a 100-degree angle. The keyboard should be slightly below elbow height. The wrists should not be bent when typing. A wrist pad will increase comfort and may help prevent carpal tunnel syndrome. Position the monitor 20 to 26 inches away from the eyes.

The knees should extend 4 to 6 inches off the edge of the seat and bend at a 90-degree angle. Use an adjustable chair with full back support. Raise it so your knees are slightly below the level of your hips. Get a taller or shorter chair as needed. The VDT screen should be 20 to 30 inches away from your eyes. You should be looking slightly down at a 15-degree angle.

A frequently seen problem is people placing the monitor on top of the computer. This usually results in the monitor being too high. It's better to place the monitor on the computer desk and place the computer on a shelf or next to the computer vertically. If the user puts the computer in a vertical orientation, he or she may want to reformat the hard drive. If the user also has to see printed material, it should be put on a typing stand next to the screen so it's at the same distance as the monitor screen.

Electrostatic attraction attracts dust to the screen and eventually hinders visibility. Clean the screen often. A flickering screen also strains the eyes. Sometimes screen flicker can be reduced by plugging other appliances and lights in different outlets to prevent electronic interference. Also, make sure all your electrical cable connections are tight. Every once in a while readjust your monitor's brightness and contrast.

SUMMARY

In conclusion, CVS is a term used to describe eye strain; tiredness; temporary weak vision; dry, irritated eyes; light sensitivity; and muscular problems that stem from using a computer. The prevalence of using computers is growing, and it is imperative that doctors recognize this syndrome and offer possible preventive strategies.

Key Points

1. CVS is the complex of eye and vision problems related to near work that are experienced during or related to computer use.
2. It is estimated that over 100 million working suffer from computer eyestrain in the United States alone.
3. Glare from surrounding lamps and lights can lead to eyestrain. Removing direct light sources; moving computer station; or installing blinds, screens, or shades can reduce glare. In addition, reflection also make it difficult to focus and cause eye strain. This can easily be eliminated by using an anti-reflection computer screen.
4. Full time computer users should take a 10-minute break every hour to reduce eyestrain problems according to experts. Part-time users should take frequent breaks after sitting in front of their display for more than 1 hour.
5. To minimize strain and eyestrain you should sit at a 90-degree angle, with arms reaching to the keyboard at a 100-degree angle. The keyboard should be slightly below elbow height. Wrists should not be bent when typing. A wrist pad will increase comfort and may help prevent carpal tunnel syndrome. Position the monitor 20 to 26 inches away from the eyes.

REFERENCES

1. Acosta MC, Gallar J, Belmonte C. The influence of eye solutions on blinking and ocular comfort at rest and during work at video display terminals. *Exp Eye Res.* 1999;68:663–669.
2. Bachman WG. Computer-specific spectacle lens design preference of presbyopic operators. *J Occup Med.* 1992;34:1023–1027.
3. Bauer W, Wittig T. Influence of screen and copy holder positions on head posture, muscle activity and user judgement. *Appl Ergon.* 1998;29:185–192.
4. Berg M, Arnetz BB, Liden S, et al. An occupational study of employees with VDT associated symptoms—the importance of stress. *Stress Med.* 1996;12:51–54.
5. Bergqvist UO, Knave BG. Eye discomfort and work with visual display terminals. *Scand J Work Environ Health.* 1994;20:27–33.
6. Berman SM, Greenhouse DS, Bailey IL, et al. Human electroretinogram responses to video displays, fluorescent lighting, and other high frequency sources. *Optom Vis Sci.* 1991;68:645–662.
7. Best PS, Littleton MH, Gramopadhye AK, et al. Relations between individual differences in oculomotor resting states and visual inspection performance. *Ergonomics.* 1996;39:35–40.
8. Bockelmann WD. Optimal ocular correction for computer operators. *Klin Oczna.* 1995;97:95–97.

9. Butzon SP, Eagels SR. Prescribing for the moderate-to-advanced ametropic presbyopic VDT user. A comparison of the Technica Progressive and Datalite CRT trifocal. *J Am Optom Assoc.* 1997;68:495–502.

10. Campbell FW, Durden K. The visual display terminal issue: a consideration of its physiological, psychological and clinical background. *Ophthalmic Physiol Opt.* 1983;3:175–192.

11. Carter JB, Banister EW. Musculoskeletal problems in VDT work: a review. *Ergonomics.* 1994;37:1623–1648.

12. Cheu RA. Good vision at work. *Occup Health Saf.* 1998;67:20–24.

Disclaimer of financial interest: The authors have no financial or proprietary interest in any product mentioned in this chapter. Presented in Part at the Royal Australian and New Zealand College of Ophthalmologists meeting; Hobart; November 2005. Supported in part by an unrestricted grant from Research to Prevent Blindness, Inc, New York, NY.

Index

WAIT
...There's More!

SLACK Incorporated's Book Division offers a wide selection of products in the field of Ophthalmology. We are dedicated to providing important works that educate, inform and improve the knowledge of our customers. Don't miss out on our other informative titles that will enhance your collection.